Puberty in Crisis

Puberty has long been recognised as a difficult and upsetting process for individuals and families, but it is now also being widely described as in crisis. Reportedly occurring earlier and earlier as each decade of the twenty-first century passes, sexual development now heralds new forms of temporal trouble in which sexuality, sex/gender and reproduction are all at stake. Many believe that children are growing up too fast and becoming sexual too early. Clinicians, parents and teachers all demand something must be done. Does this out-of-time development indicate that children's futures are at risk or that we are entering a new era of environmental and social perturbation? Engaging with a diverse range of contemporary feminist and social theories on the body, biology and sex, Celia Roberts urges us to refuse a discourse of crisis and to rethink puberty as a combination of biological, psychological and social forces.

CELIA ROBERTS is Senior Lecturer and Co-director of the Centre for Gender and Women's Studies in the Department of Sociology at Lancaster University. She is a long-standing editor of the journal *Feminist Theory* and author of *Messengers of Sex: Hormones, Biomedicine and Feminism* (Cambridge, 2007).

Puberty in Crisis: The Sociology of Early Sexual Development

CELIA ROBERTS

CAMBRIDGE
UNIVERSITY PRESS

CAMBRIDGE
UNIVERSITY PRESS

University Printing House, Cambridge CB2 8BS, United Kingdom

Cambridge University Press is part of the University of Cambridge.

It furthers the University's mission by disseminating knowledge in the pursuit of education, learning and research at the highest international levels of excellence.

www.cambridge.org
Information on this title: www.cambridge.org/9781107104723

First published 2015

A catalogue record for this publication is available from the British Library

Library of Congress Cataloguing in Publication data
Roberts, Celia, 1968-
Puberty in crisis : the sociology of early sexual development / Celia Roberts.
pages cm
ISBN 978-1-107-10472-3 (Hardback)
1. Puberty. 2. Hormones, Sex. I. Title.
QP84.4.R63 2015
612.6′61–dc23 2015006505

ISBN 978-1-107-10472-3 Hardback

This book is dedicated to my parents, Hugh and Hilary Roberts, in grateful recognition of the care and love with which they saw me through my childhood and beyond.

Contents

Figures

Acknowledgements

Working on this book I have been helped and encouraged by my family, friends and colleagues and supported by my employer, Lancaster University, the European Research Council and Cambridge University Press. It's difficult to parse the complex network of people who should be thanked, and I hope I have not left anyone out.

Firstly, I want to acknowledge the support of my partner, Adrian Mackenzie, who kept our shared life on a steady and enjoyable course, as well as reading numerous drafts and listening to my attempts to speak my argument out loud. His 2014 gig in Copenhagen made finishing this book an exciting adventure. Our sons, Connor and Callum Mackenzie, arrived in the early days of this research. Kindly, they have sometimes been a little bit interested in what I am doing. Much more marvellously, they have made life beyond the computer as compelling and exciting as possible: I will always be grateful to them for that. My wider family, Hugh and Hilary Roberts and Moya Mackenzie, my brother, my sisters- and brothers-in-law and my uncles and aunts, have been endlessly supportive and generous. Other 'family' friends – in Australia and the UK – have encouraged and helped me. I want to mention Ruth and Rex Burgess, Suzanne Eastwood, Sally and Dylan Bushell, and Mark Westcombe in particular.

My academic friends, students and colleagues – from Lancaster and elsewhere in the UK, from Australia and from Scandinavia – will find themselves in many places throughout this book. Academic research is always work-in-conversation: I could not have written this book without their multiple contributions. I want sincerely to thank Imogen Tyler, Maureen McNeil, Marja Vehviläinen, Lutz Sauerteig, Natalie Gill, Sung-Yueh Perng, Bruce Bennett, Katrina Roen, Jackie Stacey, Karen Throsby, kylie valentine, Robbie Duchinsky, Hilary Hinds, Anne Cronin, Maggie Mort, Debra Ferreday, Stacy Gillis, Sarah Kember, John Law, Pedro Pinto, Ericka Johnson, Cecilia Åsberg, Sari Irni, Kate McNicholas-Smith, Ali Hanbury, Brigit McWade, Becky Fish,

Li-Wen Shih, Claire Waterton, Anne-Marie Fortier, Lucy Suchman, Vicky Singleton, Suzanne Fraser, Cron Cronshaw, Joann Wilkinson, Mette Kragh-Furbo, Oscar Maldonado, Andrew Sayer, Catherine Waldby, Anni Dugdale, Mette Nordahl Svendsen and Brit Ross Winthereik for reading drafts, discussing ideas, inviting me to present this work and/or giving me particular assistance to get this book done.

Part of this work was supported by a grant from the European Research Council awarded to Ericka Johnson of Linköping University under the Seventh Framework Programme, entitled 'Prescriptive Prescriptions: Prescribing Healthy Subjectivities' (FP7/2007–2013 / ERC grant agreement no. 263657, PPPHS.) I have benefited enormously from Ericka's generous inclusion of me in her inspiring research group. A large chunk of the book was written whilst I was on sabbatical leave in 2011. These extended periods of relative peace are essential and I am grateful to Lancaster University for maintaining this important academic tradition.

Three emerging scholars worked as research assistants for me during this project: Sung-Yueh Perng prepared an extensive scientific database; Natalie Gill helped me with the bibliography and permissions; and Brigit McWade did some heroic reference formatting work right at the very end. Their cheerful professionalism and high-quality work inspired me to get on with mine.

Earlier versions of some of the work in this book have been published in the *European Journal of Women's Studies*, *Subjectivity*, *Feminist Theory* and *Sexualities*. I would like to thank the anonymous reviewers and the editors of these journals for their help in sharpening my arguments. Similar heartfelt thanks go to the anonymous readers of the draft manuscript of this book. I was fortunate to receive excellent, detailed feedback from each of them, and I have really tried to respond to their comments in this revised version. I want also to thank John Haslam, Carrie Parkinson and Frances Brown from Cambridge University Press for their encouragement and assistance.

1 *Puberty in crisis? Sex, reproduction and the loss of future*

Long figured as a disturbing and upsetting process for individuals and families, puberty is today widely described as itself in crisis, reportedly occurring earlier and earlier as each decade passes. Early onset or 'precocious' pubertal development now heralds new forms of temporal trouble in which sexuality, sex/gender and reproduction are all at stake. Children, it is claimed, are growing up too fast and becoming sexual too early. This out-of-time development indicates both that their futures are at risk and that we are all living in a new era of environmental and social perturbation. Something, experts, parents and journalists urge, must be done to stop this precocity.

This book describes and analyses a diverse set of discourses articulating early onset puberty as crisis, tracking their movements across a range of sites. Engaging with and (re)telling stories of sexual development, I both take seriously the scale and potential significance of the changes described and direct a critical feminist gaze to the allegiances, omissions, emotional registers and logics therein. Reading accounts of early onset puberty as entangled with broader historical and contemporary stories of sexual development, my argument challenges normative assumptions about sex/gender, sexuality and reproduction whilst paying careful attention to matters of physical and psycho-social health.

Stories of a crisis in pubertal timing started to appear in the late 1990s, with the publication of an epidemiological study by Marcia Herman-Giddens and colleagues (1997) which found that, although in the 1960s only 1 per cent of American girls started pubertal development before they turned 8, in the 1990s 48 per cent of girls in some sub-populations had this experience. The heated scientific debate around this study generated news media articles in high-circulation journals, including a cover story in *Time* magazine in October 2000. In this article, entitled 'Teens before their Time', journalist Michael Lemonick and colleagues informed readers that amidst a cloud of scientific and cultural confusion 'all anyone knows for certain is that the signs of sexual development in girls are appearing at ever younger ages' (Lemonick *et al.* 2000: 2). In December that year, journalist Lisa Belkin interviewed Herman-Giddens for a *New York Times* article entitled 'The Making of an 8 Year Old Woman'. Citing Herman-Giddens' finding that 'girls in otherwise normal health are entering puberty more than a full year earlier, on average, than was previously thought', Belkin writes,

> And this change, she warns, demands attention. "These are second-grade girls, some first-grade girls," she says, as she flashes a graph on the wall. "Is it going to keep getting lower? Are kids going to get to be 5 and 4 and 3? And is this supposed to be happening? I don't think so. I don't think that's what nature intended." (Belkin 2000)

Debates around the meaning and significance of contemporary changes to puberty timing continue to this day. In 2012, for example, *The New York Times* printed another piece entitled 'Puberty before Age 10: A New Normal?' that had earlier been published in *The Sunday Magazine* under the headline 'The Incredible Shrinking Childhood' (Weil 2012). Both titles reveal profound concern about changes in the timing of sexual development: like Lemonick *et al.* and Belkin, Weil writes that early onset puberty is increasingly common amongst girls and highlights the lack of scientific consensus about the causes of this change. Although more soberly articulated, concerns about boys also appeared in American and British newspapers in 2012 under titles such as 'Boys Now Enter Puberty Younger, Study Suggests, but It's Unclear Why' (Belluck 2012; see also Pearson 2012).

All of these journalists describe the consequences of early sexual development as negative, particularly for girls. Citing scientific research and clinical evidence about the relationship between early development, early sexual activities and other risk-taking behaviour, they highlight the social difficulties of early onset puberty. As feminist researcher Kristina Pinto writes, 'if puberty is cast as a crisis, early puberty is popularly considered to be psychologically and behaviourally endangering, akin to the sexualizing of a child' (2007: 532).

A gendered and gendering problem

The data underpinning these news media articles comes from a number of scientific fields, including paediatric endocrinology, public health and psychology, which for the most part study female sexual development (Herman-Giddens *et al.* 2012: 1059). As I explain in Chapter 4, Herman-Giddens' initial study focused on girls in part because of an interest in the development of sexually abused children. Subsequent studies across the globe followed this lead, centring their attention on female bodies: rare attempts to trace changes in male puberty found little evidence of widespread change (Euling, Herman-Giddens and Lee 2008). In 2012, however, Herman-Giddens' research group made a related argument about American boys, claiming that age of pubertal onset had decreased by six months to two years, depending on ethnic group (Herman-Giddens *et al.* 2012). Although sometimes noting this recent finding, public and media debates in this area have overwhelmingly focused on female development. As I will show, these debates resonate powerfully with wider public concerns around 'sexualisation' and the loss of childhood innocence, which similarly focus on girls and young women.

The lack of attention given to boys' development highlights the complexities of crisis articulations of puberty. Herman-Giddens argues that male puberty is more difficult to study: 'Data on male puberty are more difficult to obtain than female data because of the absence of an easily determined marker such as menarche. Male pubertal stages are harder to assess visually than girls' stages, and orchidometry [the measuring of testicular volume], an intrusive procedure, is not part of well-child exams' (Herman-Giddens *et al.* 2012: 1059). Although instructive, these justifications are barely credible in my view. As I discuss in Chapters 3 and 4, studies of female puberty often focus on breast and pubic hair growth rather than menarche; and assessment of girls' breast growth is arguably no less intrusive than orchidometry – both involve visual inspection and/or palpation (touching) of intimate parts of the body.[1] That measuring breasts is routine in some clinical settings is the result of entrenched historical practices that literally expose female bodies to more medical scrutiny than those of males. As Nelly Oudshoorn (1994) and I (Roberts 2007: 44–50) have argued in the case of early twentieth-century sex hormone research, these kinds of clinical norms both articulate existing cultural ideas about sex/gender and materialise new forms of difference. Contemporary

[1] Additionally, some research analyses voice break as a later sign of puberty in boys (Juul *et al.* 2007).

science's focus on early developing girls, in other words, both speaks to a long history of medical interest in female sexuality and enacts girls' bodies as problematic in new ways.

As discussed in Chapter 3, girls' sexual development has historically been figured as intrinsically more problematic than boys'. For girls, as cultural studies theorist Catherine Driscoll (2009: 235) argues, puberty has been figured as 'less straightforward' and as having 'more pervasive social implications'. Even today, girls are seen to need more information and active management during this time than boys. This historical difference is reiterated in contemporary concerns about pubertal timing: exploring and resisting this reiteration is a strong motivation for my concentration on girls in this book. My decision to use the term 'early onset puberty' rather than 'precocious puberty' similarly indicates my desire to problematise and resist connections between early sexual development and teen sexuality: 'precocious' carries a pathologising sexual connotation that I want to avoid.[2]

Hurried childhood and reproductive futures

Importantly, scientific work on early puberty also reports significant changes in the pace of sexual development once it starts: whilst the preliminary stages such as breast and pubic hair growth are appearing much earlier in many children, the later stages, including menarche and spermarche, are thought to be more stable. As a process, then, puberty is being temporally stretched. These changes raise difficult questions about the life course, sex, sexuality and health: how long is a normal childhood? Does the onset (or completion) of puberty end childhood? At what age is it normal or healthy to enter into puberty? What are the links between physical and psycho-social-emotional development? What might be the long-term

[2] Technically the two terms are not clearly differentiated. In current North American and British clinical contexts, 'precocious puberty' commonly refers to sexual development occurring at 6–9 years, although as I explain in Chapter 4, such classifications are highly contested and differ according to 'race', ethnicity and national location. Mul and Hughes (2008: 3) draw a distinction between 'early' puberty (that occurring at ages 8–10 for girls and 9–11 for boys) and 'precocious' puberty (that occurring earlier than these ages), but this is not a distinction consistently applied in medical or scientific literatures or in popular accounts. Nor is it a functional distinction: children with early onset puberty may also be treated with hormonal medications.

effects of early sexual development? And what, if anything, should be done about early developing children?

These questions resonate with a broad set of contemporary debates about what some call 'hurried childhood'. In the following sections I explore media, environmental, public policy and feminist accounts of recent changes to childhood and their potential effects on reproductive futures. Detailing a highly contemporary set of concerns, these explorations set the scene for this book's analysis of early onset puberty.

Media accounts: the tragic loss of childhood

News magazine headlines such as 'The Making of an 8 Year Old Woman' (Belkin 2000) and 'Teens before their Time' (Lemonick *et al.* 2000) figure early onset puberty as a loss of childhood, resonating with broader cultural concerns about contemporary children's lives. In *The Disappearance of Childhood*, media theorist Neil Postman argued that in late twentieth-century America, 'Everywhere one looks, it may be seen that the behaviour, language, attitudes, and desires – even the physical appearance – of adults and children are becoming increasingly indistinguishable' (Postman 1994: 4). First published in 1982, this claim remains culturally resonant today; indeed, as Postman wrote in his preface to the 1994 second edition, 'What was happening then is happening now. Only worse' (1994: viii). Building on Philippe Aries' (1962) seminal history, Postman describes childhood as a 350-year-old phenomenon that is in a process of rapid decline: American children no longer play their own games, have age-specific styles of clothing, or speak in a language unique to their age group.[3] Somewhat more contentiously, he argues that the birth of childhood occurred when printing was invented and the written word replaced the importance of oral cultures: this process produced categorical differences between adults and children, particularly in the labour market, because children needed education to become literate. In more recent times, Postman suggests, the rise of electronic communications (radio, cameras, telephones, cinema and television) has decimated such categories: television, he argues, produces three stages of life, infancy, senility and

[3] Other scholars have criticised Aries' work as historically inaccurate and/or intellectually unconvincing (see for example Pollock 1983 and Buckingham 2000).

'the adult-child' (1994: 99). Computers, he adds later, have a different potential: 'the only technology that has this capacity [to sustain the need for childhood] is the computer: 'In order to programme a computer, one must learn a language' (1994: 149). Such learning, he adds, demands levels of literacy requiring a childhood to achieve.[4]

Postman's argument is technologically determinist and fails to account for a diversity of other influences in the (re)production of childhood (see also Jenks 2005). The significance of his work here, however, is the power of its broader claim about the changing nature of childhood experiences across twentieth-century America. This is a claim that has strong cultural purchase today: worries about the loss of childhood, as I will show, are ubiquitous in the US, UK and Australia. (Related scientific and biomedical concerns about early sexual development, as I demonstrate in Chapter 4, are more widespread, found commonly in both developed and developing countries.)

Interested in technology rather than bodies, Postman has relatively little to say about sex and sexuality. In his final chapter, however, he briefly mentions scientific debates around biological changes in sexual development, stating that he 'rather fanc[ies]' the statistic that the average age of menarche has dropped from 14 in 1900 to 12 in 1979 (1994: 121). This appealing fact, he states, 'suggests that the contraction of childhood began to occur in physiological terms shortly after the invention of the telegraph; that is, there is an almost perfect coincidence of the falling age of puberty and the communications revolution' (1994: 121). Later Postman cites increased and earlier sexual activity as one of many negative outcomes of 'the disappearance of childhood'. Again electronic media take the brunt of the blame:

> We may safely assume that media have played an important role in the drive to erase differences between child and adult sexuality. Television in particular not only keeps the entire population in a condition of high sexual excitement but stresses a kind of egalitarianism of sexual fulfilment: sex is transformed from a dark and profound adult mystery to a product that is available to everyone – let us say, like mouthwash or underarm deodorant. (1994: 137)

[4] As it turns out, today most computer users do not learn these languages, remaining relatively 'illiterate' when it comes to programming (see Montgomery 2009 for an analysis of childhood in the age of the internet).

Like deodorant or mouthwash, this new mediatised sex hides something unsanitary, even dirty (yet profound) that is too easily available for Postman's liking. Children should have been protected, he suggests, from such early and free exposure: sex, to put it bluntly, is not for them.[5]

Postman's concerns about the loss of childhood and the consequential exposure of the 'child-adult' to sexuality speak to a widespread cultural anxiety about contemporary children's lives. Stories of early onset puberty found in popular television shows (such as Channel 4's *Embarrassing Bodies* and *Sex Education Show* in the UK), in the print news media and on internet sites for mothers and for young people both express and evoke these anxieties. In such accounts, the very idea that 'children' might go through puberty seems unnerving: puberty has long been seen as signalling the end of childhood, so its occurrence in middle childhood (6–8 years) disturbs twentieth-century western understandings of the life course.

As in Postman's book, worries about the loss of childhood expressed in popular media are commonly linked to moral concerns about precocious 'sexualisation'. News reports of population changes in the timing of sexual development often refer to the possibility of sexual predation and abuse. On a US-based online news media webpage, for example, journalist Carol Wang (2009) cites endocrinologist Kevin Corley describing girls going through early puberty: "They're not going to be emotionally ready to deal with it in many cases," expounds Corley. He also expresses concern with the kids fitting in with their peers because this change can be isolating. But there is an even more sinister concern, according to Corley. "It may also predispose some of these children to early molestation." He cites studies that suggest that the girls whose bodies develop early get unwanted attention and warns parents to keep their daughters wearing baggy clothing that doesn't emphasize their bodies.

Girls' vulnerability is also figured in magazine editors' choice of images for articles on this topic. The October 2000 issue of *Time* magazine mentioned above, for example, featured early puberty as its lead story, using as its front cover a rear-view photograph of an alarmingly thin girl wearing only a white bra (shop tag still attached)

[5] See for example, his comments on the role of the Moral Majority in preserving childhood (1994: 147–8).

and silver necklace, gazing despondently in a mirror. Large-font text positioned across the girl's back reads: 'EARLY PUBERTY: Why girls are growing up faster.' Higher on the page and in smaller font, a set of questions attempt to engage the reader's attention: 'Is it hormones? Is it fat? Is it something in the water? How parents and kids are coping' (*Time*, 2000: front cover). In the article, Lemonick and colleagues describe early puberty as an increasing problem for American girls. After outlining the physical symptoms and associated risks of early development (breast budding, pubic hair growth, increased risk of breast cancer, loss of adult height), the authors focus most strongly on the psycho-social consequences of this experience:

> Even more troubling than the physical changes is the potential psychological effect of premature sexual development on children who should be reading fairy tales, not fending off wolves. The fear, among parents and professionals alike, is that young girls who look like teenagers will be under intense pressure to act like teenagers. Childhood is short enough as it is, with kids bombarded from every direction by sexually explicit movies, rock lyrics, MTV videos and racy fashions. If young girls' bodies push them into adulthood before their hearts and minds are ready, what will be forever lost? (Lemonick *et al.* 2000)

The tone here is both moralising and nostalgic: the authors mourn a version of childhood that may be 'forever lost'; a childhood in which girls had suitable interests (in fairy stories rather than sex) and looked like children rather than teenagers. In the same vein, they later describe childhood as 'a time when life should be less about Eminem and more about M&M's' (2000).

This article articulates a high degree of ambivalence about early developing girls. Featured throughout as a sassy young woman who insists that her real name is used because the kind of sexual attention she receives is 'such a source of pride', for example, 'Angelica Andrews' laughingly describes boys as 'like dogs' in their amorous pursuit of her. The journalists remain uneasy about this sexual pride and confidence. Although quoting her boasts ('Says Angelica: "The boys tease me. They ask me, 'Have you had plastic surgery?' My friends get kind of jealous"'), they ultimately position Angelica as requiring parental surveillance to manage the effects of her developed body:

> Angelica Andrews also has her parents watching out for her. Recently, the teenager experienced her first French kiss – but her family knew all about it, and the boy was immediately instructed not to call again until she was 16, or

maybe 18. It's unfortunate that such vigilance has become necessary for the families of many 12- and 13-year-olds, whereas a generation ago, most parents could relax until a girl was 16 or 17. But as Angelica puts it, "Welcome to the 21st century!" (2000)

This uneasy mixture of old-fashioned sexual mores (the idea that parents can determine an age at which boys can 'call' girls) and a realist sense of humour (Angelica's 'Welcome to the 21st century!') is typical of mainstream American media accounts of early onset puberty. The choice of image for the front cover, however, is confusing. The featured girl does not seem sexually developed but rather underweight: at first glance readers might expect an article on anorexia rather than early development (which, as described in Chapter 4, is more often associated with obesity). The image denotes fragility and vulnerability, rather than sassy sexuality in need of parental control.

The anticipated futures in media accounts of early onset puberty also include physical problems. Wang (2009) lists a series of alarming physical outcomes of early development that underpinned one parent's decision to seek treatment:

Then there are the long-term physical consequences of precocious puberty. Among them, an increased risk of breast cancer, early menopause, brittle bones and stunted growth. It was the stunted growth that pushed Kate into seeking treatment for her daughter.

These concerns come from the clinical literature, which describes early maturing girls' loss of adult height and increased risk of cancer (this literature is discussed in detail in Chapter 6). In most popular accounts, however, these concerns about physical effects are secondary: the broader issues about the loss of childhood remain paramount. In *Time* magazine, Lemonick *et al.* (2000) speak of unknowable loss consequent on the hurried nature of childhood: 'If young girls' bodies push them into adulthood before their hearts and minds are ready, what will be forever lost?' Developing early, in these accounts, entails unknowable future risk for girls.

Popular environmentalist accounts: toxins and the loss of reproductivity

Publicly available environmentalist literatures including popular books, websites and campaign materials also figure early onset puberty as an unfathomable loss and share some of the strong emotive rhetoric of the media accounts described above. The significant difference is their concentration on links between precocious sexual development and the ubiquity of toxic chemicals. Books like Theo Colborn, Dianne Dumanoski and John Peterson Myer's widely cited *Our Stolen Future* (1996) describe early puberty as a tragic outcome of industrial pollution of rivers, air and soil and the use of toxic chemicals in manufactured objects; an outcome that steals 'our future' by thwarting human (and animal) reproductive potential.[6] On the book's accompanying website, Colborn and colleagues cite the key American study undertaken by Marcia Herman-Giddens and colleagues (mentioned above and discussed in detail in Chapter 4), which found high rates of early onset puberty particularly amongst African-American girls, insisting that, despite the study's methodological weaknesses, its findings 'cannot be dismissed'. 'It is important', they argue, 'to understand why such a notable percentage of very young girls are showing signs of sexual development' (ourstolenfuture.org/newscience/reproduction/Puberty/pubertydebate.htm).

Summarising the scientific literature, Colborn *et al.* list the three main explanations for the rise in early puberty:

> (1) increases in the prevalence of obesity; (2) changes in social factors, particularly the absence of the biological father in the home and the presence of a male other than the biological father; and (3) contamination effects, particularly in the womb. (ourstolenfuture.org/newscience/reproduction/Puberty/pubertydebate.htm)

Although noting in bold type that '**There are no certain answers on any of these issues**', Colborn *et al.* turn their attention to the issue of contamination, suggesting in passing additionally that the rise in obesity may also be caused by exposure to endocrine disrupting chemicals:

> **Contaminates can both speed and slow the rate of sexual development.** In general, it would appear from existing data that estrogen mimics speed sexual development in females, while anti-androgens slow sexual development in males. This story is far from complete. For example, we could find no report of a test of an androgen mimic (such as tributyl tin) on the rate of

[6] For an analysis of the significance of *Our Stolen Future* to the growth of public debate on endocrine disruption, see Krimsky (2000: 74–9).

sexual development in males. Androgen mimics should speed the onset of puberty in males. (ourstolenfuture.org/newscience/reproduction/Puberty/contaminant_table.htm; emphasis in original)

A table beneath this text lists fourteen chemicals thought to affect puberty (speeding it up or slowing it down), including PCBs, dioxin, DDT and bisphenol A, all of which have been the subject of serious campaigning by leading environmentalist groups such as Greenpeace and the World Wildlife Fund (see Roberts 2007: ch. 6; Krimsky 2000). This list connects readers back to *Our Stolen Future*'s central theme: that environmental contamination is affecting hormonal systems in animals and humans, and threatening ('stealing') our reproductive futures. Early puberty, then, is figured as but one negative outcome of widespread contamination; one whose effect on reproduction cannot be clarified (there is no evidence that early puberty affects reproductive capacity in later life) but which is figured here as obviously bad.

Other popular environmentalist accounts pay closer attention to early onset puberty. In her book *Raising Elijah: Protecting Our Children in an Age of Environmental Crisis*, for example, biologist and environmentalist Sandra Steingraber devotes a chapter to the topic.[7] Describing her reaction to scientific papers on the effects of environmental toxins and sexual development, Steingraber argues that early onset puberty threatens the loss of children's connections to 'life itself'. Invoking the spectre of sexual molestation, she writes,

> Surely, what makes these topics so profoundly disturbing is the juxtaposition of something public, noxious, and invasive (chemical contaminants) with something that verily defines the words *private*, *innocent*, and *off-limits* (the reproductive organs of infants and children). We are talking here about threats to that part of my children that I am charged, above all else, with safeguarding: their sexuality, their fertility, their connection to future generations, and thus to the abiding, ongoingness of life itself. These are the body parts about which the necessary motherly refrain is *This is private. This is just for you. No one else is allowed to touch you there.* (Steingraber 2011: 239, italics in original)

In a similar popular book entitled *Hormone Deception*, environmentalist writer D. Lindsey Berkson begins a chapter entitled 'Children' by

[7] For a feminist analysis of Steingraber's style of environmentalist memoir, of which *Raising Elijah* is just one example, see Alaimo (2010: ch. 4).

describing a friend 'quietly' telling her that her 9-year-old daughter was 'physically ahead of her age, already developing breasts' (Berkson 2000: 103). Berkson recounts the treating physician's 'hypothesis' about this early development:

> [N]umerous chemicals in our environment, especially in our food, are mimicking estrogen hormones and thereby causing a more rapid maturation process. She explained that nowadays, during their first five years of life, children are exposed to the same level of endocrine disruptors that used to be considered safe lifetime exposures for seventy-year-old adults! (2000: 103).

This alarming statement is not referenced. The following section of the chapter goes on to address the question 'Why are children so susceptible to hormone disruptors?' rather than to substantiate this claim (2000: 104). Five pages on, Berkson returns to the issue of early onset puberty, citing the Herman-Giddens *et al.* (1997) study. Like Colborn *et al.*, Berkson (2000: 108) accepts the results of this research, moving on quickly to discuss issues of cause. Again like her counterparts, she highlights the potential effects of endocrine-disrupting chemicals, mentioning high levels of phthalates (found in perfumes, fingernail polish, dyes and some plastics). Problematising scientific claims about the role of obesity in early puberty, Berkson (2000: 108–9) refers to an American study that found that high PCB exposure led to increased body weight in 14-year-old girls. Might the correlations between high weight and early puberty also be a consequence of endocrine disruption, she asks?

Aimed at a general audience, this book includes smaller font textbox case studies. The textbox accompanying the section on early onset puberty, entitled 'Another factor in school violence?', tells notably gendered stories about early onset puberty: for boys, Berkson suggests, early or late puberty can lead to challenging behaviour in school, whilst for girls early puberty 'can result in' behaviour problems. Early sexual activity is not specifically mentioned:

> The timing of puberty is another factor to consider in adolescent behaviour and possibly the rise we are seeing in school violence. Research on boys . . . is suggesting that 'off-time maturers,' those who go through puberty either too early or too late, have a higher level of crime, unruly behaviour in school, and greater frequency of delinquent acts. Another study on girls . . . documents that premature puberty can result in poor mental health, more behaviour problems, and lower IQ when compared to children with normal age of puberty. (2000: 110)

I analyse these kinds of stories about early maturing young people's behaviour in detail in Chapter 6. What I want to note here is the ways in which worries about early sexual development spill into concerns about 'appropriate' forms of masculinity and femininity. In these environmentalist accounts, both reproductive and gender futures seem to be at stake for early developers.

In contrast, the potential actions proposed to prevent early onset puberty seem trivial, even banal. Berkson's chapter ends with a list of 'Helpful Hints for Protecting Children', including buying wooden toys, not allowing children to chew on plastic, negotiating non-toxic treatments with dentists, frequent hand-washing and the avoidance of particular head lice shampoos (2000: 127–8). Such activities seem rather minimal in the face of violent schoolyard behaviour and the massive increases in toxic exposures described earlier. Berkson's concluding chapter, however, refers to broader policy and political issues around environmental estrogens, advising readers how they can effect change through careful consumption, personal behaviour change and 'citizen action' (2000: 293).

In each of these examples, environmentalist literatures figure early onset puberty as an outcome of children's (and foetuses') excessive exposure to endocrine-disrupting chemicals. Authors strategically and often uncritically cite scientific studies outlining the negative effects of early onset puberty on young people, arguing that early sexual development is linked with worrying (even criminal) behaviours and, in Steingraber's book, increased risk of sexual predation by others. Popular environmentalist writing thus echoes media concerns about early puberty but is much more political in its strategic approach to, and citation of, scientific studies of puberty. Early sexual development appears as a consequence of contamination rather than figuring as an issue of concern in its own right. The loss of childhood described in environmentalist books is politically connected to a loss of reproductive futurity and the survival of the human species.

Public debate and policy discourses on early 'sexualisation'

Concerns about the loss of childhood are reflected in quite different ways in public debate and related policy documents on the 'sexualisation' of girls. There is, however, notable resonance with both environmentalist and media discourses around early puberty: both rely on emotive rhetorical figurations of loss combined with minimal and uncritical use of scientific data to back up claims underpinned by normative views of sex/gender, sexuality and reproduction.

In the UK, USA, Australia and other wealthy countries, public debate on early sexual development takes place in print and electronic media, in street campaigns, in parliamentary debate and in popular books. Like the environmentalist literature described above, books such as Melinda Tankard Reist's edited collection *Getting Real: Challenging the Sexualisation of Girls* (2009) and Tanith Carey's *Where Has My Little Girl Gone?* (2011) contain a mix of 'facts', energetic polemic and advice for personal and political action. Both responding to and stimulating further media debate, these popular books are linked to the development of public policy documents: Carey's book, for example, is endorsed on the front cover by Linda Papadopoulos, author of the British *Home Office Review on the Sexualisation of Girls* (2010).

Notably, in all of these texts anything more than passing reference to scientific debates around early onset puberty is rare. The sexualisation of girls is described as a culturally produced phenomenon that has little or nothing to do with physiological development (Roberts 2013). An article in Reist's collection provides an example: producing evidence of 'inappropriate' sexualisation, author Maggie Hamilton refers to 'sexualised pre-schoolers' who engage in 'unacceptable … inappropriate and determined' sexual activities. Quoting 'Debra, a community liaison officer and mother of two girls' she writes:

> Puberty issues are happening much younger. Some girls are now fashion-conscious as young as three or four … We're now seeing six, seven and eight-year-olds involved in coercive, manipulative sexual behaviours, because there's a confusion about what sexuality means. (Hamilton 2009: 60)

In this quote early onset puberty morphs into 'puberty issues', constituted by a concern with fashion and a desire to engage in sexual activities. No mention is made here or in the fourteen other chapters of population changes in the timing of sexual development.

Practices of mass consumption are absolutely central to these discourses, which frequently focus on the availability and promotion of 'sexualising' products. In the UK, certain products aimed at pre-teen girls have been subject to fierce public debate, gaining notable media coverage and provoking comment from senior political figures. In

2010, for example, high street fashion store Primark sold padded bras for 7-year-old girls. After a public campaign led by online support and lobby group Mumsnet, soon-to-be Prime Minister David Cameron described the sales as 'completely disgraceful'.[8] With haste, Primark removed the bras from their stores, donating profits from their sale to a children's charity. Since then, however, other stores have marketed similar products, provoking more 'outrage' in the news and other media. In 2011, for example, Channel 4's *Sex Education Show* staged televisual protests against high street retailers such as Primark, Matalan and WH Smiths, admonishing them to '*Stop Pimping Our Kids!*' Related campaigns have been undertaken in other countries. In 2007 Australian writer Tania Andrusiak set up her one-woman lobby group 'Kids Free 2B Kids', which has successfully campaigned against a range of 'sexualising' products and images including children's underwear and T-shirts, mobile phone advertisements in teen magazines and representations of teenage girls in pornography sold in newsagents (Andrusiak 2009).

Listed as but one example of the contemporary 'sexualisation' of girls, these marketing practices have been the subject of governmental inquiries and taskforces, most of which figure the sexualisation of children (particularly girls) as a problematic social and commercial phenomenon that should and could be resisted. In 2006, an independent thinktank, The Australia Institute, published two linked discussion papers by Emma Rush and Andrea La Nauze, the first entitled 'Corporate Paedophilia: Sexualisation of Children in Australia' and the second 'Let Children be Children: Stopping the Sexualisation of Children in Australia'. Defining 'sexualisation' as the process of capturing of children's sexuality and 'mould[ing] it into stereotypical forms of adult sexuality' (Rush and La Nauze 2006a: 1), Rush and La Nauze argue that 'the most significant sources of premature sexualisation are girls' magazines and advertising. Television programmes . . . also play a role' (Rush and La Nauze 2006b: 7). Using child models performing 'adult' actions and poses, these media teach children how to act in a 'sexualised' way and lead them to believe that 'being sexy is the way to be successful and to feel good about oneself' (2006b: 7). Like the popular media accounts discussed above, Rush and La Nauze link 'sexualisation' to a risk of sexual predation: 'The sexualisation of

8 http://news.bbc.co.uk/1/hi/uk_politics/8521403.stm.

children also risks normalising and possibly encouraging paedophilic sexual desire for children' (2006a: 2; 2006b: 8). These articles and a subsequent law suit in which a major Australian retailer sued the Director of The Australia Institute in relation to claims about its advertising practices led to an intense media and public debate that culminated in a 2008 Senate Inquiry into 'The Sexualisation of Children in the Contemporary Media Environment' that recommended more education and discussion around these issues.

Rush and La Nauze pay only scanty attention to the physical elements of sexual development. Their longer paper includes a section on the 'Physical harm' caused by early sexuality with a comment on changes in pubertal timing, citing media reports and popular literature rather than the extensive scientific literature in the area:

> In discussion of the sexualisation of children it is often noted that in developed nations children now reach puberty earlier than they did in the past. For example, Odone cites a UK study of 1,150 eight-year-old children called 'Children of the Nineties' that found that one-sixth of all eight-year-old girls show some signs of puberty, compared to one in 100 a generation ago. Also, one in 14 eight-year-old boys have pubic hair, compared with one in 250 a generation ago (2002, p. 19). To place these physical changes in context, however, experts in childhood development often note that children's emotional and cognitive development has not advanced at the same pace (Levin and Linn 2004; Linn 2005). As a result, children's bodies are maturing before they are psychologically mature. Children are thus ill-equipped to deal with sexualising pressure which implies that only a limited range of mature body types are attractive and desirable. An increasing emphasis on a particular body type as the ideal is central to the evidence of sexualisation presented in the previous section. (2006a: 35)

This quotation leads into a discussion of the risks of anorexia and bulimia, which the authors feel are increased by sexualising media. Such risks are not mentioned in the scientific or clinical literature on early onset puberty, which tends, as noted earlier, to focus instead on the role of obesity in early sexual development. Rush and La Nauze, in other words, make no direct links between changing patterns of sexual development and 'sexualisation'.

In 2007, the American Psychological Association published their *Report of the APA Taskforce on the Sexualization of Girls* examining 'the psychological theory, research and clinical experience addressing the sexualisation of girls via media and other cultural messages, including the prevalence of these messages and their impact on girls and the role and impact of race/ethnicity and socioeconomic status' (American Psychological Association 2010: 1).[9] This report takes a more precise, academic approach, defining sexualisation as occurring when

- a person's value comes only from his or her sexual appeal or behavior, to the exclusion of other characteristics;
- a person is held to a standard that equates physical attractiveness (narrowly defined) with being sexy;
- a person is sexually objectified – that is, made into a thing for others' sexual use, rather than seen as a person with the capacity for independent action and decision making; and/or
- sexuality is inappropriately imposed upon a person. (2010: 1)

Like Rush and La Nauze, the APA apportions blame for early sexualisation to mass media (magazines, television, the internet) and advertising but also pays serious attention to toys and fashion. The APA is more critical of parents than are Rush and La Nauze, discussing the negative effects of parents' encouraging children to focus on their appearance (entering them into beauty pageants or permitting them to have cosmetic surgery for example) (American Psychological Association 2010: 15). The APA also grapples with more direct forms of sexualisation, discussing children's involvement in prostitution and trafficking and the effects of sexual harassment and abuse (2010: 16). Finally, the authors also address the question of children's own psychological and material investments in becoming sexual, arguing that 'there is ample evidence that self-objectification is common amongst women and girls' (2010: 17): indeed, they suggest that 'girls sometimes participate in and contribute to their own sexualization' (2010: 18). Unlike Rush and La Nauze's papers, however, the report makes no mention of population level changes in timing of onset of puberty.

Four similar investigations took place around this time in the United Kingdom. In 2007, media studies theorist David Buckingham prepared a report on 'The Impact of the Commercial World on Children's Wellbeing', which mentions the Australian Senate Inquiry and the APA Report and discusses popular debates in the UK and elsewhere.

[9] I cite the 2010 reprint of this report, which includes some updated references but is otherwise the same as the 2007 version.

Buckingham is refreshingly critical of these debates: 'The debate on sexualisation and body image has been conducted in rather sensationalised and moralistic terms. This can make it difficult for children in particular to discuss and come to terms with the range of messages they are bound to encounter' (Buckingham 2007: 113). He argues that 'it is not always clear whether the concern is with sexual representation of any kind, or with material that is defined as sexual*ised* – and indeed what this distinction might mean' (2007: 114), suggesting that public debates tend to position children as passive receptacles and to define any content that adults could read as sexual as problematic. In 2010, Buckingham and colleagues prepared a similar report for the Scottish Parliament's Equal Opportunities Committee entitled *Sexualised Goods Aimed at Children* (Buckingham *et al.* 2010), which included a report of their own focus group research in this area with young people and parents. This report is similarly critical of the existing debates, arguing that they conflate 'sexualised' with 'sexual' representations and position children, particularly girls, as passive recipients of harmful media content.

In the same year, popular psychologist Linda Papadopoulos (2010) prepared a more targeted report for the Home Secretary entitled *The Sexualisation of Young People Review*. Papadopoulos builds on the APA Report, defining sexualisation as 'the imposition of adult sexuality on to children and young people before they are capable of dealing with it, mentally, emotionally or physically' (2010: 6). Like the APA and Australian reports, the document focuses on mass media and advertising as well as products aimed at younger children, asking questions about how increasing emphasis on 'sexiness' is affecting girls' and boys' self-esteem, body image and understandings of sexuality, gender differences and relationships. Links are also made to reported increases in sexualised violence, schoolyard bullying and sexual harassment, with sexual abuse described as 'the extreme end of the spectrum of consequences of sexualisation' (2010: 13). 'Sexualising children', concludes Papadopoulos, 'prematurely places them at risk of a variety of harms' (2010: 14).

Until 2011, scientific and biomedical debates around early sexual development were almost entirely absent from these policy documents: the word 'puberty' is mentioned only once in Papadopoulos' 104-page review, whilst Buckingham's 2009 report flatly refuted claims of increasing rates of early onset puberty (citing a popular book by Levin and Kilbourne 2008 and one early scientific study, Eveleth 1986): 'Despite popular beliefs, young people are not maturing earlier than 50 years ago, although there was a significant fall in the age of menarche in the first part of the twentieth century' (Buckingham 2009: 116). In 2011 the new Coalition government somewhat controversially commissioned yet another report entitled *Let Children Be Children* by the Director of the Conservative lobby group, the Mothers' Union, Reg Bailey. Otherwise covering the same empirical and conceptual ground as Papadopoulos' report, brief mention is made here of the potential significance of changes in age of pubertal onset. Citing Buckingham's at that time forthcoming position, Bailey writes,

12. Since most attention is paid to the sexualisation of clothes for girls, it is important to be especially aware of girls' physical development. Girls are, on average, reaching puberty at an earlier age now than ever before. In the UK, girls can now expect to reach puberty, defined as the development of breast buds, around their tenth birthday, and, on average, girls have developed more evident breasts by 11.6 years of age. That means that today these developmental stages are reached a year to 18 months sooner than at any time over the past 60 years (Rubin *et al.* 2009).

13. We need to see concerns about the premature sexualisation of children through inappropriate clothing and other products against this backdrop. Professor David Buckingham, in a book to be published in 2011, considers the issue of whether, as well as society being increasingly sexualised, this lowering of the age at which children reach physical and sexual maturity provides a biological driver towards them seeing their potential as sexual beings at a younger age (Phoenix, 2011) (Bailey 2011: 44).[10]

[10] The *Bailey Report* relies heavily on a literature review by Ann Phoenix (2011) in which she writes: 'In his 2011 book, David Buckingham raises the question of whether the apparent "sexualisation" of children might partly be accounted for by decreases in the age at which they reach physical and sexual maturity. In other words, society is increasingly sexualised, but are children drawn into sexualisation partly for biological reasons? The age of menarche (onset of menstruation) in the United States and Europe dropped by around 2.5 years in the first part of the twentieth century, and has levelled off in recent decades. However, the onset of puberty (for example, as indicated in breast development and the growth of pubic hair) appears to be occurring ever earlier (although affected by body mass and ethnicity (Aksglaede *et al.* 2008; Kaplowitz *et al.* 2001). From the evidence available, Buckingham suggests that around one-third of seven-year-old girls are now showing pubertal characteristics, which means that they might, for biological reasons, be becoming aware of themselves as potentially sexual beings at an earlier age. This may also mean that some might

As I note elsewhere, the language of 'biological drivers' is not one I would use (Roberts, 2013): nevertheless, asking about relations between physical development and 'sexualisation' seems very important to me. This is a central theme of this book.

Feminist theorists have both selectively endorsed and criticised public and policy concerns about the sexualisation of young girls (see, for example, papers in Renold and Ringrose 2013). In an edited collection on the concept of the 'tweenie', sociologist Anita Harris writes:

> [W]hat have caused considerable disquiet amongst feminists, social commentators, teachers, and parents are the secularization of children's identities and the commodification of their cultures. In other words, tweenie is criticized for inappropriately sexualizing girls and drawing them into a world of feminine display, artifice, and the imperative to attract male attention at far too young an age. (Harris 2009: 213)

Such concerns, Harris (2009: 214–15) critically notes, echo earlier debates bemoaning the impact of adult sexual cultures on teenage women. Citing Nancy Lesko (2001) and Valerie Walkerdine (1998), Harris argues that we need instead to analyse how normative ideas about growing up are produced and to question desires to control girls' bodies and sexualities: such ideas, she shows, are linked to the reproduction of class and racialised privileges. Concerns about tween-age girls may 'have more to do with anxieties about social change and the loss of predictability as represented in conventions about linear adolescent development and the loss of the innocent girlhood reserved for the middle classes' (Harris 2009: 217). These comments have great significance for analysing debates around early onset puberty, which similarly articulate norms and anxieties around raced and classed sexual embodiments.

Although mostly running in parallel with debates on early onset puberty, public debates around the 'sexualisation' of girls constitute an important element of the cultural scene through which discourses of puberty in crisis are articulated. Throughout this book, I argue that scientific, medical and environmentalist literatures on early puberty articulate (in the sense of both speaking and being connected to) wider

need some of the products (such as 'training bras') that have attracted criticism for being sexualised (Phoenix 2011: 9–10).'

cultural concerns about sex/gender, sexuality and reproduction. The 'sexualisation' debates are a key site in which these are articulated today.

Sexual futures: feminism and early development

As Michel Foucault argued in *The History of Sexuality*, volume 1, the 'precocious and already exhausted' child became a key figure in modern European discourses of sex from the nineteenth century onwards. Although, as I discuss in Chapter 3, the sexually developing child has triggered cultural concern since that time, the early developing girl is a more contemporary problem enacted within and through an astonishingly wide set of scientific, medical and popular discourses. Such enactments should, in my view, be of concern to feminists: discourses articulating and worrying about early sexual development play significant roles in making sex in all its senses today and are tightly implicated in figurations of femininity and female sex as threatening individual and social futurity.

This threat is articulated with characteristic heavy irony by British activist and journalist Laurie Penny in her feminist manifesto for our time, *Meat Market: Female Flesh under Capitalism*. Beginning a chapter entitled 'An Anatomy of Modern Frigidity,' she writes,

> The sexual bodies of women are out of control. Look around: teenagers who should be drinking lashings of ginger beer and going on picnics are wearing thongs and listening to Lily Allen. Children delinquently rummage in each other's pornographic pencil cases. Even babies are now born with the Playboy Bunny image tattooed onto their eyeballs. Their fault, the little tarts, for daring to look at the future. (Penny 2011: 5)

The telescoping of temporalities figured in public concern about girls' sexuality (mocked here in Penny's reference to babies as 'little tarts') is, I suggest, materialised both in the bodies of early developers and in discourses articulating early development. As Penny's manifesto makes abundantly clear, such materialisations speak to core concerns of contemporary feminist body politics and demand careful theorisation.

Despite the rather obvious relevance of sexual development to thinking about girlhood and sexuality, pubertal processes and timing are usually mentioned only in passing in feminist work on girls. None of the papers in recent special issues of *Feminist Theory* (Burman and

Stacey 2010a) and *Australian Feminist Studies* (Spongberg 2008) on the child or in Ros Gill and Christina Scharff's (2011) excellent collection of essays on 'new femininities', for example, focus on puberty, menarche or sexual development. Instead, they concentrate on cultural representations, social experience and subjectivities.

Introducing a 2009 edited collection on the rise of 'tween cultures', however, Claudia Mitchell and Jacqueline Reid-Walsh do rather tentatively mention early onset puberty as a response to neoliberal consumer cultures' sexualisation of 6–10-year-old girls. Although the point is not elaborated, Mitchell and Reid-Walsh bring media representations of early sexual development into the frame, suggesting possible connections between reports of early puberty and the marketing of products for 'tween-age' girls:

> It appears that a market construction has somehow anticipated or is at least paralleling a physiological one. In some cases, western concerns about 'death of childhood' and 'hurried childhood' seem to be coming true for some western and westernized girls, as they have always been for the majority of girls in developing countries throughout the world. (Mitchell and Reid-Walsh 2009: 14)

Passing reference to the significance of population level changes in onset of puberty to the development of the 'tween' category is made in two other essays in this volume (Cheu 2009: 298–9; Harris 2009: 210) but these authors do not develop an argument around early development per se. Elizabeth Seaton's chapter goes further, engaging directly with the scientific literature on early onset puberty and its take-up in popular media. Using Bourdieu's notion of habitus and citing some of the scientific debates on the decline in age of pubertal onset, Seaton argues against the desire to find determinist explanations of early puberty. Instead she develops a fascinating question: 'Does early puberty involve a habituated and strategic response to the uncertain terrain of neoliberalism?' (Seaton 2009: 38). Her answer is a qualified 'yes':

> Precociousness may be read as a type of strategic reaction – a 'becoming adult', becoming self-possessed – for a society that no longer has time for children. Perhaps precocious sexual development can be understood in a similar way. (2009: 41)

Seaton's note of caution is rather specific: she notes (as is discussed in detail in Chapter 4) that the scientific literature on sexual development mostly argues that it is only the early stages of puberty (breast and pubic hair growth) rather than menstruation that are occurring sooner. Seaton finds theoretical mileage in this:

> Girls are not becoming women earlier – in terms of reaching menses – but rather become pubescent earlier and remain that way for extended durations. The distinction is important – as one signifies an attainment of adulthood (at least in a physiological respect) while the other signifies an anticipation of adulthood. (2009: 41)

Early onset puberty, in other words, may be a 'strategic' response to a culture that values anticipation of adulthood rather than adulthood itself. Seaton does not address the biological materialities of development. What remains to be explored, then, is how we might think about puberty as a bio-psycho-social process. How might we understand early sexual development? Should we be concerned about it as a biological phenomenon? How might feminists theorise the role of biological actors in early sexual development alongside consideration of social and psychological forces? And how can we resist articulations of girls' sexual development as negative? My aim is to provide answers to these questions. As described in the following chapter, I do this through attending to findings, feelings and figurations; refusing to draw distinctions between bodies and discourses, I speak in terms of flows and foldings, conceptualising sexual development as an embodied temporal process.

What does it mean to invoke crisis?

Across a range of sites, puberty is today seen to be either in crisis itself (starting too early for too many girls) or evidence of wider crisis (environmental and/or social disaster). *Guardian* journalist Joanna Moorhead articulates this sense of doom in her 2010 article 'Should We Be Worried about Early Puberty?' in which she writes, 'It's not, on any reading of the situation, good news for today's little girls.' But what is entailed in the term crisis? And is it a good idea for me to invoke it here?

'Crisis' comes from the Ancient Greek verb *krinō*, meaning to separate, to choose, judge or decide, to measure oneself, to quarrel or to fight. In Latin and modern European languages 'crisis' becomes a term that describes both a problem and the attempt to address it. In his scholarly history Reinhardt Koselleck (2006: 358) writes: 'For the

Greeks, the term "crisis" had relatively clearly demarcated meanings in the spheres of law, medicine and theology. The concept imposed choices between stark alternatives – right or wrong, salvation or damnation, life or death.' In medicine, for example, the term referred to both an observable condition and a judgement about what to do about it. This judgement – the crisis – would determine whether the patient would live or die:

> Depending on whether or not the crisis led to a full restoration of health, the distinction was made between a perfect crisis and an imperfect crisis. The latter left open the possibility of a relapse. A further distinction, between acute and chronic crises, had led – since Galen – to a temporal differentiation in the progression of illnesses. (Koselleck 2006: 360)

Until the seventeenth century, Koselleck shows, this medical meaning maintained dominance, and uses in law and theology were less strong. In the early modern period, however, the term was taken up in politics, economics, history and psychology. In 1792 a German dictionary brought the three meanings together: 'change in a course of illness', 'decisive point of time' and 'alarming situation', but it was not until 1845 that a dictionary listed it as a word used in ordinary parlance and as describing a personal experience in daily life (Koselleck 2006: 366). In the eighteenth century, 'crisis' regained some religious and theological connotations, but was also widely used to discuss the French and American revolutions and so acquired a secular apocalyptic meaning. The description of these revolutions as crises indicated the need for action: as in the original medical meaning, naming a crisis both described the event and was a prescription for therapy. Koselleck argues, then, that the term became important in the eighteenth and nineteenth centuries because of its 'metaphorical flexibility' (2006: 358). Indeed, he suggests that its multiple and flexible meanings meant that 'from the 1770s on, "crisis" becomes a structural signature of modernity' (2006: 374). This signature remains very powerful for the next 200 years: 'In our century there is virtually no area of life that has not been examined and interpreted through this concept with its inherent demand for decisions and choices' (2006: 358).

Used to denote moments in history, 'crisis' in modern times describes two kinds of events placed at opposing ends of a continuum. Firstly, there is crisis that is singular, existential and absolute: 'nothing will be the same after this'. Secondly (a version that arguably predominates today), there is crisis that is recurring, even cumulative. This latter usage tends to belong to economic arguments, such as Marx's theory of over-production as that which constitutes the core crisis at the heart of capitalism. The emotional weight conveyed in contemporary uses of the term is built more on the former history of devastating change, whilst its ubiquity in academic and media accounts stems from the latter (crises are repetitive and to be expected). For Marx and Engels the term had an inherently positive meaning politically: economic crisis produced the moment for revolutionary action. In 1857, for example, Engels wrote, 'The crisis will make me feel as good as a swim in the ocean' (cited in Koselleck 2006: 394).

The twentieth-century expansion in usage of the term does not result in clarity or precision. Koselleck (2006: 397) argues that '"Crisis" remains a catchword, used rigorously in only a few scholarly or scientific contexts.' In 1935/6 Edmund Husserl famously described the 'crisis of European sciences' as a symptom of a crisis of European civilisation, arguing that phenomenology would alleviate this. In the later part of the century the term was increasingly used to describe intellectual events and changes: within feminism, for example, the rise of poststructuralist approaches in the 1970s and 80s led to what Linda Alcoff (1988) described as 'the identity crisis in feminist theory'.

Today, the term is widely used to describe both economic and environmental situations: outlining contemporary descriptions of these two forms of crisis, for example, Noel Castree (2010: 185) asks whether 'the recent profusion of "crisis talk" in the public domain presents an opportunity for progressive new ideas to take hold now that "neoliberalism" has seemingly been de-legitimated'. In the health field, mention of crisis is similarly widespread. Public health commentators link global health problems with contemporary problems in economics and the environment, describing an 'unstable world' and an increasing gap between rich and poor that has devastating effects on poorer people's health (see, for example, Benetar, Gill and Bakker 2011). In all these cases, crisis is used to figure something serious and requiring action but that may be recurrent and/or enduring (environmental or economic crises) or singular (epidemics or shortages of health care workers in particular places and times, for example).

'Crisis' is also a term deeply loved by contemporary news media (see, for example, Triandafyllidou, Wodak and Krzyzanowski 2009). Koselleck writes,

> In all the human and social sciences, crisis appears as a key concept; in history, of course, to characterize epochs or structures. Political science tries to operationalize the term and distinguish it from 'conflict.' From medicine the concept has spread to psychology and anthropology, ethnology, and the sociology of culture. Above all, it is the media which have inflated the use of the term. (Koselleck 2006: 399)

In all this contemporary 'crisis talk', as Castree puts it, there is much less of the original meaning of the imposition of harsh alternatives. 'Crisis' can now be used to speak of an enormous range of kinds of issues or problems, recurrent or unique, local or global, interior to a person or to one body or in the public domain. There is a 'tendency towards imprecision and vagueness' that may, Koselleck argues, itself 'be viewed a symptom of a historical crisis that cannot as yet be fully gauged' (2006: 399). 'Crisis', he warns, is a word that scholars should be careful about: it means too much and too little.

Despite this learned warning, I have chosen to use the word in this book's title. Puberty has long been thought of as an individual crisis but is now also framed as a dramatic environmental and population-health problem. Early onset puberty is understood in environmentalist discourses as signalling a crisis for the continued existence of the human race by threatening healthy sexual reproduction. The original connotations of the Greek term are present in contemporary public and scientific debates about puberty: not only do these describe a situation (in a set of bodies and/or in the wider environment), they constitute a demand for action. This book makes a critical argument about this demand for action. Whilst I am convinced that epidemiological changes in the timing of puberty are significant and demand exploration and explanation, I contend that the figuring of early onset puberty as crisis leads in many cases to unwarranted and potentially harmful actions for individuals.

Instead, I argue, we need to develop alternative actions that rely less on medical and pharmaceutical intervention and are oriented towards facilitating and acting upon an understanding of human bodies as bio-psycho-social – as situated, lived and always in process. This may mean refusing processes of medical assessment and surveillance and/or medicating and moving instead towards experiments in articulating early onset puberty in more open and accepting ways.

The structure of this book

Puberty in Crisis provides an interdisciplinary account of early onset puberty, exploring medical, scientific, environmental and news media figurations of 'out of time' sexual development. Exploring and resisting crisis articulations and consequent demands for action, it opens up new ways of theorising sexually developing bodies. Working with a rich legacy of concepts and tools gleaned from feminist theory, cultural studies, sociology, and science and technology studies, I suggest that puberty be reconceived as bio-psycho-social folding: a situated, material-semiotic temporal process in which sexed bodies change, flow and temporarily (if often stickily) congeal.

Chapter 2 addresses questions of method and introduces the book's conceptual framework. Exploring contemporary debates in feminist science studies and feminist work on the biological body, it situates the book in an intellectual and political trajectory that attempts to address sexed embodiment as simultaneously material, semiotic and 'lived'. I introduce the three threads of bio-psycho-social folding that I trace throughout the book, namely findings, feelings and figurations and describe my ethnographic approach to textual analysis.

Chapter 3 provides a historical account of scientific work on puberty, narrating its coming into being as an object of scientific interest. It tells a story about the ground-breaking mid twentieth-century longitudinal research – J.M. Tanner's Harpenden Study – that underpins the measurement of pubertal stages in most scientific and clinical contexts today. Here I make an argument about the figuration of Tanner's child subjects, suggesting that, in his vigorous attempt to measure pubertal development, Tanner both articulates and disavows the bio-psycho-social complexities of sexual development.

Chapter 4 builds on this historical account, analysing contemporary scientific literatures describing global changes in sexual development, particularly amongst girls. Critically engaging with the key scientific publications in this field, I explore the ways in which 'race', social class, gender and sexuality are articulated in biomedical and scientific engagements with children's bodies and biological actors such as genes and hormones. Epidemiological discourses around early puberty are highly contested. They also hold profound implications for clinical practice, involving the re-ordering of clinical guidelines for the treatment of early maturing children through altering the very definitions of 'normal' and 'abnormal'. This chapter demonstrates the material-semiotic nature of clinical norms and the complexities of their establishment and contestation.

Chapter 5 addresses questions of causation: what are the arguments made in scientific and other literatures about the possible causes of early onset puberty? What assumptions, logics, omissions and feelings do these debates enact? Here I engage with debates in a wide range of scientific fields, from genome-wide association studies to developmental psychology; from physiological studies of nutrition and weight to environmental research into contamination and toxicity; exploring the multiplicity of early maturing bodies which are figured as vulnerable in so many different sites. Engaging with feminist work on 'sexualisation' and feminist science studies, I suggest that early puberty could be understood as part of a complex bio-psycho-social ecology of human and non-human actors.

Chapter 6 turns to scientific and public debates around the effects of early development, which focus on early sexual activity and drug-taking, psychological effects, increased risk of cancer and concerns about height. In conversation with existing work on the 'sexualisation' of girls and feminist work on young women's reproductive bodies, I argue that many of these debates enact a supposedly pre-existing and apparently desirable sexual 'innocence' for girls. Linked with the preceding work on causes of early puberty, this chapter makes a strong political argument for destabilising the generic category of 'girls' and moving towards articulating differences. Borrowing Deleuze's concept of the fold, I argue for an understanding of sexual development as a situated, ongoing process.

Chapter 7 analyses the treatment of girls going through puberty early. This is a highly contentious field. Engaging with recent work in feminist science studies on drugs and research on pharmaceuticalisation, I consider the stakes of formulating a critical approach to medical treatments. I suggest that there is much to be learnt from existing debates on the medicalisation of atypical sexual development and height that demonstrate the serious and long-lasting effects of the pathologisation of children's bodily differences. I also explore the use of puberty blocking medications by young trans people. In promoting early onset puberty as a condition requiring medication, I argue, pharmaceutical companies powerfully contribute to new articulations of sexual development as crisis.

The Conclusion draws the threads of my argument together, highlighting key conceptual questions about children and young people's physical and psychological development, sexuality and embodiment and articulating the intellectual and political significance of understanding puberty as folding.

2 *Articulating findings, feelings and figurations: approaches and resources*

In contemporary medical textbooks and educational materials for young people, their families and their teachers, puberty is described as a series of predestined and largely inescapable biological processes involving the growth of breasts, testicles and pubic hair, changes in overall body shape and size, the deepening of voices, first experiences of nocturnal seminal emissions or menstruation. Separated from but also kick-starting the psycho-social elements of growing up normally referred to as adolescence, puberty is understood as the unfolding of dualistic physiological sexual maturity and the development of a capacity to reproduce (Roberts 2007: 69–72). As feminist theorist Catherine Driscoll notes, in puberty manuals for young people, teachers and parents, 'The "facts" of puberty are cast in disciplinary terms, with those anomalies and variations that are named as acceptable marking limits beyond which difference is by default unacceptable or normal' (Driscoll 2009: 235–6).

In contrast to this didactic emphasis on physical facts and norms, this book articulates puberty as a bio-psycho-social phenomenon, a different kind of folding process in which distinctions between the biological, the psychological and the social are continually blurred.[1] Learning from feminist theory, science and technology studies (STS), sociology, history and cultural studies, I argue that bodies develop in and through social, historical and geographical 'locations' (meaning physical, psychological and social positioning). Studying pubertal bodies involves engaging with *findings, feelings and figurations in*

[1] Throughout this book, following Haraway (1997), I use 'articulate' to indicate both a practice of speaking or accounting for, and as a way of making linkages. Christina Hughes and Celia Lury explain this approach well: 'articulation . . . is a political practice for grasping things together, of overcoming dichotomies . . . and a device for being demanding about how technologies of knowing/being are deployed in practice and being similarly demanding of raising questions about alternative figurations' (Hughes and Lury 2013: 797).

relation, rather than simply accumulating and sorting biological facts. In this book, then, I am interested in scientific findings (including numerical and visual data, graphs, statistical trends and relations) but engage with these as always-in-process outcomes of particular forms of practice including experimentation, clinical practice, calculation, representation and publication. As I will explain, for me, the word 'findings' works better than 'facts' or 'data' to signal this sense of labour and contingency.

Like many contemporary feminists, I am also interested in feelings – what others call affect (see, for example, papers in Pedwell and Whitehead 2012). As described in the Introduction, puberty is an affective subject, with early sexual development provoking intense feelings of concern. Throughout this book I explore the ways in which negative and positive feelings are entangled with sexual development, paying attention to the ways in which they are expressed in a wide range of accounts of early onset puberty. Although I do not engage with psychoanalytic accounts of puberty (which are extensive and fascinating), I do work with psychological concepts and theories in many of the chapters, exploring the significance of family dynamics and childhood experience to sexual development as a folding process. My overarching aim in addressing the feelings associated with early onset puberty is to loosen some of the tighter knots joining female sexuality, youth and anxiety.

Alongside these considerations of findings and feelings, this book explores figurations, defined by Donna Haraway as 'performative images that can be inhabited . . . [v]erbal or visual . . . condensed maps of contestable worlds' (Haraway 1997: 11). Asking how early development is described and visually represented, who describes it and where, I explore how figurations of early developing children make particular worlds. Which resources are drawn upon and what kinds of cultural freight do figurations of early onset puberty carry? How and where do these figurations circulate?

My ambition, then, is to explore how these three intertwined elements – findings, feelings and figurations – articulate sexually developing bodies as bio-psycho-social. This exploration requires a diverse archive and an interdisciplinary set of research tools. In the chapters that follow, I analyse scientific and medical texts, environmentalist, public health, activist and commercial websites, non-fiction books for lay readers, advertisements and newspaper stories, television shows, art images and scientific photography. As I will go on to describe, my analyses combine practices of critical reading developed in feminist theory, cultural studies, history and sociology with the empirical, ethnographic orientation of much science and technology studies (STS). It is through this interdisciplinary nexus of materials and methods, I argue, that the complex nature of the sexually developing body can be better understood.

Theorising bodies-in-the-making: drawing on science studies and the sociology of biomedicine

Understanding bodies as bio-psycho-social involves exploring biological processes and materialities alongside, with and through cultural stories about them. As many scholars have argued, these materialities are densely elaborated in scientific and medical texts and enacted in associated technical practices in clinics, laboratories, conference centres and journals and, I would add, through a broad network of news and online media, activist texts and practices, art and popular culture practices, and fiction and non-fiction popular writing. These are what I call findings. In all these sites, particular (non-inevitable) kinds of bodies come into being, are made or 'done'.

Existing work in STS and feminist theory provides rich resources for understanding and analysing bodies in this way. Citing and expanding actor network theory (ANT),[2] for example, Haraway (1991) famously describes bodies as material-semiotic actors, emphasising the inevitable combination of forces constituting their existence. As such, bodies are always 'situated', as are knowledges of them. Situatedness, for Haraway, refers not to fixed 'time and place' coordinates or modes of identification but rather to particular congealments in ongoing, human–non-human relations (Haraway 1997: 142 and 199; see Roberts 2007: 43–50). In later work, Haraway (2008: 163) writes of bodies 'in-the-making', arguing that they are 'always a vital entanglement of heterogeneous scales, times, and kinds of beings webbed into fleshly presence, always a becoming, always constituted in relating'.

[2] Developed most notably by Bruno Latour, Michel Callon, Madeleine Akrich and John Law, actor network theory (ANT) constitutes a set of key contributions to science studies and to the social sciences more broadly. The most relevant aspect of ANT here is its emphasis on the importance of non-human actors in the production of worlds, and hence to social scientific analyses.

This orientation has practical, conceptual and political consequences. Most importantly, bodies in all their richness become objects and subjects of social scientific practice and discourse. Exploring a wide range of sites, times and actors, Haraway brings human and non-human bodies into the centre of feminist theorising as simultaneously both 'real' and 'made'; vital and becoming; material-semiotic.

Although the bulk of her research materials are written and visual texts, Haraway (1997: 191) describes her work as ethnographic. Working with a wide range of texts as well as accounts of her own practice (for example of dog agility training in Haraway 2008), she ranges across a diverse set of materials from different places and times, creating a different articulation of situatedness that both recognises the broad and diverse connections or 'diffractions' constituting an object of study (such as 'the gene' or 'the foetus') and emphasises her position as reader, writer, story-teller and political actor. In her classic book on primatology *Primate Visions* (1989), for example, Haraway reads cartoons, pharmaceutical advertisements, novels, television shows, scientific accounts of field and laboratory work and museum curatorial practices, amongst other texts. Exploring particular figurations of 'the human' and 'the animal' (specifically the primate), Haraway opens the commitments, assumptions and politics of technoscience to debate and contestation.

Dutch STS scholar Annemarie Mol (2002) takes a more strongly ANT-influenced approach, arguing that bodies are 'multiple' – brought into being or 'enacted' through the practices of any particular time and place. In slicing, measuring, counting, probing and walking, for example, medicine 'does' bodies with atherosclerosis. This is an ontological argument. Mol suggests that bodies are 'brought into being, sustained, or allowed to wither away in common, day-to-day, socio-material practices. Medical practices among them' (2002: 6). Moving away from the now commonly used 'performed', Mol introduces the less familiar word 'enactment' to describe this coming into being in activity that is not driven by an actor (2002: 32–3).

Interested in material practices and thus relying methodologically on ethnographic observation and interviewing, Mol tries to avoid semiotics. Attending to the 'logics' of medical care for Mol does not mean exploring cultural figurations (see also Mol 2008). Although heavily indebted to anthropology, she describes her research as 'empirical philosophy', reflecting her core focus on philosophical questions

(Mol 2002: 1).[3] This approach leads to rich accounts of particular diseases and bodies in a mode described as praxiographic (writing focusing on practice). Her ethnographic accounts take readers into particular clinics, homes and laboratories in order to explore the enactments of bodies taking place there and thereby to theorise the body as ontologically multiple.

Although influenced by both scholars' theorisations of bodies-in-the-making, my approach in this book remains methodologically closer to Haraway's situated story-telling than to Mol's empirical philosophy. Rather than undertaking a specifically located ethnography of early onset puberty – following practices in a particular clinic, for example – I have focused here on texts, exploring a wide range of intersecting and distinct accounts of sexual development. This expansive approach allows me to investigate the findings, feelings and figurations constituting early onset puberty as crisis and to locate scientific and medical accounts of sexual development amongst broader cultural articulations of sex/gender, sexuality, age, race and social class. Learning from Mol and Haraway, I theorise bodies as coming into being in relational activities of humans and non-humans, including textual practices.

This book's argument about developing bodies is also strongly influenced by Anne Fausto-Sterling and to a somewhat lesser extent Evelyn Fox-Keller who, like Haraway, are both feminist scientists *and* analysts of science. Both writers undertake detailed readings of scientific and/or medical texts, exploring how biological actors such as genes and hormones are said to be involved in the making of bodies (Fausto-Sterling, 1985; 2000; 2004; 2008; 2012; Fox Keller 1984; 2000; 2010). Although neither would identify as ethnographers, Fausto-Sterling and Fox Keller bring embodied histories of scientific training and work to their critical readings of texts, writing as critical insiders within scientific discourses. Fox Keller (1983) also uses interviewing in some of her work. In contrast to Haraway, however, they both draw rather clear boundaries around their objects of analysis, focusing on scientific arguments and practices without also analysing other texts. I engage with their work in several ways in this book. Using their

[3] Coming out of the Netherlands, empirical philosophy now constitutes an important strand of science studies, see for example Willems and Pols (2010), Pols (2012) and Mort et al. (2013).

arguments about hormones and genes to underpin my own, I also attempt to replicate the precision of their readings of scientific literatures. I am inspired by their relentless exploration of the ways in which sex and gender are articulated through scientific knowledges and practices and their orientation towards science, which is engaged and respectful but also intrinsically critical.

In researching biomedical and scientific accounts of early onset puberty, I am also influenced by contemporary sociological and STS work on contemporary medical technologies and practices. The work of Adele Clarke and colleagues (2010), for example, provides both conceptual and methodological tools for exploring the ways in which medical practices delineate their objects of study. Although less interested in ontological arguments about bodies or sex/gender, these and other North American scholars – including, for example, Jennifer Terry, Michelle Murphy, Joseph Dumit and Steven Epstein – lead the way in demonstrating how to tell detailed stories about science and medicine that expose and critically examine the ways in which expert knowledges come into being, shaping and delimiting bodies, health and disease. Their powerful critical emphasis on questions of race and ethnicity as well as sexuality and sex/gender is instructive. In this book I explore the ways in which class, race, age, sex/gender and sexuality are articulated and move across a range of early puberty discourses.

Engaging with biological bodies: corporeal and new materialist feminisms

Critical investigations of scientific and medical knowledges have recently been problematised both by feminist scholars working within what can be broadly conceived as corporeal feminism and by those identifying as new materialists and/or post-humanists (see McNeil 2010; Dolphijn and van der Tuin 2012). Indeed, as is now common within literary studies and feminist queer theory (Wiegman 2014), critique per se is sometimes rejected as a mode of feminist engagement with science and medicine (usually, ironically, as itself a form of criticism of others). In a recent interview, for example, feminist physicist Karen Barad (whose work I discuss below) states: 'I am not interested in critique. In my opinion, critique is over-rated, over-emphasized, and over-utilized, to the detriment of feminism' (Barad, in Dolphijn and van der Tuin 2012: ch. 3).[4] Both Elizabeth Grosz (2010) and Elizabeth A. Wilson (1998) have similarly argued that the feminist tradition of work on biology has been overly negative and suggested that feminists have shied away from meaningful engagement with biology as both a science and a set of material forces (see also Kirby 2011). Acknowledging the work of Fausto-Sterling and Fox Keller as counter-examples, Grosz writes that 'feminist theory has protected and insulated itself from any incursions into biology through the fear indeed paranoia surrounding the question of essentialism, though biology is one of the few disciplines able to adequately contest essentialism' (Grosz 2010: 50). In 2004, Wilson similarly argued that feminist theories of the body 'have usually been reluctant to engage with biological data; they retain, and encourage, the fierce antibiologism that marked the emergence of second-wave feminism' (Wilson 2004: 13). Her counter-suggestion, and the direction of her own work, has been for feminism to 'be more affectionately involved with neurobiological data' (2004: 14).

Like Fausto-Sterling and Fox Keller, a range of scholars in feminist science studies and anthropology do, in my view, undertake the fearless and/or affectionate engagement with biology as knowledge and practice that Grosz and Wilson advocate (see, for example, Rapp 2000; Franklin and Roberts 2006; Fujimura 2006, 2011; Franklin 2007; Landecker 2007; Rosengarten 2009; Murphy 2012).[5] Situated within this lineage of feminist engagement with biology, and worrying about the potential losses involved in moving away from critical reading practices and their associated pleasures, this book remains critical in many ways. Although of course not wanting to occupy the superior, hypervigilant position that is often associated with what Wiegman (2014: 7; see also Stacey 2014), following Eve Sedgwick's appropriation of Melanie Klein, calls paranoid reading, I remain unable to

[4] Such rejections of critique, as Robyn Wiegman argues, take place within a political and economic context in which the value of academic criticism has been seriously undermined. The shift away from critique towards affirmative engagements with texts of all sorts arguably constitutes an attempt to reconfer value onto intellectual analysis and interpretation, particularly those arising from the humanities (Wiegman 2014: 16). For commentaries on this argument, see Hemmings (2014); Lewis (2014) and Stacey (2014).

[5] For an introduction to this work, see McNeil and Roberts 2010.

engage non-critically with science and medicine. True to my training in poststructuralist feminist theory and women's studies, I want to engage with these powerful discourses in a somewhat diagnostic way, looking for trouble (Butler 1990) and sometimes remaining ambivalent (Stacey 2014: 47), even furious, about them. This is not to say, however, that I am not also looking for positive accounts and useful, hopeful figurations. My overarching aim is to explore the ways in which sexually developing bodies are articulated and to demonstrate the relevance of such articulations to feminist politics and theory.[6]

Despite disagreeing with their assessment of feminist work on biology, I find both Grosz's and Wilson's analyses of bodies inspiring. Engaging with traditional and more recent psychoanalytic theory and the writings of Jacques Derrida and Gilles Deleuze amongst others, and sharing a great interest in evolutionary theory, both theorise bodies as inextricably cultural and material and also psychological. Both bring feeling or affect to the analysis of bodies-in-the-making within science: something that Haraway and Fausto-Sterling, for example, do not.[7] I have discussed Grosz's contribution to feminist theories of embodiment elsewhere (Roberts 2007) but want to note here her insistence on theorising sexual and racial differences as both material and psychological. As evident in the following quote, her understanding of difference is influenced by psychoanalysis (emphasising the impossibility of conscious control) and by Darwin (differences are 'evolutionary'):

> Sexual difference (the acquisition of at least two radically different types of subject position according to at least two different morphological structures)

[6] In this aim, I demonstrate the characteristic trait of feminist academics, according to Wiegman, which is the resolute clinging to interpretation as sustaining. Acknowledging this, I find myself in agreement with her that 'the widely heralded distinction' between critical and positive approaches (what she calls paranoid and reparative readings) 'is not really one, as both practices are engaged in producing, confirming, and sustaining critical practice as a necessary agency, no matter the different object relations and analytic itineraries that govern each' (Wiegman 2014: 18). For responses to Wiegman's argument, see Hemmings (2014), Lewis (2014) and Stacey (2014). For a related argument about feminist science studies, see McNeil (2010).

[7] In her early work Fox Keller also engages with psychoanalytic theories in thinking about scientists investments in their work (see for example Fox Keller 1984; 1995).

and racial difference (the acknowledgement of a multiplicity of corporeal and cultural variations) are neither constrained to the forms in which we currently know them, nor are they open to self-conscious manipulation, identification, or control by subjects. They are material, evolutionary forces through which we work but which we do not control, which we cannot rise above but which nevertheless direct us toward the possibilities of change. (Grosz 2005: 88–89; see also Grosz 2012: ch. 9)

This emphasis on possibilities for change signals Grosz's desire to theorise both biology and science in a positive, affirmative mode. Although, wanting also to read scientific texts in a more 'paranoid' mode, I find Grosz's emphasis on material, biological and evolutionary forces as processes that 'we do not control' but 'through which we work … towards the possibilities of change' a helpful framing through which to think sexed bodies-in-the-making. Understood as a bio-psycho-social process, sexual development is a compelling example of the ways in which evolutionary and biological forces, in inextricable relation to cultural and social ones, 'direct us to the future' (Grosz 2005: 89). Grosz's acknowledgement of the impossibility of conscious control of corporeality seems to me an essential element in any attempt to understand puberty. Sexual development – moving towards what Grosz describes as 'the acquisition of at least two radically different types of subject position according to at least two different morphological structures' – usually lies outside conscious control; it 'happens' in and through our bodies-in-the-world. But this is not to say that it is 'simply' biological: such events are experienced; 'worked through' to use Grosz's words. They are also, as I describe in Chapter 7, increasingly open to pharmaceutical intervention and control. Our bodies are neither free to develop in any way, nor constrained to develop in the way they often do. I learn from Grosz that this paradox constitutes a hopeful site for feminist corporeal politics.

Although in dialogue with similar philosophical trajectories, Wilson spends more time than Grosz investigating the specific claims of particular scientists around bodies and feeling, notably in the fields of neurology (1998; 2004) and artificial intelligence (2010). Engaging with scientific theories and findings, Wilson tells stories that challenge conventional thinking about bodies both in science and medicine and in feminist theory. In describing the neuroendocrinology of the human gut, for example, she argues that depressive states could be figured as bodily (rather than only mental or central nervous system) ones:

> The nervous system extends well beyond the skull, and as it so travels through the body it takes the psyche with it. The transferential nature of the nervous system (i.e. its obligatory relations to other systems biochemical, psychological, enterological) has yet to be grasped in either psychoanalytic or gastroenterological frameworks. (Wilson 2004: 47)

Putting scientific findings about neurotransmitters in the gut into conversation with psychoanalytic theory, she contends, could change the way we understand mental illness and associated behaviours such as refusing to eat (2004: 45).

In recent work, discussed in more detail in Chapter 7, Wilson (2011) uses concepts from feminist theorist and physicist Karen Barad to explore the actions of antidepressants in children's bodies. Barad's contribution to feminist theories of embodiment is an example *par excellence* of the new approach that uses scientific work as a conceptual interlocutor rather than treating it as an object for feminist critique. Most notably in *Meeting the Universe Halfway: Quantum Physics and the Entanglement of Matter and Meaning*, Barad (2007) concentrates on quantum physics, specifically the theoretical and empirical work of Niels Bohr. In painstaking engagements with this highly valorised scientific field (one that is much less frequently explored by feminists than biology due in large part to its less obvious connections to feminist politics) Barad introduces several concepts that help feminists to think differently about the ontology of bodies (human and non-human, living and non-living); specifically intra-action, agential realism, agential cuts and entanglements.[8] Each of these concepts signals Barad's argument – following Bohr – that entities come into existence in specific material arrangements of practices, which she calls apparatuses. Entities – including human and non-human bodies – are 'entanglements of matter and meaning' (Barad's intellectual debt to Haraway's 'material-semiotic' is clear here). Like Mol, Barad is careful to argue that entanglements do not mix or put into relation pre-existing entities; rather, entities are made, or come to matter as they

[8] As she notes elsewhere, Barad also hopes that her work will alert physicists to the significance of feminist theory to their work (Barad in Dolphijn and van der Tuin 2012).

form apparatuses.[9] This difference is referenced in her neologism 'intra-action', which is used instead of 'interaction' to indicate a different understanding of causality. Like many earlier STS accounts, Barad insists on the role of non-human forces in the making of human and other bodies. In contrast to what she calls 'performative accounts' of embodiment – Judith Butler (1993) is the key reference here – 'agential realism takes account of the fact that the forces at work in the materialization of bodies are not only social, and the bodies produced are not all human ... [A]gential realism clarifies the nature of the causal relationship between discursive practices and material phenomena' (Barad 2007: 33–4).

Both this critique of Butler and the use of the term 'realism' speak to Barad's desire to move away from an analysis of language as constitutive social force (what Haraway [1988: 579] would call a 'semiotic technology'). Although also deeply invested in thinking about the materiality of human and non-human bodies, I want in contrast to continue to pay attention to language's materialising power when considering human bodies in development. Barad's careful explications of quantum physics experiments and theories as argumentation trouble me insofar as they marginalise the question of language's performativity, using scientific stories to speak about ontology in modes that – even if they are not strictly 'dutiful' (as she claims in Dolphijn and van der Tuin 2012) – rhetorically resonate with the specific scientific tradition that inspires her and in which she was trained. For me, Haraway's more irreverent writing, mixing scientific discourses with those from popular culture and everyday life, works better to highlight the inescapable performativity of words in relation to things. Perhaps what is at play here is partially a historical distinction between biology and physics as discursive and experimental traditions: Haraway's examples (plants, insects, dogs) speak to excess, exuberance and the impossibility of control; Barad's (the two-slit experiment; Schroedinger's Cat) to precision, repetition and proof; although it should be noted that both scholars delight in their examples' capacity to surprise, and that Barad sometimes writes in more experimental ways about these materials (see for example, Barad 2010).

[9] Mol also uses the term 'entanglements' in theorising ontology (see, for example, Mol 2002: 156–7).

Like Haraway, Barad insists that the scientist is part of the making of bodies or worlds that she calls apparatuses. (Bohr's work on the effect of scientists' presence on the outcome of physics experiments is fascinating in this regard.) This is highly significant for feminist theory, as it implies an ethical responsibility and demands that scientists relinquish the traditional role of the disinterested objective observer in favour of a position Haraway (2007) names 'modest witnessing'. Of course the social scientist or cultural critic should similarly understand themselves as part of the scene of analysis. The choices I make in this book – to explore some areas and not others, or to put particular theories and examples into conversation – are always consequential. I have done my best here to be clear and explicit about this but cannot simply render my investments transparent either to readers or to myself. My main goal in this book is to explore the complex flows between social, biological, psychological and environmental events constituting bodies-in-the-(sexual)-making. Such exploration, I argue, provides parents, clinicians, policymakers and others with a more adequate basis for decision-making and action when it comes to early development. Given the importance of science and medicine in articulating bodies as developing early, much of the work in this book focuses on technical discourses, exploring modes of explanation and forms of data as well as their affective charge. But how, given the rich feminist tradition I have just described, do I do this work?

Reading science: engaging 'the literature' as ethnographic informant

The question of how to engage with contemporary scientific discourses remains fraught within feminist research, as debates in the *European Journal of Women's Studies* (*EJWS*) on 'the new materialism' (Ahmed 2008; Tuin 2008; Davis 2009) and in *Feminist Theory* on non-human feminisms (Roberts and Hird 2011) indicate. Despite their significant differences, and in tune with Grosz and Wilson, the three authors involved in the *EJWS Open Forum* (and many they cite) all praise 'careful attention' to biology and biological processes within feminism. They disagree strongly on feminists' success in doing this: Sara Ahmed (2008: 27) points to the work of feminist science studies scholars such as Haraway, Fox Keller, Emily Martin, Sandra Harding and Sarah Franklin in 'engag[ing] with the question of biology, materiality, life itself'; Noela Davis (2008) argues that this work tends to view the biological and the social as two distinct domains; domains that can be mixed but are not inseparable.

In both cases, the authors spend too little time elaborating their call for 'careful attention' to the biological: Ahmed cites early feminist writer Deidre Janson-Smith's (1980) description of metabolic and other changes during the menstrual cycle (Ahmed, 2008: 30) but this description is rather far from the presentation of biological data Ahmed claims it to be. Similarly, the example of Anne M. Briscoe's (1978) work on hormones provides a basic factual description of hormonal processes rather than a discussion of data or biological debates (Ahmed 2008: 37). Davis similarly argues that such texts are indicators only of 'restricted and conventional' engagements with biological processes, but offers few examples of how feminists might do better. Her key counter-reference is Wilson's *Psychosomatic* (2004), a book that does pay serious attention to biological explanations of symptoms of psychological distress. Davis cites Wilson's rereading of Freud's analysis of Fraulein Elisabeth in which she argues that the physiology of the patient's paralysed legs is inseparable from the death of her father and the words of Freud as analyst. Davis contends that 'the biology that Wilson is describing is social – it converses, it suffers, it yearns. Its functioning cannot be confined to an outside of sociality as is conventionally done' (Davis 2008: 71). Again, however, this example stays rather a long way from 'biological data'; Davis gives little sense of how one might approach the analysis of any field of contemporary biology or physiology. (It should be noted that Wilson's book does engage with biological findings and argumentation, but this work does not figure in Davis' analysis.)

This problem seems to hinge, at least in part, on the definition of 'data'. In a recent conversation with Vicki Kirby in *Feminist Theory*, Wilson provides a helpful discussion. Although asserting that: 'Feminist work is at its strongest . . . when it is able to work with, rather than against, scientifically generated theories and data', she notes that she is 'increasingly concerned that there is now a tendency to simply flip these politics around, and to side with scientific data in a very literal kind of way' (Kirby and Wilson 2011: 233). Elaborating a path that avoids either of these responses, Wilson argues that 'data given empirically or experimentally are mobile, contradictory, and contingent, rather than fixed. Those contingencies can be highly stable – spreading out over long periods of time and across a large number of places – but they are contingencies nonetheless, and as such warrant neither refusal nor reverence' (2011: 234). Here, then, data are not factual descriptions (like those to which Ahmed points) and they do not describe fixed, asocial domains (as Davis suggests they do in much feminist work). Instead, biological data are part of the argument: something to be valued, worked with and critiqued. Aligning myself with this view, I have chosen here to refer instead to 'findings' in order to highlight the contingent, always-already 'worked up' nature of the data presented in scientific publications. As many ethnographic studies of scientific practice have shown, published scientific findings are the result of complex networks of skilled labour, institutional arrangements and rhetorical, statistical and experimental traditions, and must be understood as outcomes or 'results', not as 'raw' facts. The exhortation to engage *directly* with biology, then, makes little sense; even if the encouragement to engage openly or energetically with scientific findings is embraced (see also McNeil 2010).

Studying scientific findings, scientists and/or scientific work as a social scientist or humanities scholar involves significant methodological challenges. For some projects, it means spending time in laboratories and clinics, sometimes even learning to perform scientific work (see, for example, Rapp 2000; M'charek 2005; Franklin and Roberts 2006; Hird 2009). In others, it means careful reading of historical archives and published papers (see, for example, Terry 1999; Kay 2000; Landecker 2007; Wilson 2010), interviewing scientists (see for example, Fox Keller 1984; Reardon 2004) and/or working with a wider range of texts (see, most significantly, Haraway's work). In each case engaging with science involves ethical responsibilities, not only to engage well with scientific content and practice but also to explore broader questions relating to justice, power and politics as well as feeling.

One important way to act responsibly in studying science is to figure its multiplicity and to understand science as extending well beyond the laboratory walls (Roberts and Mackenzie 2006). In current work on neuroscience and parenting, for example, Mackenzie and I figure science as enacted by a range of experts and non-experts; neuroscientific models of parenting, we show, are lived by children and adults in consequential ways. Studies of parents' and children's brain chemistry do not simply provide 'data' but, in intra-action with other findings and practices, articulate modes of embodied interaction and understanding. In this, like Amade M'charek (2010: 309), we learn from 'scholarship in feminist technoscience [that] has urged us to not only study the scientific citadels (laboratories and related scientific institutions) ... but also to pay attention to popular science and other everyday practices in a world that is populated by science and technology'. In this book, similarly, I range across scientific papers, press releases, news media articles, websites, parental guides, environmentalist websites and campaigns, and young people's blogs and vlogs. The science of early sexual development and the enactment of pubertal bodies, I argue, occur in all these places.

Despite this breadth, much of this book addresses scientific and biomedical discourses. Several chapters contain detailed discussions of scientific data and arguments, putting scientific and medical knowledges and practices under a social scientific microscope not in order to prove them wrong or misguided but to open up a space of sustained engagement in which social scientific concepts and research (about bodies, gender, racialisation, images and language) come into critical contact with scientific discourses about biological processes, bodily changes in populations and the biochemical effects of pharmaceuticals. This focus on primary scientific and biomedical texts is somewhat unusual, even within science studies. As Nikolas Rose (2013: 4) argues in his review of social scientific literature focusing on the life sciences, 'when those from the social and human sciences do turn to biology, there is an understandable tendency to draw upon books about the life sciences written for non-specialists, and to select those themes that match their theoretical or political aspirations'. I have tried to avoid this tendency here, engaging directly with scientific literatures as much as I can.

In doing so, I am inspired by Christopher Kelty and Hannah Landecker's call for social scientists to treat '*The Literature as an informant*' in attempting to understand large-scale change in particular scientific fields (as opposed to undertaking detailed case studies of particular people or places) (Kelty and Landecker 2009: 177, emphasis in original).[10] Kelty and Landecker make several suggestions for

[10] Kelty and Landecker (2009: 176) argue that the vast scale of twentieth-century science means that new methods have to be developed to produce 'synthetic accounts of long-term, large-scale changes in thought and practice'. This certainly accords with my experience of working on early puberty: my database

undertaking such ethnographic work on scientific texts: scholars should read for practice (analysing the depictions of particular methods across a set of papers); read for plot (observe patterns of story-telling); and attend to problematisation (ask what is the problem posed and what is its solution). In this book I follow this advice, additionally, learning from Haraway, taking these methods into a wider range of cultural texts. I am concerned here with the ways in which scientific and biomedical discourses appear in, resonate with, use or contradict other discourses, specifically those coming from environmentalists, journalists, and feminist and other activists.

Importantly, this book does not require an existing understanding of any particular scientific or biomedical field: I explain and situate the knowledges under discussion, albeit only as an engaged 'outsider'. Although most of my engagements in this project have been with texts – the literature is my key informant – for a decade or more I have discussed early puberty with a range of experts, including clinicians, scientists, historians, sex educators, environmentalists and parents. My 'ethnographic readings' (Kelty and Landecker 2009: 185) are informed by these engagements and I sometimes refer to them directly here. My analysis of scientific and other literatures is a form of conversation with interested others: the version I present here is but one iteration formed after receiving years of multi-disciplinary comment on spoken and written drafts.

Figurations of childhood: drawing on feminist theory and cultural studies

As noted in Chapter 1, there is much public talk today about the changing nature of childhood. A body of recent work coming from feminist theory and cultural studies illuminates this talk, helping to situate my more specific concerns about early developing children in a wider cultural frame (see, for example, papers in Burman and Stacey 2010; Spongberg 2008).

The core thesis of this corpus is that modern childhood is a gendering, racialising and classing process articulated through scientific

of scientific articles has 1,500 entries, expanding rapidly each year: 'the literature' in this case, as in most others scientific fields, has become 'something far larger than anyone can digest' (Kelty and Landecker 2009: 177).

conceptualisations of 'the child' as a (sexually) developing being. Originating in late nineteenth- and early twentieth-century sexology, psychoanalysis, anthropology, sociology, economics and politics, amongst other disciplines, these discourses enact childhood as a transitional stage between birth and adulthood, something to be scientifically studied and managed across different sites. Such theories, as Erica Burman (2008) and Claudia Castañeda (2002) both show, produced normative understandings of gendered, classed and racialised childhoods against which all children are potentially measured. Puberty, as I will argue in Chapter 3, has a particular place in this modern version of childhood, emerging as a set of physical changes heralding the beginning of adolescence, a period of highly problematic social and emotional change. As Driscoll writes, 'Puberty constructs dichotomous body types as social meanings that enable particular functions tied to patriarchal, capitalist late modernity' (Driscoll 2002: 104).

Feminist and queer debates around the child also raise important questions about the relation between representations or imaginings of the child and the historical actors we might describe as embodied children. In queer debates, as Karin Lesnik-Oberstein (2010) argues, discussions of the child focus on the symbolic as opposed to 'real' children.[11] Whilst emphases on the powerful place of the child in cultural and psychological imaginings are important, attempts to mark these out from embodied human actors are unconvincing and conceptually and politically limiting, tending to delimit children's physical and psychological experiences as authentic and difficult, even impossible, to speak (Lesnick-Oberstein 2010: 318–19; see also Bray 2009). In other frames, as Daniella Caselli (2010: 244) points out, children and childhood are closely linked to arguments about the importance of theorising that which is 'extra-discursive' and 'extra-textual' in the production of human subjectivity, often figured as 'affect'. Such links, Caselli argues, rely on childhood's historical connection to nature and 'its allegedly instant accessibility from an affective point of view' (Caselli 2010: 245). Caselli exhorts feminists to problematise this connection and to admit that 'childhood ... cannot simply heal the wound of language and restore fullness' (Caselli 2010: 251).

[11] Lee Edelman, one of the key theorists in this field, capitalises 'the Child' to signify this difference (Edelman 2004).

Feminist science studies scholar Claudia Castañeda (2002) addresses a similar set of issues, suggesting that discussing figurations of children bridges the (supposed) gap between representations and imaginings of children and the child and embodied children. Relying on Haraway and other science studies theorists' understandings of the activity of non-human actors, Castañeda argues that children are material-semiotic entities, their lives always 'the effect of the agency of nature and the discursive matrix through which it is formed and reformed' (Castañeda 2002: 171). Figurations of particular children are 'the effect of a specific configuration of knowledges, practices, and power, such that providing an account of the child's figuration entails generating accounts of necessarily powerful and yet still contestable worlds' (2002: 4). The approach I take here is very much in line with Castañeda's position: as in my earlier work on sex hormones (Roberts 2007), I describe the activity of both human and non-human actors in articulating or enacting sexed bodies.

In this rich body of work, feminist theorists describe the racialisation, gendering and classing of the child. Burman (1994) argues that within developmental psychology the child is figured as white, male, active, spontaneous and bourgeois (playing rather than working). Such representations leave untheorised the millions of children globally who, for example, work, live on the streets, are sex workers or fight in wars (Burman 1994: 53).[12] Castañeda also articulates the silences around certain children's lives, arguing that normative western models of childhood permit and support problematic practices and interventions in the lives of some non-western children (international adoption in particular). The universalising of a particular model of 'good' childhood renders differences between children opaque and leads to cultural and material forms of erasure: contemporary children are seen as archetypal flexible subjects. As Burman and Stacey (2010: 231) argue, for Castañeda, it is precisely the incompleteness and accompanying instability that renders the child so appealing and available to adult discursive production (making and re-making).

This figuration of children as flexible subjects of mutable potentiality is echoed in recent analyses of scientifically oriented discourses of hope. Vincanne Adams, Michelle Murphy and Adele Clarke (2009), for

[12] See also Mayall 1995; Balkishori Team of VACHA Women's Resource Center with Jackie Kirk 2009; Moletsane 2009.

example, describe medical and cultural practices around contemporary childhood as exemplary sites of the over-valuation of and intense desire to control the future (see also Edelman 2004). Girls in particular, Adams *et al.* argue, function as sites for investment and the production of future capital:

> Girlhood is one site among many where distinctively gendered anticipatory regimes are at stake. In neo-liberal development regimes coalescing since the early 1990s, 'girlhood' has been identified as a crucial site for the creation of 'human capital'. Human capital is intrinsically an anticipatory form, calling for investment in the skills and health of humans for the sake of greater returns towards GDP in the future. (Adams *et al.* 2009: 253)

These calls include exhortations to invest in the education and health of poor girls globally, practices of vaccinating girls against future STDs (the HPV vaccine) and educational discourses aimed at increasing awareness of the potential of domestic (endocrine-disrupting) chemicals to increase future cancer risk. Each of these calls focuses on girls' future fertility: either to reduce that of poor and/or young girls or to ensure the reproductive capacity of other girls so they can reproduce at 'the right time'. As I argued in Chapter 1, puberty is another key site of such investment, understood culturally and scientifically as a process in which girls' reproductive capacity comes into being.

Feminist work on children and childhood highlights the importance of attending to historical, class, gender, racial and geographical specificities when analysing accounts of sexual development and sexuality. The stories of alarm and concerns about sexualisation that characterise media, environmental and public debates around girls' early puberty need to be read as situated, historically and geographically specific (albeit international) knowledges. These discourses, as I will argue throughout this book, enact particular groups of girls in specific ways. Even references to 'all girls' or 'girls globally' do this; discourses can never be universal in their reach. Understanding such debates as contributing to the making of girls' bodies – rather than additional to or inscriptive of them – increases their significance to my argument. Whilst most of the work undertaken for this book focuses on scientific and medical accounts of pubertal bodies, I do not want to separate these accounts or findings from figurations or from feelings. It is the mutual enfolding of these that for me constitutes sexual development.

Why bother with science and biomedicine in exploring early onset puberty?

Sustained engagement with scientific and biomedical debates is both politically and conceptually useful to feminist projects around girls, sexual development and adolescence more broadly. As in other health-related fields, technoscience and biomedicine are at the heart of existing debates and are central to the enactments of contemporary bodies (Clarke *et al.* 2010). As Rose writes, 'To live well today is to live in the light of biomedicine' (Rose 2013: 7). There is much to learn from technoscience and biomedicine and much that social science and feminist theory can contribute in trying to develop new lines of thought and new enactments of pubescent bodies. I see this book, then, as part of what Haraway somewhat provocatively calls a 'successor science' project: one that 'offers a more adequate, richer, better account of a world, in order to live in it well' (Haraway 1988: 579).

This book brings together a set of analytic practices and conceptual tools from feminist theory, cultural studies, sociology and STS, in order to speak of and to scientific and medical worlds, and wider public and 'lay' debates about developing bodies. In each chapter, I attempt both to render the specificities of the knowledges and practices under discussion and to explore their wider significance. My attitude is curious and fascinated, sometimes appalled; and I am driven by a desire to explore and to come to know better. I hope this attitude provokes readers' interest in the details: there is so much more to know than I can tell here. I am heartened by Wiegman's writing about feminist research, in which she argues that both paranoid (critical) and reparative (positive or affectionate) approaches ultimately affirm the value of interpretation: '*No one will read this*, a thousand scholars murmur, as we chew on the world in ways that have everything to do with finding interpretations that can sustain us' (Wiegman 2014: 19). Telling stories about early sexual development, engaging with findings, feelings and figurations, is for me part of a feminist project to understand the world better and, in so doing, to contribute to making it differently, for all of our sakes.

The following chapter tells a story about the history of the scientific study of puberty, arguing that, from their inception, scientific articulations of 'normal' and 'early onset' puberty have been inextricably entangled with historically specific figurations and enactments of sex, sexuality, race and class. Such entanglements, I suggest, continue to underpin and limit much contemporary thinking around sexual development. Critically analysing these relations is a prerequisite for opening up space to explore alternative findings, feelings and figurations of sexual development.

3 *Telling histories: the scientific study of puberty*

I don't want to inherit these violent histories . . .; that's why I have to tell them.

(Haraway 2003: 82)

Today puberty is widely understood to be both itself in crisis and indicative of a broader environmental and/or social crisis. Children's bodies are said to be changing at previously unknown rates with as yet unclear but potentially dramatic effects. Such assessments are based on historical comparison. This chapter narrates a history of scientific studies of physiological sexual development, articulating how puberty has been defined and made in modern science and medicine. As outlined in the previous chapter, I rely on an understanding of scientific work as culturally, geographically and historically situated practice: building on a critical science studies tradition, 'science' and 'biomedicine' are understood as activities involving humans and non-humans that enact bodies and worlds. A wide range of discourses and activities constitute the apparatuses of technoscience: as embodied actors working with and through a range of materials, ideas and feelings, scientists and clinicians make bio-psycho-social worlds through their work. Telling stories about scientific history is one route to exploring the articulations of differences that are simultaneously material and conceptual or 'material-semiotic' to use Donna Haraway's term.

Since late modern times, puberty has been figured in Euro-American cultures as a difficult period in a person's life, fraught with emotional and physical risk and requiring careful negotiation.[1] From the mid nineteenth century, such management increasingly came to involve medical knowledge, with advice manuals written by doctors suggesting both spiritual and physical techniques to assist young men and women to weather the transition between childhood and adulthood

[1] For discussion of puberty in early modern times, see Toulalan (2011).

(Moran 2000: ch. 1). Puberty was thought to consume immense reserves of nervous energy, leaving girls in particular in a vulnerable state, unable, for example, to participate in education (see for example, Maudsley 1874). Puberty was conceived as a crisis. As historian Julie-Marie Strange writes,

> At the end of the nineteenth century, female puberty and menstruation were clinically described as 'critical epochs'; moments in the female reproductive life-cycle thought to excite physiological and psychological instability ... The influence of such 'crises' was overwhelmingly thought to be detrimental, rendering the female sex periodically incapacitated. (Strange 2001: 249)

In this chapter, I provide a historical account of scientific understandings of puberty as biological crisis. My key questions are: how did puberty come to be an object of such intense concern and investigation? How were the modern norms of puberty against which all children are now measured established? How did children become involved in these scientific activities? Which non-humans were important and how did scientists and others figure sex/gender, 'race'/ethnicity, class and age in this work? What are the resonances of historical scientific work on puberty that should be considered in thinking through contemporary debates on puberty in crisis?

Adolesence and puberty in the nineteenth and twentieth centuries

The nineteenth-century view of puberty and menstruation as crisis facilitated a popular argument that women were unable to participate in many elements of public life: 'From adolescence to the menopause ... the sophisticated language of empiricism and scientific objectivity defined women as incapable of competing with men on account of their biology' (Strange 2001: 249). Such definitions were fiercely contested by American and British first-wave feminists and women physicians such as Celia Mosher, Elizabeth Garrett Anderson and Mary Putnam Jacobi, who argued that menstruating women did not need rest but rather to be educated about reproductive physiology (Bland 1995: 67–70; Brumberg 1997: 6–25; Strange 2001: 253–7).

Notably, these debates took place in the very early days of a 'glandular' model of sex and sexual reproduction, when the physiology of ovulation and menstruation were poorly understood and sex hormones as yet 'undiscovered' (Roberts 2007: ch. 1). In 1905 G. Stanley Hall devoted only one short paragraph to the 'glands' in his seminal two-volume work, *Adolescence: Its Psychology, and its Relation to Physiology, Anthropology, Sociology, Sex, Crime, Religion, and Education*,[2] presciently arguing that developing understandings of the 'sex glands' would fundamentally change scientific understandings of the body:

> We shall never understand many of the deepest problems involving the relation of the mind to the body until we can write a new chapter of psycho-physiology on glandular physiology. Secretions and excretions, both internal and external, including the functions of what we may still call the sexual glands, although unlike others, they secrete only living cells, condition many psychical states in a way hardly less basic than they do all other physiological processes, and for fundamental feelings and instituting that are probably quite as important as the brain itself. (Hall 1905: 114)[3]

Widely viewed as instituting the scientific study of adolescence, Hall's text collated a stream of nineteenth-century thinking about sexual development and, although quite backward-looking in its physiological and moral orientation, made many claims that remain pertinent to psychological literatures today (Arnett 1999; Moran 2000: ch. 1; Driscoll 2002: 53). Most famously, Hall described adolescents (particularly young men) as being at risk of suffering a period of biologically caused 'storm and stress' involving mood disruption, conflicts with authority figures and risk behaviour.[4] Hall was a man of his scientific times. Both a eugenicist and a Lamarckian, he argued that child development was a 'recapitulation' of the origins of humanity ('phylogeny') and that the adolescent period of storm and stress must be a recapitulation of a highly stressful period in ancient human history. Adolescents required strict control to avoid the perils of development,

[2] This was also the year that the term 'hormone' was coined and that Freud published his ground-breaking 'Three Essays on Sexuality' (Roberts 2007: ch. 1).

[3] It was not clear to Hall and his contemporaries, for example, whether the pubertal body and facial hair at puberty were 'the products of sexual secretion' or not (Hall 1905: 416) or how sexual development related to bone growth: Hall describes the relation as 'mysterious' (1905: 425). Similarly he writes, 'Precisely what menstruation is, is not very well known' (1905: 480).

[4] Here Hall borrowed a German term 'Sturm und Drang' describing literature that expressed the psychological difficulties of young men, most famously Goethe's *The Sorrows of Young Werther* (1774).

most notably masturbation, which could permanently weaken their bodies and reproductive capacities (Hall 1905: 432–71). Young people, Hall asserted, should be guided carefully towards a Christian and moral set of beliefs and behaviours (abstinence followed by reproductive marital sex)[5] in order to maintain the rightful dominance of white middle-class people in European and North American societies.[6]

Hall was also deeply interested in the biological aspects of puberty, with long sections of *Adolescence* describing the physical changes of sexual development that he argued took place at around 11–12 years of age (1905: 420). The first chapter of his book, entitled 'Growth in Height and Weight', contains nineteenth-century data on children's growth gathered by anthropologist Franz Boas amongst others (Hall 1905: 1–50). These data make comparisons across and within nations (comparing countries and cities) and across social groups (urban boys versus 'peasants') (1905: 9). As I will explain, most of these studies describe relatively few subjects (data on length and weight at birth is much more extensive) and many are methodologically poor. Hall agrees: 'there is very often lack of uniformity in taking measurements ... age determinations are often too inaccurate, and frequency of measurements vary' (1905: 12). Descriptions of single individuals, Hall argues, are often 'the most valuable measurements' (1905: 14); case studies often analysed the growth of the scientists' own children.

Later chapters describe pubertal changes to breasts and genitals, menstruation, seminal emissions and the production of ova and sperm. Hall writes extensively of menstruation, arguing in explicit agreement with Havelock Ellis in *Man and Woman* (1894) and with the wider nineteenth-century view of sexual difference (Laqueur 1990; Schiebinger 1991), that:

> A woman during her reproductive life is always engaged in menstruating. Everything she does or says must be judged by its exact position in this cycle which permeates her whole physical and psychical organism. (Hall 1905: 491)

[5] 'True conversion is as normal as the blossoming of a flower. The superiority of Christianity is that its corner-stone is love, and that it meets the needs of this most critical period of life as nothing else does ... Sex is a great psychic power which should be utilized for religion' (Hall 1905: 464).

[6] For detailed analysis of this aspect of Hall's argument, see Arnett (1999; 2006).

This view, Hall admits, 'is in distinct opposition to views like those of Miss F.P. Cobbe and Mrs Fawcett', leading British feminists at the time (1905: 491). For Hall, like many of his contemporaries, women are more difficult than men to understand scientifically because they are closer to nature and more profoundly oriented towards reproduction:

To understand a woman's body and soul is a larger problem than to understand a man's. It is true of her more than of him, that to know a part we must know the whole; first, because her nature is more generic and less specific, and, second, because reproduction, the deepest secret of animate nature, plays a larger role in her life. (1905: 506)

Sexually developing girls are figured as vulnerable to interior and exterior forces and, if 'weak or unadvised', to ruinous, unspecified danger. Using an extended aquatic metaphor, Hall writes:

In fine, puberty for a girl is like floating down a broadening river into an open sea. Landmarks recede, the water deepens and changes its nature, there are new and strange forms of life, the currents are more complex, and the phenomena of tides make new conditions and new dangers. The bark is frail, liable to be tossed by storms of feeling, at the mercy of wind and wave, and if without chart and compass and simple rules of navigation, aimless drifting in the darkness of ignorance, amidst rocks and shoals, may make of the weak or unadvised wrecks or castaways. (1905: 507–8)

Hall was also interested in the physiological effects of class and 'race' on pubertal growth. Citing research supporting the 'long held' belief that 'increase of comfort increases stature and weight' (1905: 31), he describes the effect on growth of 'hard conditions during ... earlier years' and discusses contemporary thinking about whether such retardation can be 'made up or compensated for later' if conditions improve (1905: 24). Hall suggests that interruptions to later periods of growth are more likely to be enduring: 'It is not unlikely, too, that as a spent ball is more easily stopped or turned, so the later stages of growth are more easily prevented by improper diet or hygienic conditions, excess of defect of exercise, excitement, overpressure in school, vice' (1905: 27–8). Like many of his nineteenth-century peers, Hall also argued that differences between the sexes (relating to height in this case) are greater in the 'civilized races' than 'among savages' ('a fact against the theory of progressive equalization of the sexes', in his view). Members of the 'civilised races' were also generally taller in his view (1905: 30). Such highly valued differences come to the fore in sexual development: 'racial influences upon both weight and height seem to assert themselves strongly at puberty' (1905: 30–3).

Such ideas were anathema to first-wave feminists and other educated and/or politicised women. In 1916, a group of English women doctors founded the Medical Women's Foundation and worked against the pervasive view of female puberty and menstruation as intrinsically negative (Strange 2001). Distributing leaflets and promoting better sanitary conditions for girls in schools, they encouraged mothers to talk to their daughters in more detail about puberty. Although aiming to 'emancipate women from a heritage of menstrual disability', as Strange puts it, however, 'female practitioners remained tied to a culture of menstrual discretion' (2001: 248). Some working-class women also decried the notion that girls should remain ignorant of puberty, as letters published by the Women's Cooperative Guild (1915) suggest (2001: 251). Addressing puberty was but one part of a move towards providing sex education for young people and promoting a more positive view of sexual development and desire (Mort 1987).

As endocrinological models of sexual difference developed in the 1920s and 30s, puberty came to be understood as a hormonal process within medicine (Oudshoorn 1994; Sengoopta 2006). Medical information became increasingly available to young people and their parents, and policy and public talk of sexual and social 'hygiene' developed in government documents, youth magazines and in young people's associations and clubs. Despite this, sex education remained rare in British schools. Historian Lesley Pilcher (2005: 154) calls it an 'absent presence':

> In fact, given that virtually every other bodily system, function and process, from the frequency of bowel movements to the proper way to breathe, are specified, the human sexual and reproductive body is conspicuous by its absence from the handbooks of health education in the first four decades of the twentieth century, then, official guidance on the health education curriculum did not explicitly encourage or advise schools to provide sex education to children. (Pilcher 2005: 156)

Towards the end of the Second World War, however, this situation changed, with the British Department of Education more strongly advising schools to provide sex education that included discussion of the biological underpinnings of sexual development. The 1956 handbook of health education included a chapter on sex education, covering puberty and menstruation: indeed, as Pilcher notes, 'the onset of puberty is noted to prioritise sex education, making it "the single most immediate problem to be considered from the point of view of health education"' (Ministry of Education 1956: 43–4, cited in Pilcher 2005: 159).

Joan Jacobs Brumberg similarly shows that by the post-war period American girls were 'routinely prepared for menstruation' through 'conversations with mothers and peers, as well as reading materials and corporate-sponsored films provided at home and at school' (Brumberg 1997: 31; see also Moran 2000). Although in Germany hormonal explanations of puberty became common amongst non-medical educators from the 1950s (Sauerteig 2012: 6), it was not until 1968 that the British Department of Education confirmed that it was important for young people to understand the hormonal processes of human reproduction: this was partly driven by the advent of the contraceptive pill (Pilcher 2005: 161).

By the mid twentieth century, the experience of puberty was also irrevocably changed by the creation of 'the teenager' as a social identity (Savage 2008: ch. 29) and then by the first rumblings of the sexual revolution (Hall 2000: 166). The publications in 1948 and 1953 of the *Kinsey Reports* on male and female sexual behaviour had inaugurated a new sexually explicit yet scientific public discourse on sexual practices and desire in both the USA and in Europe (Moran 2000: chs. 5 and 6). The troubles of adolescence were given new form through an explosion of personal accounts in film, song, magazines and television programmes and avenues for the promulgation of medical advice multiplied, with young people receiving state-sanctioned sex education in schools and many other forms of information through the print media and, more recently, television. From the late 1960s, German advice manuals commonly included explicit images of bodies in development (Sauerteig 2012: 7), although resistance to explicit content in sex education was strong in the United States in the 1970s and 80s (Moran 2000: ch. 6) and in Britain in the 1980s (Pilcher 2005; Holland and Thomson 2010).

Across the developed world, the experience of adolescence also became entwined with consumption. As Savage writes:

> The many possible interpretations of youth had been boiled down to just one: the adolescent consumer ... This new type was the ultimate psychic

match for the times: living in the now, pleasure-seeking, product-hungry, embodying the new global society where social inclusion was to be granted through purchasing power. The future would be Teenage. (Savage 2008: 465)

As discussed in the Introduction, contemporary concerns about the 'loss of childhood' and the 'sexualisation' of girls are closely linked to worries about consumption: arguably, young people today are living through the collapse of this consumerist version of social inclusion (see Giroux 2012; 2013; Tyler 2013: ch. 7).

The scientific work I explore in this book is articulated with wider scientific and cultural understandings of childhood, adolescence and puberty. Although Hall's particular concerns with sex, 'race' and class are of their time, they are also folded into contemporary thinking in a range of ways: older ideas about sex/gender, for example, echo in contemporary concerns about the effect of early development on girls' sexual behaviour. The extraordinary development since Hall's time of popular and scientific debate around adolescence, sex/gender and sexuality is an important backdrop for the more specific set of concerns about the timing of sexual development that I address here.

The early science of growth

During the modern period (~1750–1950), the science of puberty was advanced most notably not through endocrinology but via auxology, the interdisciplinary scientific study of growth. The study of human growth has its roots in mid eighteenth-century attention to measurement and recording. The first textbook on growth, written in 1729 by Prussian physician Johann Stöller, contained no measurements of children; it was entirely theoretical. In 1754, however, physician Christian Jampert presented a thesis based on measurements of children in a Berlin orphanage, probably relying on methods used to measure soldiers. In 1777 the first longitudinal study of growth was reported by George LeClerc Comte de Buffon in his important volume, *Natural History*. This study was based on measurement of his assistant Philippe Guéneau de Montbeillard's son from birth to adulthood (1759–77). This study confirmed the concept of a 'pubertal growth spurt' and seasonal changes in growth rate. Some sixty years later Belgian mathematician Adolphe Quetelet (who introduced the Normal Curve into statistics) combined a mathematical approach with empirical data on children's growth. Quetelet was interested in ideals of growth and beauty and is now thought to have been highly selective in his use of data (he did not, for example, find any girls taller than boys and failed to discover a pubertal growth spurt: his curve is of a continuously falling velocity of growth from birth to maturity) (Ulijaszek, Johnston and Preece 1998: 448).

In the nineteenth century a new style of growth research involving a more systematic study of groups of children gradually developed in Europe and the United States. The nineteenth-century sentimentalisation of childhood saw rising interest in *some* children's health, campaigns to promote their interests and the establishment both of paediatrics as a speciality and institutions to care for destitute children (Lederer and Cooter 1992: 96; Lesko 2012: 72–4). Interest in children's wellbeing was strongly articulated with discourses of race, class and sex: black American children in the first part of the century, for example, were most often measured in attempts to protect them from post-slavery child smuggling (Tanner 1981: 165).[7]

In the second half of the century, new measures to protect and care for young people on both sides of the Atlantic ironically produced particular groups of children – those living in newly formed care institutions due to disability, neglect and/or poverty – as readily accessible research subjects. As historian Susan Lederer shows, 'orphans' (children living in orphanages who may or may not have living parents elsewhere) frequently served as 'research materials' for American scientists from the late nineteenth century and into the next century. Consent to perform experimental interventions, which were sometimes

[7] Although the importation of slaves was outlawed in the US in 1807, slaves remained a marketable commodity until the 1860s. In his history of auxology Tanner writes, 'It turns out that the greatest number of children in the first half of the nineteenth century were measured for purposes of identification and prevention of smuggling rather than for the investigation of social ills and the conditions of factory life' (Tanner 1981: 165). 'Manifests' or lists of slaves were made to prevent new slaves being smuggled in during inter-state voyages: these lists recorded height and age and in the later part of the twentieth century, became important resources for economic historians who, with the help of auxologists, use them to make arguments about the treatment of slaves, particularly in relation to reproduction: 'The chief interest of this group for economic historians has been in determining the mean age at menarche and at first birth of a child, to confirm or refute suggestion that slave owners deliberately manipulated their reproductive behaviour of the female in order to increase their stock of slaves for use or sale' (Tanner 1981: 166).

dangerous and often unpleasant, needed only be obtained from the institution (Lederer 1992; Lederer and Grodin 1994; Lederer and Davis 1995). The regimentation of life in such institutions provided practical and scientific 'benefits' to researchers.[8] Lederer cites Alfred Hess, a New York physician who carried out multiple experiments on children at the Hebrew Infant Asylum in New York City in the first two decades of the twentieth century:

> It is probably also an advantage, from the standpoint of comparison, that these institutional children belong to the same stratum of society, that they have for the most part been reared for a considerable period within the same walls, having the same daily routine, including similar food and an equal amount of outdoor life. These are some of the conditions which are insisted on in considering the course of experimental infection among laboratory animals, but which can rarely be controlled in a study of infection in man. (Hess, cited in Lederer 1992: 116)

This element of control was also appealing to early European auxologists: in late nineteenth-century Italy, for example, Luigi Pagliani compared the growth of 'orphans' (including abandoned children) and wealthier schoolchildren; similar studies were undertaken in France by Paul Godin. This kind of control was also, as we will see, of utmost importance to scientific work on puberty.

In the early to mid twentieth century, researchers such as anthropologist Franz Boas, psychologists Bird T. Baldwin, Nancy Bayley and Frank Shuttleworth, and auxologist Howard Meredith argued the growth curves obtained from cross-sectional samples were quite different from those obtained by following individuals over time. Studying growth from the 1890s to the 1940s, Boas (who had worked with Stanley Hall) coined the term 'the tempo of growth' to describe individuals' varying speeds of development, arguing that the pubertal spurt came at various times for different children. In the 1920s and 30s, several large-scale American longitudinal studies, including Baldwin's pioneering study based at the Iowa Child Welfare Research Station (results published by Meredith in the 1930s), the Harvard Growth

[8] Lederer (1995) and others argue that such research was not motivated by cruelty but by desires to understand children's bodies and to make progress in scientific and medical careers (Goodman, McElligott and Marks 2003). Such research was strongly resisted, particularly in the United States, by anti-vivisectionists (Lederer 1995).

Study, and the Ohio-based Fels Longitudinal Study, tracked the growth of groups of children recruited from schools and local families. Initiated during the Great Depression, these studies had a strong focus on the impact of poverty on child growth. Both this focus and their methods inspired the subsequent English research. In 1948 British biologist and physician James M. Tanner visited these studies, learning Meredith's techniques of measurement in order to reproduce the first American-style study of growth and development in Europe (Tanner 1981).[9]

Building the Tanner Scale: engaging the children of Harpenden

In 1948, Tanner was approached by E.R. Bransby, a nutritionalist at the Ministry of Health who had undertaken a study of children's nutritional requirements at the National Children's Home, Harpenden, just outside of London. Bransby thought a long-term study of children's growth should be carried out and had money from the Ministry for this purpose (Tanner and Inhelder 1956: 18; Tanner 1981: 349).[10] Rather immodestly, Tanner writes, 'Tanner, who had graduated in medicine from London in 1945 and had recently begun to lecture on growth at Oxford, was the obvious, indeed only, candidate' (1981: 349).

Later that year, Tanner travelled with his military-trained assistant, Reginald H. Whitehouse, to the Highfield Branch of the National Children's Home, Harpenden, to begin the detailed, longitudinal study of children's growth that was ultimately to form the basis of clinical norms around growth in general and particularly puberty. In the birth moment of modern molecular science, then, just four years before Watson and Crick described the helical structure of DNA, these men

[9] The surveying of school age children continues to this day. Although mostly cross-sectional, some countries, including the UK, now continuously collect data on whole populations.

[10] One of Tanner's friends described this event rather differently, emphasising its fortuitous nature: 'By 1948 he was a lecturer in Physiology at the Sherrington School and following a presentation on his travels to the Royal Society, and a fortuitous meeting with a Dr. Bransby who was in the audience and had spent the war years using a National Children's Home in Harpenden to develop appropriate rationing levels for children, Jim's Harpenden Longitudinal Growth Study started in 1949 and was to continue for the next 25 years.' (www.theirhistory.co.uk/70001/info.php?p=7&pno=0).

were about to engage in a vigorous programme of the rather more old-fashioned activity of measuring (Hall 2006: 18).[11]

A group of children living at Harpenden were studied from 1949 to 1971. Tanner and Whitehouse visited the institution every three months, measuring each child every six months from the age or 3 or 4, and then every three months during puberty. These measurements were meticulously taken and recorded, forming the basis for several ground-breaking papers, the development of the Tanner Scale of pubertal changes (1955) and in 1982 the publication of the *Atlas of Children's Growth: Normal Variation and Growth Disorders.*[12] Inescapably intertwined with but also challenging both the accumulated knowledge of the two centuries of research and broader cultural figurations of adolescence described above, this study today underpins most research-based measurements of child growth and pubertal development.

It is significant that Tanner and Whitehouse's study took place between World War II and the 1970s: this was a period both in which meticulous scientific research was well funded and highly valued and in which institutionalised children's bodies remained rather freely available as 'research materials'. The post-war period saw the rise of controlled experimentation and the quantification of human bodies in medical science (Epstein 2007: 48). Tanner and Whitehouse's study was exemplary in its elaboration of modern scientific methods and approaches, including the systematic employment of disadvantaged children as research subjects. Institutions like the British National Children's Home (founded by a Methodist minister in 1869 as a caring alternative to state-run workhouses and renamed the 'National Children's Home and Orphanage' in 1908)[13] provided exciting

[11] Tanner writes of his colleague with whom he worked for the rest of his life: 'Whitehouse was innocent of any academic training but had handled without difficulty the job of Regimental Sergeant-Major at the Royal Army Medical Corps training school; the Harpenden Growth Study seemed scarcely more exacting' (Tanner 1981: 349–50).

[12] In 1956 Tanner and Whitehouse moved their work from St Thomas' Hospital in London to the Institute of Child Health, University of London, to study disorders of growth using the same techniques (these are also reported in the *Atlas*). The Institute of Child Health became a major centre for treating children with growth hormone deficiency.

[13] The New Poor Law of 1834 had required English and Welsh parishes to provide basic shelter, food and clothing for the destitute in return for their labour. In these workhouses, children over the age of 7 were separated from their mothers,

possibilities for scientists and clinicians wanting to understand more about children's bodies. Accessing such children in the 1940s to 1970s was relatively straightforward in the United Kingdom. It was not until the 1960s, following the Nuremberg Trials, which lead to the 1947 Nuremberg Code of informed consent precluding research on children because they could not consent, and the 1964 Helsinki Declaration of the World Medical Associations which allowed adults to give proxy consent for children, that such research became much more tightly controlled (Epstein 2007: 42; Brierley and Larcher 2010).

Rules and practices around child experimentation are nationally specific. Germany, for example, had had regulations that restricted the use of children in non-clinical research since the early twentieth century (Maehle 2009). In 1974, American legislation compelled researchers to ensure that human subjects were not put at undue risk and to document their procedures of acquiring informed consent from participants (Lederer 1995: 142). This legislation focused particularly on vulnerable populations including prisoners, children and the poor (Epstein 2007: 44) but it was not until 1983 that specific regulations were published for child research subjects in the USA (Glantz 1994: 123) and health care ethics committees became common (Larcher 2009). In the UK, the Committee on the Safety of Medicines established in 1964 and the Medicinal Act of 1968 controlled the use of medicines in clinical trials but there was no specific legislation on the use of children in non-therapeutic research: researchers were left to make their own ethical decisions. Although clinical research ethics committees were established in the UK in the mid 1990s, researchers are still not legally obliged to consult them or follow their advice (Larcher 2009; Brierley and Larcher 2010). Publications from the Harpenden Study do not describe a process of obtaining either participants' or their parents' consent to involvement (see, for example, Marshall and Tanner 1969; 1970). It is hard to imagine,

and fathers were always housed individually. Children 'were at the mercy of those who ran the workhouses and many children suffered cruelty and malnutrition' (Kellett 2011: 11). Although workhouses were not abolished until 1930, institutions like the National Children's Home were meant as a more caring alternative, a move later followed in the establishment of the welfare state.

as I will discuss later, that such a study would today be approved by an NHS ethics committee.

During visits to Harpenden, Whitehouse made fifteen measurements of each child according to standardised protocols. Over the period of the study this amounted to fifteen measurements on 9,000 child occasions: a vast archive of data (Ulijaszek, *et al.* 1998: 451). Children were required to hold their bodies in particular ways during each test: for height measurements, for example, they had to stretch up, 'assisted by the measurer applying upward pressure under the ears' (Tanner 1981: 352; see Figure 1). The anthropometrist used verbal encouragement and held down the child's heels if they came off the ground (Tanner and Whitehouse 1982: 2). For seated measurements children 'stretched up as much as possible, aided by gentle pressure under the chin', whilst for supine measurements, children lay on their backs with knees bent up to a right angle: 'One measurer held the child's head in the Frankfort plane and applied gentle pressure to bring it into contact with the fixed headboard. A second measurer supported the child's legs and brought the moveable footboard to rest against his buttocks' (Tanner and Whitehouse 1982: 2) (see Figure 2). The unique anthropometric instruments devised by Whitehouse to make these measurements, including a stadiometer, a skinfold-measuring caliper and an anthropometer, are now standard across the world. Manufactured in Wales, this range of instruments is named 'Harpenden' and remains available from the original company (www.anthropometer.com/).

Scientific photography and the measuring of children's bodies

During measurement sessions, Tanner took photogrammetric pictures of each child: 'pictures so made that enlargements remain dimensionally accurate to the extent that measurements can be taken off them' (Tanner 1981: 352). These also involved strenuous control from the young children and the scientists themselves:

> The child stood motionless on a turntable placed 10 metres from the camera and was posed in the standard position recommended for somatotyping . . . The turntable was then turned (electronically, in later models) to give side and back views . . . All the pictures were positioned and taken by Tanner. (1981: 352).

A large selection of these images is reproduced in the *Atlas of Child Development*, which contains two oversize pages per child: one

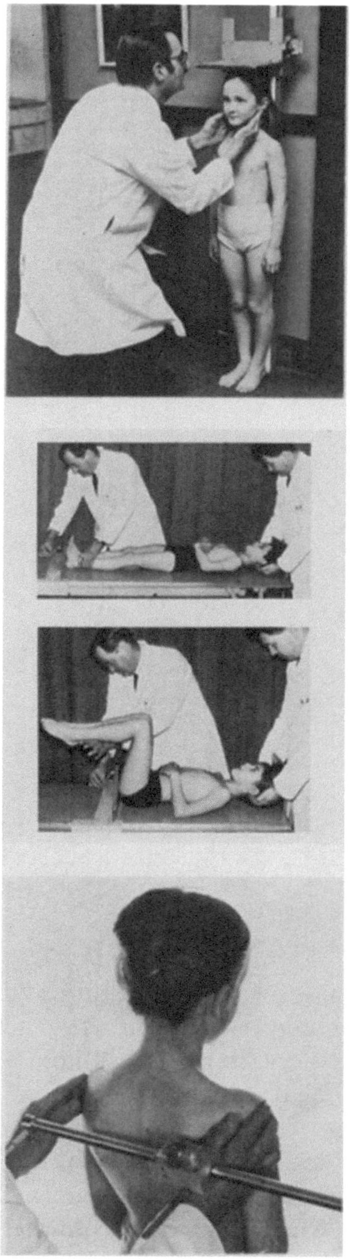

Figure 1 Tanner and Whitehouse's anthropometric devices in action.

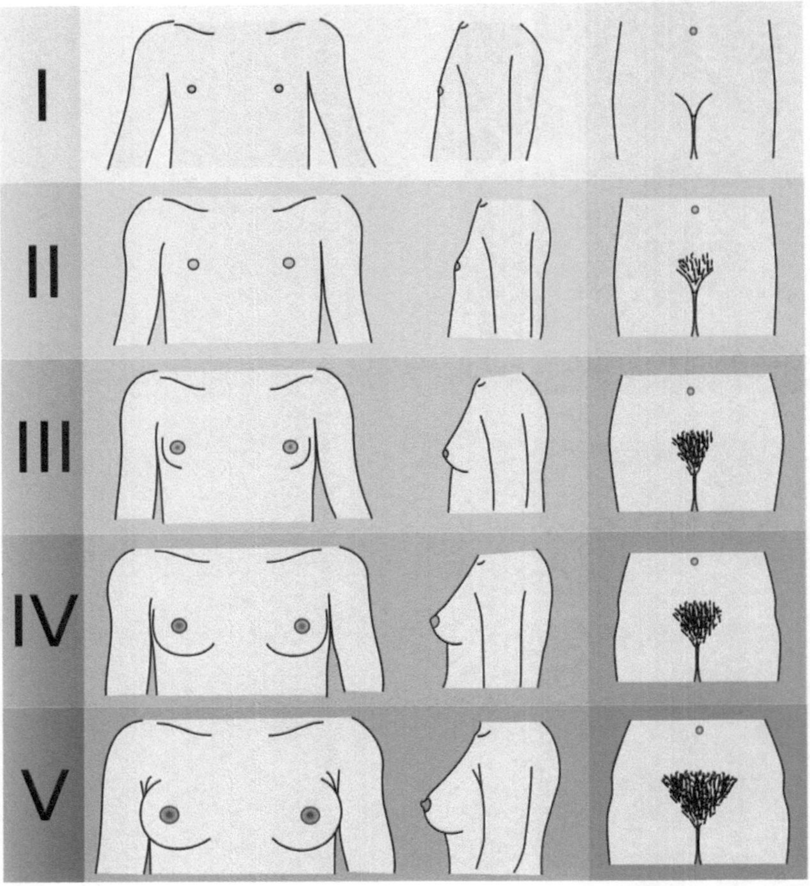

Figure 2 The Female Tanner Scale.

displaying growth charts and giving a short written history and description, and the other a set of photographs following the child from early childhood to adulthood. These black and white images are unnerving: the children are naked, their eyes covered with two black triangles. The bodies, shown in frontal, side-on and back profiles, are placed in front of a set of grid lines. The eye covering does little to hide the children's identities: their bodies are otherwise profoundly exposed (indeed, one part of the book contains images of children's faces without eye covers to demonstrate the facial features common to particular genetic conditions). As a recent analysis of similar images used in medical texts suggests, such coverings do not protect anonymity (Creighton *et al.* 2002: 68). Although in the *Atlas* the children's facial expressions and bodily deportment are usually highly controlled and 'neutral', several of the younger children (aged between 3 and 5) appear to be distressed and/or unable to follow the strict instructions: they are turning away, leaning or slumping.

Tanner's images build on a tradition of medical photography stemming from the mid nineteenth century in which photographs, in contrast to engravings, represented accuracy and scientific dispassion (Tagg 1988; Maehle 1993; Jackson 1995; O'Connor 1995). Building on earlier studies of criminals, this tradition developed in the later decades of that century alongside an increasing emphasis on the collection of statistical data about children's bodies and the detailed analysis of the different bodies of pathologised groups, such as 'mental defectives' (Jackson 1995: 323). Following Foucault, historian John Tagg argues that the new institutions constituting modern networks of power were founded on a coupling of photography and evidence: practices of record-keeping and observation 'enabled ... an unprecedented expansion and integration of social administration, amounting ... to a new strategy of governance' (Tagg 1988: 5). Photographs were thought to provide incontrovertible evidence of pathology, and pictures of particular individuals were used to exemplify 'cases' and thus constitute typologies (Jackson 1995: 324, 332). Charles Darwin's cousin, Francis Galton, used blurred photographic sequences to depict 'types' (army officers, private soldiers, criminals convicted of murder, non-violent felons, Jews) as part of his eugenic project (Hacking 1990: 183). These photographs were drawn from both his *Life History Album* project promoted by the British Medical Association in which he asked parents to document their children's development through photography and writing and his collection of photographs from American prisons (Kemp 1997: 131–2).

Sometimes individuals – including 'cretins', people suffering from anorexia nervosa and other mental illnesses, and intersexed individuals – were photographed naked (Jackson 1995: 325). These images were used in 'before and after' comparisons, intended to demonstrate the effectiveness of particular treatments. Maehle notes that images of naked female obstetric patients caused offence to some physicians at the turn of the century. As they pointed out, taking such photographs was not only a question of decency, but also of ethics. It was believed that these women had often been photographed without their consent or that of their friends while they were unconscious under anaesthesia. (Maehle 1993: 574; see also Kemp 1997: 125–6)

In 1895 concerns about consent came to the fore when the Board of Guardians of a London hospital resolved that no photographs should be taken of patients 'of weak intellect' (cited in Maehle 1993: 575). The *British Medical Journal* expressed concern about this decision, arguing that the permission of friends should be enough in that case, and reaffirming the clinical value of photographs to both doctors and patients (Maehle 1993: 576).

Revealing a patient's identity by unnecessarily photographing their whole body also raised concerns in medical communities. 'In fact', Maehle (1993: 574) states, 'around 1900 the practice of taking anonymous photographs of patients set in'. This involved covering the patients' eyes or photographing only parts of the body (see also Kemp 1997: 148). Maehle (1993: 583) argues that such practices also reflected 'a more somatic and localistic [rather than a social or psychological] concept of disease, due to the growing influence of the natural and basic sciences on nineteenth-century medicine'. The move away from conventional portrait-style backdrops towards plain black ones is also part of this trend.

Tanner's use of whole body nudity (albeit with eye covering) had a highly specific goal: his images were intended as objects for measurement and the construction of statistics. Rather than revealing the outcomes of an intervention, these images documented an unfolding physiological process. Published in the *Atlas* as chronological sequences, they are also visual 'examples' of an individual's change over time. In this respect, Tanner's images also reference Eadweard Muybridge's late nineteenth-century stop-motion images of naked men moving (jumping, throwing, mounting a bicycle), which were originally published in the atlas-like *Animal Locomotion* (1887) and republished in *The Human Figure in Motion* (1901) (Braun 1997; 2010; 2013: 47–50).

Like Tanner, Muybridge's aim was accurately to record human (and animal) bodies in movement in order to promote scientific understanding, although, as historian of photography Marta Braun (2013) points out, he also regularly retouched, resized, cropped and moved his images before printing (Braun argues that this did not constitute a transgression of rules about objectivity as it would today).[14] Muybridge's work for *Animal Locomotion* was overseen by a committee including founding members of the American Society of Anthropometry, who introduced a grid background (similar to Tanner's) to the work, based on English ethnologist J.H. Lamprey's work (described below). Muybridge's images of male workers and hospital patients demonstrate the use of photography to explore 'his committee's concerns with health, class and race at the end of the nineteenth century' (Braun 2013: 49). Although such images were limited as scientific texts, photography was soon accepted by many as the ideal medium in which to record medical conditions. Indeed, as Cooper states, 'Many hospitals employed photographers, most still do have a photographic department, but full-length nudes are rare' (Cooper 1995: 43).

Photography was also widely used in the nineteenth and twentieth centuries in scientific work on 'race'. The sciences of anthropometry and anthropology used standardised photographic techniques to document the 'differences' between 'races' and to document different bodily 'types'. Like Tanner's, such images were often taken in front of a grid with the subject standing next to a measuring device. Muybridge borrowed the Lamprey method, devised in 1899 and published by the Ethnological Society of London. In this, Lamprey 'placed the naked figure in front of a grid made up of 2 inch squares formed by placing fine silk thread on a wooden frame. So the lines of the grid enabled "the study of all those peculiarities of contour which are so distinctly observable in each group"' (Lamprey, in Cooper 1995: 57). Lamprey's method allowed for measurement and analysis: in contrast to Muybridge's mobile subjects, the figures are immobilised by metal stands and other devices. This method was used in Australia, South Africa, British Columbia, Ceylon and India as part of British colonial projects into the early twentieth century. In the late nineteenth century, governors of British colonies were specifically instructed to take such images of those they governed, although, due to strong local resistance, images tended to be taken of slaves or prisoners rather than free citizens (Cooper 1995: 60).

[14] Unlike Tanner's, Muybridges' images have been extensively analysed by historians of photography and other cultural critics: see Braun (1997; 2010) and Cartwright (1995).

Tanner's production of a visual atlas also built on earlier American auxological work. Shuttleworth's 1938 two-volume *The Adolescent Period: A Graphic and Pictorial Atlas* contained images similar to those made by Tanner but these were used only to illustrate differences ('retarded, average and advanced' puberty) rather than as photogrammetric presentations of data: models were neither posed against grid backgrounds nor stabilised by equipment (Shuttleworth 1938: 51–2).

As a genre of scientific publishing, atlases had a long history, dating from the eighteenth century, in which they gradually came to be seen as accurate representations of reality. In fact, Roberta McGarth argues, they 'created new objects of study and formed new realities; it was a radical reconfiguration of knowledge that disturbed any idea . . . of real that precedes its representation' (McGarth 2002: 29). Tanner's atlas was unique in its creation of child growth and sexual development as a quantifiable object of study. The images in his atlas were literally scientific objects – they were not intended as illustrative representations but were themselves to be measured.

The historical literature on scientific photography illuminates the ways in which cultural understandings of bodies are articulated through visualising practices intended to ensure objectivity. Tanner and Whitehouse's precise techniques constitute a highly elaborated version of the attempt to represent bodies as physiological entities. Such precision does not, I suggest, successfully reduce bodies to mere objects. The practices with which Tanner and Whitehouse engaged the children of Harpenden articulate a wide range of social relations: of class, dis/advantage, health, race and sex/gender. Situating these practices and the resulting images in a history of scientific photography illuminates the material-semiotic relations that make possible this particular rendering of 'objective facts'. Most notably, perhaps, it underlines the significance of the disadvantaged social position of these children: living in a children's home made it difficult (although, as we will see, not impossible) to resist Tanner and Whitehouse's scientific figurations of development.

What to measure? Accuracy, choice and expertise

The Harpenden Growth Study focused on physiological measurements of subjects' bodies using Whitehouse's custom-made tools, and of the photogrammetric images. In their pursuit of accuracy, Tanner and

Whitehouse also used calipers to record fat in children's skin and X-rays to record internal as well as external growth: 'Radiographs were taken of arm, calf, and, for a time, thigh, delineating bone, muscle and fat' (Tanner 1981: 352). In 1982 Tanner and Whitehouse argued that the radiation to which children were exposed during the study was 'the same amount that a child living at sea level inevitably receives during a 2-week holiday in the mountains, since natural radiation increases with altitude' (Tanner and Whitehouse 1982: 5) and somewhat defensively stated that although such experimental exposure would probably no longer be permitted, 'this was not the case when the X-rays reported here were taken' (1982: 5).

Some clinical and orthodontic examinations were also undertaken (dental development is a standard measurement of age). In subsequent writings, Tanner describes his decisions about which data to collect. In a resigned yet humorous tone, he states, 'No psychological work was undertaken, nor any physiological research, after an early disappointment over the accuracy of 24-hour urine collections (bottle-sharing and beer-substitution being excessive)' (Tanner 1981: 353). Here, I suggest, we can see the effective resistance of some Harpenden children.

Introducing himself to a 1953 meeting of experts in Geneva (described in more detail below), Tanner described the lack of physiological and biological data on the Harpenden children as 'a very grave gap in our investigation', stating that 'it is a matter of money and space as usual' (Tanner, in Tanner and Inhelder 1956: 19). He also affirmed that 'we do not have at the present time any psychiatric or psychological studies in progress, and this is a field about which I wish to be informed, and know, practically speaking, nothing' (Tanner, in Tanner and Inhelder 1956: 19). This failure to take account of the psychological aspects of the children's development was, I suggest, underpinned by the historically situated figuration of institutionalised children as convenient – albeit sometimes resistant – research materials. Itself a legacy of the history outlined earlier, this figuration's central role in the Harpenden research has important ethical and scientific implications for the study of puberty today.

Who were the participants in the Harpenden Study?

Overall, 450 boys and 260 girls participated in this research, of whom 85 boys and 48 girls were studied for ten years or more

(Tanner 1981: 353). Some were parentless children who had lived in the home since they were babies. Others – in increasing numbers as the study went on – were taken into the Home 'as the result of family breakdown' (1981: 353). They were all from working- or lower-middle-class families. Some of these children may well have been suffering from abuse and/or neglect and all of them had experienced (potentially traumatic) separation from familiar carers and surroundings. Despite this, all the children in the study are described by Tanner as 'healthy' and 'well nourished'. In the first paragraph of the *Atlas*, Tanner and Whitehouse write: 'The children we studied from 1949 to 1970 were healthy, well-nourished boys and girls attending the usual schools, playing the usual games, and up to the usual activities' (Tanner and Whitehouse 1982: 1). Tanner and Whitehouse did not elaborate on the fact that these were children living outside 'the usual' familial care arrangements. Any difficulties the children might have encountered whilst living at the National Children's Home are effaced. Their atypicality is constrained to their backgrounds which might, Tanner argues, affect the timing of their development (and hence the numerical values of their growth curves) but not its overall pattern or shape:

The Harpenden Growth Study data were used to determine the shape of the individual height and weight curves at adolescence, *but they are not suitable as figures on which to base standards*. For one thing, they are obviously too limited in number, and for another they come from boys and girls living in a children's home. The home is an extraordinarily good one, in which the children live in 'family units' consisting of a dozen boys and girls of all ages supervised by a housemother and her younger assistant. Most of the children are from broken homes, usually manual working class. Most enter at between 3 and 5 years and stay in the home till between 15 and 18. The home is well situated in extensive grounds, the food is excellent, and the children attend the schools in the town in the ordinary way. *We think it very unlikely that the shapes of these children's adolescent growth curves are in any way unusual*, but menarche does occur slightly later than in the London County Council children. For this reason in making the standards we have moved the age of peak velocity of height and weight earlier by 0.2 yr. in both sexes. This means that the average age of menarche in the standards is 13.0 years, and peak height velocity 11.9 years in girls and 13.9 years in boys. These figures are probably closely representative of urban children of average economic status in Southern England in the early 1960's. (Tanner, Whitehouse and Takaishi 1966: 465; emphasis added).

The representation of these children as 'normal' was also pursued by the National Children's Home (NCH, now 'Action for Children') in promotional activities. In films and media releases, the occupants of homes like Harpenden were described as healthy and psychologically robust. The aim of the NCH was to provide children with a home-like setting and a parental-style care relationship: after the Second World War children lived in houses in family-style groups and were educated in local schools.[15] Many of these children had some contact with their birth parents or other relatives, and some were placed in sibling groups within the NCH setting (in the earlier part of the twentieth century, boys had been separated from girls). From a present-day point of view these children would be assumed to be at high risk of attachment difficulties or other stress-related or developmental difficulties or trauma (Hughes 2006; Schofield and Beek 2006).

Although keen to represent the majority of children in their study as typical (if 0.2 years slower than their peers), Tanner and Whitehouse sometimes stressed the developmental effects of deprivation and neglect: indeed, Tanner is today highly regarded for his emphasis on the social aspects of growth (see, for example, Ulijaszek *et al.* 1998: 455). Tanner was well aware of the potential effects of neglect and separation on children's psychological development. In 1953–6 he had participated in a series of four meetings funded by the World Health Organization Study Group on the Psychobiological Development of the Child, held in Geneva and London, and later co-edited the four volumes documenting these discussions (Tanner and Inhelder 1956; 1957; 1958; Inhelder and Tanner 1960). At these meetings, John Bowlby had presented his seminal work on the effects of children's separation from their parents during hospitalisation (Tanner and Inhelder 1957: 213–34) and the effects of deprivation and trauma had been debated in detail (other participants included Margaret Mead, Konrad Lorenz and Jean Piaget).

In the *Atlas*, Tanner and Whitehouse briefly broach the question of the interrelationship of the physiological and psychological, presenting three cases of 'short stature . . . due to psychosocial stress' (Tanner and Whitehouse 1982: 1). Subject 99 demonstrates what they (1982: 179)

[15] Films made to promote the NCH in the 1950s follow the progress of children entering Harpenden and acclimatising to life there (see for example www.youtube.com/watch?v=9brSkv1lWDo).

describe as 'short stature due to psychosocial stress with catch-up on change of environment'. His history is described as follows:

> Subject 99, a boy, was the third child out of four in a fireman's family. His mother brought him to the clinic with the complaint of short stature ... [Subject 99's birth and birth weight are described] ... his appearance was not that of Silver-Russell syndrome, and his mother admitted that his behaviour was different from that of her other children, in that he stole, "but only food, Doctor". His feeding pattern was grossly disturbed. At times he ate little and at others he ate voraciously ... He was anxious and slept badly ... Mother readily agreed that the child was probably 'delicate' (a designation we fiercely oppose when mothers apply it to small children with growth hormone deficiency, Silver-Russell syndrome ... [etc.]). In consequence, the boy was sent to a special boarding school for delicate children where this growth showed a marked and sustained catch-up. Height reached the 15th centile after 3 years of this 'treatment'. No drugs were given at any time ... We presume he had reversible growth hormone deficiency with a disturbance of the nearby appetite centre, both for psychosocial reasons. (Tanner and Whitehouse 1982: 178)

Similar narratives are composed about Subjects 100 (a boy) and 101 (a girl). Subject 100 'had a very disturbed home background and was sent to boarding school immediately after the first measurement' (1982: 178). Subject 101's 'home was very disorganized and attendance at doctors' clinics or hospitals very unreliable' (1982: 178). The pictures of this child, as Tanner and Whitehouse write, 'show an initially obviously unhappy girl, [aged 4.8 years] growing into the smiling subject of the last occasion [aged 8.4 years]' (1982: 178). In each case, Tanner and Whitehouse figure the 'change of environment' of moving into institutional life away from 'difficult' family as promoting health and happiness, as well as growth.

This figuration of life at children's homes was widespread. As Lesko (2012: 72–4) suggests, in both the USA and Europe care institutions for children (such as juvenile detention centres and orphanages) were increasingly imitating domestic settings, arguing that modelling themselves on family life improved the quality of care and better prepared children for later life. Interestingly, Lesko points out that the emphasis on maternal care was in stark contrast to discourses around middle-class non-delinquent boys who were thought to be best served by separating the sexes both in the home and at school.

Using the children at Harpenden as research subjects put Tanner in a difficult position, caught between a tradition in which 'orphans' functioned as convenient research materials and a developing scientific understanding (found in the work of Bowlby and Donald Winnicott for example) of the long-term impact of childhood trauma. This historically specific dilemma is evident in Tanner's writings: although acknowledging that the background of his sample might be physiologically consequential, Tanner underplays the possibly enduring effects of early neglect and completely ignores the difficulties of institutional life for children. He also, as I argue below, remains oblivious to the possibility that his own engagements with Harpenden residents may have been harmful.

Scaling up puberty: counting and accounting for differences

Tanner and Whitehouse were particularly interested in sexual development. During the Harpenden Study, 228 boys and 192 girls were measured every three months as they went through puberty, using manual palpation and tools such as the orchidometer to measure testicular development (Marshall and Tanner 1969, 1970; Tanner and Whitehouse 1982: 2). Tanner himself rated each child's pubertal stage (Tanner and Whitehouse 1982: 1).

It was the frequency of measurement in the Harpenden Study that constituted its main scientific contribution to understandings of puberty: this frequency allowed Tanner to test existing statistical models and 'logistic curves' articulating child development (Tanner 1981: 353–6). Tanner and Whitehouse's laborious approach foregrounded the significant differences in children's growth patterns and the importance of recognising wide variation in 'normal' development. Through the careful accumulation of detail Tanner and Whitehouse produced data that multiplied bodies and biological processes, allowing them to 'define the range of variation seen in the development of pubic hair, genitalia and breasts' (1981: 354). Their findings thus highlight both sequence *and* variation. In the *Atlas* they write:

> There are very large variations in the ages at which the various manifestations of puberty occur in girls and boys. These variations take three forms.
>
> 1. Early or late occurrence of puberty as a whole.
> 2. Differences in timing between different sequences, i.e. say, pubic hair early in relation to breasts . . .

3. Differences in the rapidity with which each individual sequence progresses; that is, between the time taken by one girl to pass from the earliest breast bud to an adult breast compared with the time taken by another who starts breast development at the same time. (Tanner and Whitehouse 1982: 122)

In contrast to Tanner's statements about the unsuitability of the Harpenden weight and height results to function as standards, the statistical analysis of the puberty measurements resulted in what is now known as the Tanner Scale (1962): a simple graphic tool used to measure and describe children's breast, or testicle and penis, and pubic hair development (see Figures 2 and 3). These 'pictorial standards' are organised in five stages, and separate the growth of breasts, testicles, penises and pubic hair to allow clinicians and researchers to distinguish different sequences and speeds of growth.

The relation of these five standards to the pubertal growth spurt and to the onset of menarche varies: Tanner also produced 'individual-type standards for distance and velocity of height and weight' using his longitudinal data to form the shape of standardised growth curves (Tanner 1981: 354). Radiological data on bone, muscle and fat growth were also used to study changes at puberty. Here the researchers found notable differences between boys and girls in the relations between bone, fat and height growth (1981: 354). In collaboration with a Scottish study of a representative sample of schoolchildren, longitudinal radiographic data were also used to establish standards of skeletal maturity (1981: 355).[16]

Sexual and physiological development, for Tanner and Whitehouse, are both measurable and delineated processes (that can be represented in simple graphical form) *and* sites of intense individual variation. In their publications, children's growth is figured as predictable and consistent. Tanner argues, for example, that the *Atlas* shows how well the somatotypes of children match their adult somatotypes. The life

[16] All of this work was mathematically complex: from 1950, Tanner and Whitehouse collaborated with biometrician M.J.R. Healy from the Rothamsted Agricultural Research Station, an institution close to Harpenden that played a significant role in the history of British statistics more broadly. Several technical papers and the first book on auxiological biometry (Goldstein 1979) stemmed from this enduring collaboration.

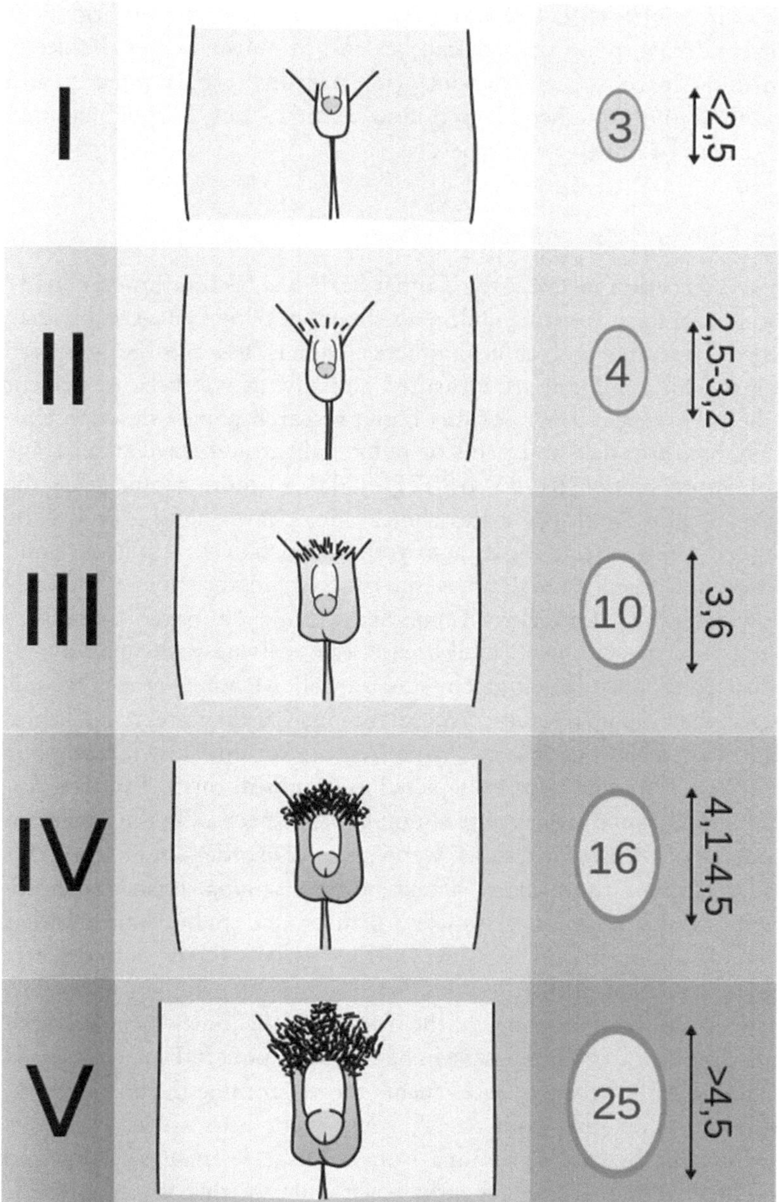

Figure 3 The Male Tanner Scale.

stories of Subjects 99, 100 and 101, however, indicate their argument that children's (poor) growth can, at least in unusual cases, be determined by 'psychosocial' factors. This paradox – that puberty and growth are both predictable and idiosyncratic – has, I argue, haunted the science of puberty ever since.

The Tanner Scale and charts travel

Since publication in 1962, the Tanner Scale has become an immensely mobile tool for measuring children's sexual development. Used widely in both research and clinical practice, it has become the standard against which children are measured globally: as will become evident in the following chapters of this book, research papers describe children's breast/testicle and penis or pubic hair growth as 'Tanner stage X' or more simply 'B1–B5' or 'PH1–PH5'. In more recent years the Scale has also developed a less clinical life. I have found it on a wide range of websites: one encourages young Christian men to understand and control their sexual urges (lavistachurchofchrist.org/LVstudies/GrowingUpInTheLord/Boys/TannerStage.htm); another reassures young women who have small breasts (www.living-with-small-a-cup-breasts.com/breast-development-stages.html). Members of teen forums discuss their Tanner results, asking anxiously if they are at the 'right' stage for their age (www.virtualteen.org/forums/showthread.php?t=31701). Although usually depicted in graphical form, Tanner's original photographs also appear in non-clinical spaces. On the American Academy of Family Physicians' webpage on 'Disorders of Puberty', for example, the authors insert a text box containing Tanner's photographic scale of breasts, testicles, penises and pubic hair in their attempt to educate and reassure worried parents (www.aafp.org/afp/990700ap/209.html).

Alongside the flourishing of the Tanner Scale comes some recognition of the cost to young people in having their pubertal stages assessed by adults. Although such assessments remain routine in clinical work, research studies now tend to ask young people to assess their own development by making comparisons with scale images (Dorn and Biro 2011). In the case of early onset puberty this is not possible due to the children's young age. Whilst sophisticated computerised imaging technologies are available for measuring general morphology

(Ulijaszek *et al.* 1998: 30–8), the standard technique for assessing pubertal stages remains direct human observation.[17]

Tanner's height and weight curves (adjusted to align with less atypical populations as mentioned above) have also been widely used in clinical and research literatures and in public health initiatives, such as the NHS 'Red Books' given to British parents at a child's birth to record their growth. In 2002, however, a working group convened by the Royal College of Paediatrics and Child Health concluded that the Tanner-Whitehouse charts were no longer suitable for use in the UK; indeed that they are now 'obsolete' (Wright *et al.*, 2002). The longitudinal 'style' of Tanner's charts, however, remains gold standard in the UK.

In recent years growth charts have become embroiled in the politics of pharmaceuticalisation.[18] Over the later decades of the twentieth century, medical and public debate around treating children's atypical growth with hormones intensified in countries including the USA, the UK and Australia (Hall 2006; Morrison 2008; Rayner, Pyett and Astbury 2010). Quoting an interview with Tanner, Stephen Hall argues in *The New York Times* that the use of cross-sectional (as opposed to longitudinal) charts promotes over-diagnosis of pathology, supporting an explosion in the medical treatment of atypical growth:

> The Tanner-inspired longitudinal charts are still sold and used in England, but he said their use had been overshadowed by cross-sectional charts distributed by drug companies or growth foundations that receive financing from companies that make human growth hormone, the use of which has exploded in recent years. (Hall 2005: 2)

Criticisms of Tanner's sample

Tanner's acknowledgement of the specificities of the Harpenden sample is sometimes mentioned in recent epidemiological research on pubertal timing. In their paper on British girls' sexual development, for example, Carol Rubin and colleagues write,

17 Biomarkers for pubertal development are generally limited in use, being technically difficult to assay, invasive and expensive (Ulijaszek *et al.* 1998: 39–41).

18 See Chapter 7 for a discussion of this term.

> As stated by Marshall and Tanner, participants came mainly from the lower socio-economic sectors of the population. A poor nutritional status and overall well-being in early childhood may well lead to a later pubertal development in these girls compared with what would have been expected in the British population at the time. (Rubin *et al.* 2009: 502)

In his 2004 parental guide to early puberty, similarly, leading US clinician Paul Kaplowitz (2004: 76) describes the Harpenden sample as 'extremely non-random', arguing that its results should not be seen as constituting a norm for today's children.

In their 2008 state-of-the-art review of the epidemiological literature on early puberty (see Chapter 4 for a full discussion), Euling and colleagues make a further criticism, arguing that the participants in the study were all white and so should not be taken as typical for non-white children, who are today seen as notably 'different' in their patterns of sexual development. They write: 'Racial differences in patterns and progressive stages of pubic hair development increase the variability in pubic hair staging measures that use a scale (Tanner staging) developed for white individuals', they write (Euling *et al.* 2008: 173). Although this criticism seems somewhat misplaced – the *Atlas* does describe some non-white participants – it is true that Tanner and Whitehouse did not make distinctions according to 'race', which today is seen as scientifically incorrect (this debate is described in more detail in Chapters 4 and 5). Such distinctions sometimes have highly serious implications: discourses around 'racial' and ethnic differences in child growth are central to contested 'age determination' techniques used in assessing child asylum-seekers' cases, for example (Hopkins and Hill 2010: 141–4).

In all these criticisms, contemporary researchers point to the limitations of Tanner and Whitehouse's English sample in terms of the *timing* of 'normal' puberty and consequent assessment of contemporary changes in pubertal development. Importantly, however, these concerns have *not* reduced international and interdisciplinary reliance on the Tanner Scale as the standard articulation of the *stages* of puberty: although sequentially ordered, these can be disarticulated from age-related norms. The children of Harpenden still literally represent 'normal' puberty: photographs of their genitals and breasts (and line drawings based on them) circulate around the globe as tools with which clinicians, scientists, parents and children measure bodies to make judgements about growth. But what does it mean for a particular group of children living in an English care institution to function in this way? And what ethical and scientific questions does their position raise?

Revisiting Harpenden: the costs of participating in research

The post-war encounters between Tanner, Whitehouse and the children at Harpenden took place at a time in which English children were expected stoically to manage psychologically challenging separations from birth families and immersion in moral regimes of institutional care that attempted to replicate 'family life' (Lesko 2012). Being part of the Harpenden Study also exposed children to strenuous regimes of measurement and exposure (to cameras, instruments and X-rays) requiring them to stand still, tall and quiet. Although reported in some of Tanner's writing, the children's labour as research subjects is mostly absent in the published reports (this is common practice in scientific research) and their detailed contributions are certainly obscured in the simple graphic representations of the Tanner Scale widely used since in paediatric endocrinology.

Although Tanner and Whitehouse described 'psychosocial reasons' for lack of growth, the general effects of war-related trauma and post-war shortages of nutritious food are not analysed in this study: as noted above, the children are described as 'well nourished'. Similarly, no concerns are expressed by Tanner and Whitehouse about the ways in which their own interventions may have been – and indeed may continue to be – experienced as traumatic by their research subjects.

Searching for more information about life at Harpenden, however, I came across an extensive website containing text and archival photographs, produced by former resident Philip Howard, both to record his own experiences and to facilitate contact between others who lived there. Here Howard documents his memories of participating in the Tanner and Whitehouse study. His generally positive account of this experience, which meant welcome time off school and a feeling of being 'special', is rather poignantly undercut by his reference to 'ordinary children' who 'might have been a little scared' of having to do the things he and his friends did. I will quote Howard at length, but encourage readers to visit his website for a rich visual and textual account of life at Harpenden. Beginning the story of his experience of the Tanner study, Howard writes:

Our regular visits for the Growth Study Tests every few months were welcomed by most of us. An entire morning off school was something of a treat. The tests took about two hours. There were not that many of us in the group, but as we were all seen individually, although there were several staff involved, much of the time was waiting to be seen. The tests took place in one part of the main hall; this part of the hall was kept locked, other than on the days of the medical tests, because of the specialised medical equipment used only for our measurement tests. *Ordinary children might have been a little scared of having to strip down to their underwear and have parts of their bodies measured in size and density; we took it as fun.* The growth studies became a major source of reference on child development. (www.theirhistory.co.uk/70001/info.php?p=7&pno=0, emphasis added)

Howard describes the embarrassment he (and others, he claims) felt when experiencing a sexual response during the measurement sessions. Here he reveals some of the more difficult elements of life at Harpenden, noting the repressive reaction to sexual arousal boys would have expected from their carers:

As well as our measurements, photographs of our body stature and growth were taken from our front, back and side. These were done naked, and as there were no girls present, we did not find any reluctance at having such photographs taken.

If a few of us were embarrassed at times, it was when the staff might have touched certain parts of our body during the tests. When it came to standing up for the photographs, on occasions a few of us experienced erections. With the others occupied with their own part of the test, it was generally only the staff that witnessed our embarrassment. At our young age, we did not understand why things like this should happen. *If this had been in front of the Sisters or a Houseparent we could have expected some form of punishment; the medical staff took little notice of us.* (emphasis added)

Participating in the Tanner study, however, also helped Howard to feel marked out in a positive way:

On most occasions when our tests were over, it was necessary to return to school for the rest of the day. On odd times it did become possible to get the entire day off if it was felt that you might miss your school lunch, or those that were taken to school by coach found that there was no transport available. *We had a souvenir to show our friends that were not on the tests – odd ballpoint pen marks that were applied to our arms and other areas, that provided accurate reference points for measurements.* If we were well behaved a souvenir photo came our way on a few occasions, but taken when we were fully dressed. (emphasis added)

Howard's attention to the details of his and his friends' experiences is instructive: he reminds us how modern pubescent bodies were enacted – literally marked – through Tanner and Whitehouse's measuring practices, which involved wearing plastic pants, being drawn on and touched by medical staff, having to pose for photographs and enduring long periods of waiting around. Howard also points to the historical specificities of this study, which was made possible by the fact that he and his friends were not 'ordinary children', but rather stoical children living in the care system, who could be expected to cope with such challenges and even to 'take them as fun'.

Howard's account demonstrates that the social production of twentieth-century clinical 'norms' of puberty were in part enacted by (and thus dependent upon) children living in an atypical situation, one that (as Howard's reference to what the Sisters and house-parents' response to an erection might have been suggests) was sometimes violent and frightening. Elsewhere Howard describes repeatedly being hit by a slipper for wetting his bed; and his website contains a photo of a boy in the rubber shorts that children who wet their pants were sometimes required to wear. Howard describes the confusion that some children felt on being asked to wear plastic pants whilst being X-rayed for Tanner's study.

The other test was a series of x-rays, this was done alone in a more enclosed area of the hall, often as our final test. We would be provided with a pair of plastic pants to put on. To children in our Home at the age six or seven, the only reason in our minds why you would be provided with such a garment was that you might wet yourself. *At this age we could understand little about the complexities of x-rays, and even if we were older learning that x-rays could be dangerous to certain parts of the body, might have introduced even more fear.* (emphasis added)

Howard describes the X-rays as the most difficult part of participating in the study: not only did children have to wait a long time, they were also left alone during the test. Here, the plastic pants helped to hide children's fear-driven 'accidents':

The x-ray session seemed to take the longest part of the tests, positioning the machine to take the x-rays of our hand & wrist, jaw, head, calf, thigh, arm, chest. The boring part of these x-rays, was standing still once positioned over the machine, whilst the doctor went away to another area. For a young child on their first session, the plastic pants hid any accident that happened during the x-rays, strong elastic in the leg area, kept this matter secret from the doctor, allowing your return to the dressing area to put your clothes back on and to try and hide the event. In future sessions you would know not to be afraid, when it came to putting the plastic pants on ready for your x-ray session, you might find they were already slightly damp.[19]

In all his writings, Tanner assumes that children's experiences of participating in the Harpenden Study were neutral and he is, as mentioned above, very positive about the lives of the children at the National Children's Home. Although Howard describes the fear associated with the X-rays and some embarrassment about the required nudity, I have not come across any direct claims that children were physically or psychologically harmed during this work. Some recent writers, however, do raise concerns about the potentially long-lasting effects of being photographed as a subject of medical research. Despite stating that 'there are no data on the impact that being photographed may have on the patient or their family', gynaecologist Sarah Creighton and colleagues (2002: 67) argue, in the *British Journal of Urology International* for example, that being photographed – particularly naked and as a child – is likely to have negative effects on at least some patients: 'Medical photography', they remind us, 'is not a "neutral" act' (Creighton *et al.* 2002: 67).

The examples offered by Creighton *et al.* are images taken in the 1960s of two intersexed children, who gave their permission for the images to be published in Creighton *et al.*'s paper because of their profound concern about the medical use of such images. Intersexed children were, and are still today, often photographed naked, with particular attention paid to their genitals. Such photography is sometimes for an explicit clinical purpose (to record a pre-surgical state of the body, for example) but other times seems to be 'simply' a record or

[19] In another place, Howard describes these accidents as pranks: 'The only other activity was to be given several x-rays that took in various parts of the body. For safety reasons, instead of wearing our ordinary underpants during the x-rays we were provided with a special pair of thick plastic pants to put on; these apparently provided protection to our gonads from the x-rays. *A trick that was played by various boys was at the very end of the x-ray session*; leaving the plastic pants slightly damp was a joke for the next boy who came along to find when he put them on' (www.theirhistory.co.uk/70001/info.php?p=7&pno=0, emphasis added).

'snapshot' taken for no clear purpose. Although the children in the Harpenden Study were not photographed for clinical purposes or even in the course of any treatment, their experiences of being photographed naked may be similar. Indeed, Creighton *et al.*'s analysis shows that even images taken of visually 'normal' bodies can upset patients. They describe an interviewee's distress some thirty years later when viewing a photograph of herself as a visually normal, naked 3 year old, standing crying against a large ruler (2002: 69). As Creighton *et al.* suggest, 'it is reasonable to assume that taking pictures of intimate areas such as breasts or genitals, or a naked full body, would be more likely to cause psychological distress' (2002: 68).

Creighton *et al.* conclude that full naked body images are intrinsically unethical and potentially so damaging that they should never be taken. A 2005 consensus conference jointly sponsored by the Lawson Wilkins Pediatric Endocrine Society and the European Society for Paediatric Endocrinology and involving two leading intersex activists similarly proposed in its *Consensus Statement on Management of Intersex Disorder* that medical photography in this field should be curtailed (Karkazis 2008: 237).

Medical photographs travel in unexpected and relatively uncontrolled ways: intersexed people reported unexpectedly coming across images of themselves as children whilst seeking information on their conditions (Creighton *et al.* 2002: 68). The images used in the Tanner study have a similar ongoing life: not only were the children and young people in this study photographed over many years, the images of their naked bodies are used over and over again in scientific and clinical texts (for example the *Cambridge Encyclopedia of Human Growth*) and are available on the internet. It is important to note that although Philip Howard reproduces some of these images on his website, he obscures the faces on the naked photographs.

Movingly, Howard's website contains a set of photographs collated from his fellow participants in the Harpenden Study. These are the 'souvenir' pictures that were sometimes taken as a treat for the children who 'had done all everything the people in the white coats had asked' (www.theirhistory.co.uk/70001/info.php?p=7&pno=0). The pictures show fully clothed children laughing or smiling at the camera, their arms around their friends, seemingly enjoying the experience of posing. Here the gridlines of the photogrammetric equipment and the turntable fade into irrelevance and the liveliness and resilience of the children takes centre stage. The stunning contrast between these images and the sombre control found in the *Atlas* speaks volumes about the work involved in being a 'child subject' of twentieth-century developmental science.

Making modern pubertal bodies

Tanner and Whitehouse's study constitutes a typically modern approach to bodies, both attempting to pin them down through processes of measurement, documentation and standardisation (through the Tanner Scale) and in so doing multiplying and enacting differences. As I will argue in the following chapter, contemporary scientific work on rising rates of early onset puberty builds on this tradition. Scientists continually try to count bodies, to plot graphs and to make international comparisons, and to build health policies and treatment protocols around such statistics, whilst at the same time acknowledging that very little is understood about the causes of such trends or indeed the processes initiating puberty in any particular child's body. As I discuss in Chapter 5, scientific research also describes children travelling on diverse paths into early puberty: they are adopted internationally; they experience racism; they are overweight; their fathers do not take care of them. Such children do not form coherent populations and their physiological experiences constitute compelling 'mysteries' for biomedicine and technoscience.

Tanner and Whitehouse's work enacts a paradoxical understanding of puberty as simultaneously measurable and predictable and individually psycho-social. For me, this paradoxical biomedical and technoscientific enactment of children's pubescent bodies demonstrates a key feature of embodiment: that it is never possible to distinguish the physiological, psychological and social aspects of bodies. These elements are always inter-implicated or entangled, moving in and out of focus but remaining constantly in productive play. Tanner and Whitehouse's Subject 99 exemplifies this most directly. Tanner describes his stature as 'due to psychosocial stress.' I suggest that a similar claim – that growth is (bio)-psycho-social – could be made about *all* the children involved in the Harpenden Study *and* about the children described in the recent scientific and clinical literatures on early onset puberty. In thinking critically about discourses of a crisis in pubertal timing, then, we need to take account of this entanglement and become aware of where, how and why particular 'cuts' are made to distinguish the physical and the social in stories of early developing bodies.

From a feminist science studies perspective, bodies are enacted in historically and geographically situated practice; they are made in the kinds of complex interactions between technologies, institutions, people and non-human actors that constitute the Harpenden Study of child development. Karen Barad (2007) introduces the term 'agential cuts' to describe the way in which any particular experimental apparatus (or knowledge-related practice) necessarily allows some actors and actions to be included whilst excluding others, thus enacting the phenomenon under study in a particular way. This is a radical argument about ontology. As introduced in Chapter 2, for Barad there is no pre-existing real that is viewed from different positions; the cut is agential because it brings the phenomenon into existence:

> The apparatus enacts an agential cut – a resolution of the ontological indeterminancy – *within* the phenomenon ... The agential cut also enacts a local causal structure in the marking of the measuring instrument (the effect) by the measured object (cause), where 'local' means within the phenomenon. If the apparatus is changed, there is a corresponding change in the agential cut and therefore in the delineation of object from agencies of observation and the causal structure ... enacted by the cut. Different agential cuts produce different phenomena. (Barad 2007: 175)

Annemarie Mol (2002) makes a related argument in her book on the multiple ontologies of bodies with atherosclerosis. Working with ethnographic materials from a range of clinical, laboratory and domestic sites, Mol argues that bodies are differently 'enacted' – brought into being in an ontological sense – through temporally and geographically specific arrangements of practices and things. Rather than 'agential cuts', Mol (2002: viii) speaks of networks of practice that enact 'an intricately coordinated crowd: the *body multiple*'. This crowd of multiples needs to be coordinated to avoid 'clashes and explosive confrontations' (2002: 6) and so that care (medical and otherwise) can take place. Although there is no singular, 'real' body, the body multiple 'hangs together' (2002: 55). In atherosclerosis clinics and labs, and in patients' homes, this is achieved partly through naming (the word 'atherosclerosis' moves across a range of sites) but also through practices that sometimes bracket and sometimes highlight the practicalities of measuring and delineating bodies and diseases: such practices allow the fiction that bodies and diseases are singular entities which can be treated. Rejecting this fiction, Mol suggests instead that we think of bodies (and diseases or conditions) as composites, emphasising their 'manyfoldedness' (2002: 84).

I have argued in this chapter that historical enactments of pubescent bodies demonstrate that puberty is not a singular, delineable process but rather a process of multiplication. Pubertal bodies, like those with atherosclerosis are 'manyfolded'. They are also made to hang together or to congeal in particular ways so that clinical practice and scientific work can go on. The Tanner Scale plays a hugely important role in this.

I have also argued here that the internationally accepted pubertal standards against which early developers are now routinely measured were produced through making certain material-semiotic cuts during the Harpenden Study: Tanner's decision not to include psychological testing; the use of Whitehouse's body-holding devices; and the choice of the National Children's Home as the research location, amongst many others. Although the effect of Tanner's work has been to make pubertal bodies quite solid – to get them to hang together – in some places and encounters, my analysis highlights the contingencies and possible points of contestation that are inevitably part of this process.

But how does my analysis – relying as it does on text, images and written testimony – speak to the biological matter of bodies in development? What can Tanner's findings tell us about how puberty happens and what it feels like? As discussed in Chapter 2, some contemporary writers, notably those identified with 'new materialism', demand a more 'direct' engagement with matter, including biological bodies. Part of a determined (and in my view problematic) shift away from critique, such demands emphasise the importance of careful listening and attention when engaging with scientific accounts and practices. This kind of care, I argue, has long been the mainstay of STS engagements with science and biomedicine which often, as discussed in the previous chapter, use ethnographic methods to get close to the objects of study (scientists, scientific work, technical research objects and practices, for example). In this chapter I have used the literature as an informant, approaching texts in an ethnographic manner and exploring the multiplicity of pubertal bodies enacted in them.

Emphasising multiplicity is central to STS accounts of bodies-in-the-making. If bodies are understood as made in practice, they are also both multiple and relational; they can never be ontologically fixed or singular. This point, according to Mol (2012), is often lost in new materialists' calls to concentrate on matter. Arguing this point and rather boldly eliding Barad's distinction between interaction and intra-action, Mol insists on the significance of matter's activity and ontological multiplicity:

> Like that of the canon, *their* [the new materialists'] 'ontology' is stable and singular – but it is *not* out of reach. They say that we should (finally!) stop fussing about language and interpretations and attend to the activities of matter itself – in its ontological essence (e.g. Coole and Frost, 2010). What they lightly skip over, though, is that matter never is 'itself' all by itself. Even when it is not being interpreted, matter is never alone. For it may well be that matter acts, but what it is able to *do* inevitably depends on adjacent matter that it may do something *with*. Action is always interaction. And it is only in interactions, or intra-actions if you prefer (Barad 2007), that objects relationally afford each other their (always local, often fluid) 'essence'. As the new materialism forgets these relational engagements and affordances it has no way of talking about what matter 'itself' does, other than naively echoing natural science textbooks and journal articles – minus the materials and methods sections. Decades of work in STS is being disdainfully discarded. (Mol 2012: 318)

As an STS scholar, I agree with Mol that the materials and methods used to produce scientific findings cannot be left aside in engagements with these findings. In this chapter, then, I have spent quite a lot of time discussing Tanner and Whitehouse's methods and tools. I am also, as outlined in Chapter 2, convinced of the importance of language in analysing pubertal bodies. Throughout this book, I discuss the material and the semiotic as conjoined in their actions. We cannot, I suggest, understand Tanner's contribution to the making of pubertal bodies without thinking about his practices of measuring and photographing *and* his textual and visual inscriptions. Inextricably linked, these forces figure pubescent bodies in particular ways.

I have also spent time considering the feelings evoked through and by Tanner's work. Exploring the ways in which the Harpenden Study relied on children's management of difficult feelings (of embarrassment, boredom, fear and excitement) I have demonstrated the intra-action of feelings, tools and discourses in auxology. I have also touched on my own feelings about viewing Tanner's photographs and explored concerns about the potential psychological effects on original study participants of the widespread circulation of these images.

Thinking about pubertal bodies as made in the findings, feelings and figurations of Tanner's Harpenden Study means understanding them as historically specific, ethically consequential and potentially contestable. Working from such a view of sexual development would, I suggest, alter current approaches to early onset puberty. Rather than figuring a crisis that needs to be solved through establishing new norms and medically intervening in children's abnormal bodies, we might instead ask how we might learn to live better with, and scientifically represent, diverse developing bodies. This argument is pursued in the following chapter.

4 *Defining early onset puberty: troubling findings about sexual development*

Puberty has been lavishly described within twentieth- and twenty-first-century science and biomedicine. As shown in the previous chapter, children's progress through the multiple and uneven physical 'stages' of development has been articulated in meticulous detail in texts that flow outside the traditional boundaries of science and medicine, becoming widely available in some forms for use by parents, teachers and young people. The hormonal cascades associated with puberty have also been intensely researched for almost a century, with an increasing emphasis in recent decades on connections between the brain, the central nervous system and the reproductive organs. Here, technical discourses are less certain: in many ways the 'interior' (endocrinological, neuroendocrinological and genetic) micro-processes of puberty remain a 'mystery' for contemporary scientists. Indeed, the 125th Anniversary special issue of the journal *Science* listed 'What triggers puberty?' as one of the top yet-to-be-answered 125 scientific questions for the twenty-first century (Anon. 2005). Much recent research focuses on genetic pathways in sexual development and gene–hormone–environment interactions in trying, as expressed in the *Science* article, to find out 'what exactly forces childhood to end' (Anon. 2005).

This chapter explores the scientific and clinical literature on early sexual development, focusing on technoscientific and biomedical research papers published in the leading journals forming the core of the mainstream debates. These papers were located through repeated searches of relevant databases and following citational trails, tracking the 'life' of particular datasets and arguments both in scientific publications and in more public domains.[1] Attempting to come to grips with

[1] This database compiles the results of systematic searches of scientific and medical literatures (1960–2012, with some later additions) using PubMed and Web of Science. Although the database ranks articles by citation frequency, we did not undertake formal citation analysis for this book. The strengths and limits of

this lively field here, I trace key scientific publications through their description in press releases cited by journalists, social scientists and interested commercial and political actors.

Inspired by Kelty and Landecker's (2009) ethnographic approach to studying scientific literatures, I explore several phenomena. Firstly, I focus on the methods, findings and framing arguments presented in the scientific papers: what kinds of findings are articulated here and how are these made? What kinds of stories are told about puberty? (In later chapters I focus on what kind of problem puberty is said to constitute and what solutions are offered in biomedical and technoscientific literatures.) Secondly, I follow the citational chains linking key papers, asking how scientists create debate around early puberty through citing or refuting each other's work. Thirdly, I document the circulation of key scientific results and arguments into popular media accounts, analysing journalists' representations of scientific debates in this field.

Ultimately, I am concerned with the pubescent bodies enacted in these publications. Pursuing a feminist science studies approach, I argue that scientific papers articulate bodily differences in highly consequential ways, enacting early developing bodies as raced and classed, sexed and gendered, normal or pathological. Scientific publications on early sexual development sort and classify 'types', figuring and reconfiguring historically specific categories in order to study processes of change. Pubertal bodies are conjured in this work and lived in relation to it. The research described in these papers always involves bodily and affective engagements: the data are the result of Harpenden-style interactions between scientists or clinicians and children (although often within clinical rather than domestic care settings). Multiple bodies and feelings are at play here, bringing these texts to life.

citation analysis are clearly articulated by Kelty and Landecker (2009) who argue that although it visually highlights the communal nature of scientific work, it does not facilitate textual interpretation or reading. As discussed in Chapter 2, in this book I treat text ethnographically. I agree with Kelty and Landecker (2009: 189) that 'an ethnographic sensibility for the literature allows interpretation back into the space opened by citation indexing, and adds an awareness of material practice to analysis afforded by rhetoric of science [approaches]. It gives new meaning to the idea of sitting down with the literature, situating individual scientists as secondary sources as, alongside the ethnographer, they too process the mass of literature that forms their intellectual and practical environment.'

Engaging with a set of diverse texts, this chapter analyses scientific stories that simultaneously constitute a set of technical discourses that are part of ongoing debate and enact material-semiotic bodies as involving particular characteristics, risks and potentials. My aim is to explore these stories, debates and enactments as a form of intervention. In thinking about young people, sex/gender and sexuality, feminists cannot afford to leave the physical elements of puberty to scientists and clinicians; to either take for granted what they argue or to assume it is wrong. Far better, I suggest, to attempt to get to grips with this research, its findings, logics and apparatuses, and to explore what kinds of resonance or 'interference patterns' might be generated through such an encounter (Haraway 1997: 16; Law 2004: 68–9). What can we learn about developing bodies through engaging with science and biomedicine? And what does a feminist science studies approach have to offer this field?

'Normal' puberty

Although it is beyond the scope of this book to provide a full account of research into 'normal' or on-time puberty, it is important to introduce the basic scientific narrative of the processes of sexual development before exploring early onset puberty in detail. In undergraduate biomedical textbooks, puberty is defined as the process that produces bodies able to sexually reproduce. In the 2013 edition of *Human Physiology: From Cells to Systems*, for example, Lauralee Sherwood (2013: 744) writes, 'Puberty is the period of arousal and maturation of the previously non-functional reproductive system, culminating in sexual maturity and the ability to reproduce.' In an era of ever-increasing rates of infertility, this is a rather uncomfortable definition: many fully developed individuals will not be able to reproduce.[2] As these high rates of infertility indicate, norms of sexual development and sexual physiology (as we will also see in the puberty case) are frequently transgressed.

[2] In a 2012 factsheet, the European Society of Human Reproduction and Embryology states that one in six couples worldwide experience some form of infertility problem at least once during their reproductive lifetime and that the current prevalence of infertility lasting for at least twelve months is estimated to be around 9 per cent worldwide for women aged 20–44 (www.eshre.eu/sitecore/content/Home/Guidelines and Legal/ART fact sheet).

For physiologists, achieving sexual maturity involves developing 'secondary sexual characteristics' (breasts, pubic hair, adult genitalia) and moving into adult cycles of production of sex cells (eggs and sperm). Although the triggers of pubertal development remain unknown, it is widely thought that maturational changes and decreased inhibitory mechanisms in children's brains, probably activated by the neuropeptide kisspeptin (a communicating protein-like molecule), increase the secretion of gonadotropin-releasing hormone (GnRH) from the hypothalamus in pulses during sleep (see, for example, Apter 1997; DiVall and Radovick 2009). These pulses become longer until an adult pattern is established. The pulses of GnRH cause increased secretion of luteinising hormone (LH) and follicle-stimulating hormone (FSH) from the anterior pituitary, which in turn increases secretion of either testosterone from the testes or estrogen (estradiol) from the ovaries as they grow. It is these well-known sex hormones that are said to 'arouse' (to use Sherwood's word) dormant reproductive systems, stimulating the development of many secondary sexual characteristics, including breast growth. The relationship between these parts of the brain and the gonads is called the HPG (hypothalamus-pituitary-gonadal) axis.

Like many hormone stories, this mainstream account of sexual development figures sexual difference as binary: descriptions of puberty in girls focus on the estrogen-producing ovaries and those about boys focus on testosterone-producing testes (Roberts 2007). In relation to boys, for example, Sherwood (2013: 744) writes that 'Testosterone is responsible for growth and maturation of the entire male reproductive system.' In a section on girls, she states:

> GnRH begins stimulating release of anterior pituitary gonadotropic hormones, which in turn stimulate ovarian activity. The resulting secretion of estrogen by the activated ovaries induces growth and maturation of the female reproductive tract as well as development of the female secondary sexual characteristics. (2013: 773)

Research into early onset puberty undermines this mainstream story. Some recent literature, for example, suggests that early breast development may not be associated with activation of the HPG axis, and occurs without increased LH or FSH levels (Aksglaede *et al.* 2009). Girls also experience changes in androgen secretions at puberty. In pubescent girls, these 'male' hormones, coming from the adrenal glands, are linked to the growth of pubic and underarm hair, overall growth and the development of libido (Ankarberg and Norjavaara 1999; Dorn and Rotenstein 2004; Wu, Zhang and Lee 2012: 341). Estrogens also play a 'surprising' role in male sexual development. 'Recent findings suggest', Sherwood notes (2013: 746), 'that estrogen plays an essential role in male reproductive health; for example, it is important in spermatogenesis and surprisingly contributes to male heterosexuality. Also, it probably contributes to bone homeostasis.' Such surprises, as I argue elsewhere, stem from a long history of understanding sexual difference as binary and even oppositional and have no basis in physiological reasoning or material evidence (Roberts 2007; see also Oudshoorn 1994; Fausto-Sterling 2012b).

In physiological accounts, puberty materializes mature forms of biological sexual difference and the capacity to reproduce. Sometime after puberty starts, it is argued, the oocytes present in the girl's body since birth begin to mature and are released from the ovaries in a cyclical manner in ovulation. Menstruation also begins. In boys, sperm production starts as testosterone triggers the development of the seminal vesicles and the prostate gland. The hormonal messaging systems established at puberty in boys involve essentially constant testosterone secretion and sperm production, while those established in girls involve the intermittent release of ova and the cyclical secretion of estrogen. 'Female reproductive physiology', Sherwood (2013: 757) writes, 'is much more complex than male reproductive physiology. Unlike the continuous sperm production and essentially constant testosterone secretion characteristic of the male, release of ova is intermittent, and secretion of female sex hormones displays wide cyclic swings.' Sherwood's use of the non-technical term 'swings' – a word often associated with emotional lability – references a widespread cultural interpretation of this difference: women are often understood as moody and fluctuating because of their sexual physiologies, whilst men are seen as constantly desiring and stable (Roberts 2007).

Increasing rates of early onset puberty and the sense of crisis around these have stimulated research into the basic biology of sexual development. The high numbers of girls entering puberty early have led clinicians to call for changes to clinical guidelines and practices. Only fifty years since their development, Tanner's norms and standards seem no longer to hold true for many girls and are also starting to come into doubt for boys. As I will show, studies indicate that sexual development starts up to two years earlier in large cohorts of girls, with the timing of early development seeming to stretch: the first stages of puberty (breast and pubic hair growth) are starting earlier and earlier, with less clear changes occurring with regard to the onset of menstruation. Recent research into puberty in boys shows similar trends, with sexual development appearing to start six months to two years earlier than in Tanner's time (Herman-Giddens *et al.* 2012). Population changes of this scale over such a short time period are extraordinary.[3]

This chapter explores claims about rising rates of early onset puberty, focusing, as do the scientific and biomedical literatures and public debates, on girls. At the time of writing debate around boys' development was minimal. Research in this field, as mentioned in Chapter 1, is said to be hampered by difficulties in nominating a definitive moment of male puberty equivalent to the onset of menstruation. Asking boys or their parents about bodily processes is figured as more invasive than posing similar questions to girls and mothers. In an article in *The New York Times*, for example, lead author of the two key American studies Marcia Herman-Giddens states that colleagues reviewing a proposal to ask boys about seminal emissions 'just freaked out' (cited in Belluck 2012). These anxieties, I suggest, also indicate reluctance to articulate male sexual development as a biomedical problem: male puberty is widely figured as a positive development rather than a matter for concern (see also Egan 2013: 64–7).

Counting pubertal bodies and establishing the limits of 'normal'

From 1969 the lower end of 'normal' age span for puberty was set at 8 years of age for girls and 9 for boys. In the 1970s to 1990s, children undergoing pubertal development before age 8 for girls and 9 for boys were referred for assessment and treatment. As described in the previous chapter, these internationally agreed markers were based on Tanner and Whitehouse's longitudinal study of sexual development (1948–70) and specifically on the 1962 book *Growth at Adolescence* and on papers that Tanner co-authored with physician and human biologist W.A. Marshall (Marshall and Tanner 1969; 1970). As

[3] Changes in levels of childhood obesity may be similar: for a comparison between discourses on childhood obesity and early puberty, see Throsby and Roberts (2010).

clinician Paul Kaplowitz writes in his book-length parental guide to early onset puberty, 'One reason why the Marshall and Tanner paper was so widely quoted in the United States was that during the period from 1970 to 1990, there was simply nothing published based on U.S. populations of girls that provided meaningful data on the onset of puberty' (Kaplowitz 2004: 67).

In the 1980s and 1990s, however, clinicians like Kaplowitz 'were seeing large numbers of girls referred for early puberty, a large proportion of whom were between the ages of 7 and 8' (2004: 67) and beginning to doubt the continued relevance of the Tanner findings. In 1988, Dr Marcia Herman-Giddens, Director of the Child Protection Team at Duke University Medical Centre, published a report on the possible association between child sexual abuse and sexual precocity, finding that one in fifteen female victims aged 10 or younger had begun sexual development before age 8 (cited in Kaplowitz 2004: 67). This finding prompted her to develop a pilot and then a large-scale study of pubertal timing in American girls.

The larger ground-breaking study (Herman-Giddens *et al.* 1997) – often referred to as the 'Pediatric Research in Office Settings' or 'PROS' study – found that rates of early onset puberty were increasing and that these increases reflected patterns of diversity in pubertal timing that had not previously been explored. Using data collected by 225 clinicians working in a network of paediatric practices (the PROS network), Herman-Giddens *et al.* examined the clinical records of 17,077 North American girls, 9.6 per cent of whom were African-American and 90.4 per cent white (children of 'mixed race' were classified as 'other' and excluded).[4] Although a clinical rather than a random sample, this was a large group to study.

Herman-Giddens *et al.*'s key finding was that the *mean* age of puberty for white girls was 9.96 and for African-American girls, 8.87. At age 8, 48.3 per cent of African-American girls and 14.7 per cent of white girls showed pubertal maturation (evidenced by breast development described as Tanner breast stage 2). At age 7, 27.2 per cent of African-American girls but only 6.7 per cent of white girls had begun development (see Figure 4). In other words, almost a third of the

[4] Constituting 2.8% of the sample, all children classified as other than White or African American were excluded from the study (Hermann-Giddens *et al* 1997: 507).

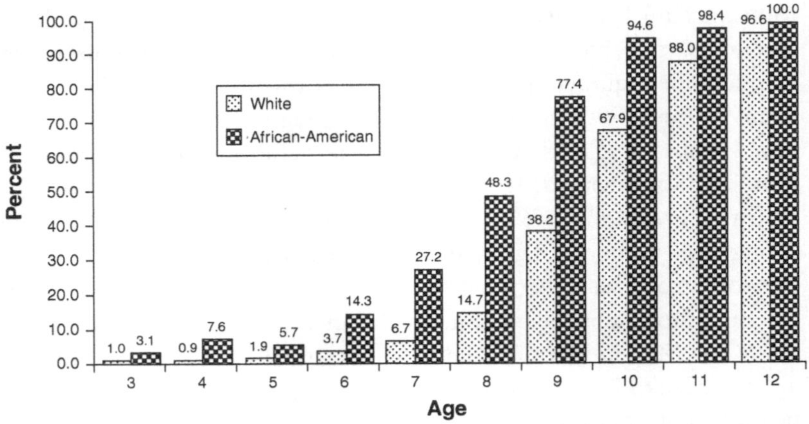

Figure 4 Racial differences in pubertal timing: Herman-Giddens *et al.*'s (1997) findings. Prevalence of breast and/or pubic hair development at Tanner stage 2 or greater by age and race (Cochran-Mantel-Haenszel x^2 = 354.8, df = 1, $P < .001$; Breslow-Day x^2 = 10.0, df = 9, $P = .354$).

African-American girls had started puberty by their 7th birthday. These figures were staggering: the 'commonly used figure' of girls going through puberty before 8 was 1 per cent (Herman-Giddens *et al.* 1997: 511). Importantly, the majority of these girls did not start menstruating earlier than their counterparts – the mean age of menarche was still 13, an average that had remained unchanged for fifty years. Instead of having two years in the first stages of puberty, then, these girls had three to five years. For scientific and clinical endocrinological communities, the consequences of these findings were profound: if such large numbers of children were going through puberty at these ages, should the parameters of 'normal' and 'early' puberty be redefined?

Collecting data between 1988 and 1994, another major study came to similar conclusions. Funded by the US government, this study – known as the National Health and Nutrition Examination Survey (Third Cycle) or 'NHANES III' – studied 7,000 subjects aged between 1 and 16, selected to make racial comparisons easier. Assessing the growth and pubertal stage of the 1,623 girls in the study, like the PROS study NHANES III found that breast and pubic hair development in 8-year-old girls was common, especially in black and Hispanic girls: 27.8 per cent of black girls and 25.4 per cent of Hispanic girls had started breast growth by 8, compared to 11.4 per cent of white girls

(Wu *et al.* 2002). NHANES III also showed girls beginning menstruation at 12.54 years, a lower average than the 12.75 of twenty years earlier (2002).

In response to the PROS study and to a letter published by a group of paediatric endocrinologists in *The Lancet* calling for revised protocols for assessing early puberty (Elders *et al.*, 1997), the American-based Lawson Wilkins Pediatric Endocrine Society undertook a comprehensive review of the published data. Publishing its recommendations in *Pediatrics* in 1999 (Kaplowitz, Oberfield and the Drug and Therapeutics and Executive Committees of the Lawson Wilkins Pediatric Endocrine Society 1999), this review made several key points:

1. that the PROS study was the first comprehensive study indicating a decline in average age of puberty for American girls (1 year for white girls and 2 years for African-American girls);
2. that this decline was not connected to significant or enduring negative psychological or behavioural outcomes or significant loss of adult height (concerns about this are described as 'overstated'); and
3. that hormonal therapies (GnRH analogs) had not been proved effective in preventing height loss in girls starting puberty between 6 and 8 years of age.

Led by Kaplowitz, the authors proposed new guidelines for defining (and therefore treating) early onset puberty: only girls with either breast development (thelarche) or pubic hair development (pubarche) before age 7 in white girls and age 6 in African-American girls should be evaluated clinically. In other words, these guidelines proposed that white girls starting puberty at 7 and African-American girls starting puberty at 6 should now be considered 'normal' and not offered treatment. Such girls were now reconfigured as 'largely being healthy girls who are the tail end of the normal distribution of the timing of puberty' (Kaplowitz 2004: 76). No proposals were made to change the age triggering evaluation in boys (beginning puberty before 9 years). These proposals were taken up in a major textbook, Wilson *et al.*'s *Williams Textbook of Endocrinology* (1998) and consequently by many practitioners, leading to a culture of 'watchful waiting' rather than intervention (Pathomvanich and Merke 2000: 115).

Despite this take-up, the proposals caused significant controversy in the field. Some senior clinicians expressed great reluctance to change the guidelines stipulating 8 as the cut-off point for 'normal' puberty for girls. Led by Robert L. Rosenfield, a group of paediatricians published a letter in *Pediatrics*, arguing that 'it is premature to conclude that the normal age of puberty is occurring earlier' or that children undergoing puberty before 8 or 9 should not be assessed (Rosenfield *et al.* 2000: 622). Herman-Giddens, Slora and Wasserman responded, stating that although they agreed that 'puberty at an early age may not be "normal" even though a large number of girls are experiencing it ... the new recommendations for the evaluation of early puberty are sound' (Herman-Giddens *et al.* 2000: 623). The pubertal development of 7–8-year-old white girls and 6–8-year-old black girls starting puberty is 'rarely found to have a pathologic cause' (2000: 623). In two articles published in *The New York Times* in 2001, science journalist Gina Kolata described ensuing tensions within the endocrine community as stultifying. Citing Kaplowitz she reported that:

> The issue has now reached the point of an acrid dispute among pediatric endocrinologists, with the experts on each side barely able to speak civilly about their opponents. 'A certain amount of dissent can be refreshing,' Dr. Kaplowitz said. "But this is not refreshing." (Kolata 2001a)

One of the key criticisms of the Herman-Giddens study focused on the assessment of breast development: gathering data from sixty-five clinics, the study included assessments of breast tissue that were made only visually, rather than through touch ('palpation'). Although the basis of Tanner's studies and a common assessment practice, experts agree that visual assessments are difficult to make: accumulations of fat can look like breast tissue. In contrast, trained professionals can more clearly distinguish between the feel of fat and glandular (breast) tissue (Euling *et al.* 2008: 175). In conducting his review of this data, Kaplowitz asked the Herman-Giddens team to reanalyse the data, comparing the visual and palpation data from the clinicians who had used both methods (accounting for 39 per cent of the sample of girls). He writes: 'It turned out that 4 percent of girls with breast development by inspection had no breast tissue by palpation, while 1.7 percent of girls who had no breast tissue by inspection were found to have breast tissue by palpation. In other words, in the great majority of cases, the inspection and palpation rating of breast development agreed' (Kaplowitz 2004: 72). This re-examination also found that 'misclassifications' of breast tissue were just as likely in thin as in fat girls, and that the data were not skewed by older girls being fatter than younger girls. Kaplowitz concludes that, 'While it would have been ideal to do visual scoring and then palpation for all the subjects, the [re-examined] ... data suggest that the results of the PROS study were not significantly altered by relying on inspection as the primary method of examining breasts' (2004: 73). The NHANES III study also used visual assessment only.[5]

In a 2003 paper, however, Midyett, Moore and Jacobson criticised the Herman-Giddens study and the consequent Lawson Wilkins Pediatric Endocrine Society recommendation, stating that:

> This recommendation seemed to us somewhat premature, considering the acknowledged limitations of the study and lack of data on endocrine evaluations performed on girls with early pubertal changes. In fact, the revision has led to extensive controversy with a number of pediatric endocrinologists issuing statements contesting the new guidelines. We share the concern expressed by other endocrinologists that liberalizing the definition of 'normal' carries with it the risk of overlooking pathology. (Midyett, Moore and Jacobson 2003: 47)

Reporting an analysis of 1,570 patient visits to their outpatient paediatric endocrinology clinic, Midyett*et al.* (2003: 47) argued that 'signs of puberty in 6- to 8-year-old girls should not be considered normal or benign' and that reducing the cut-off age for 'normal' puberty would 'result in failure to identify conditions that respond to early intervention'. Cases in which there was real endocrinological pathology[6] – evidenced by what they called 'true precocious puberty', the development of both breasts and pubic hair, as opposed to 'partial puberty', the growth of breasts or pubic hair – would be missed and girls would

[5] In 2000 and 2002, another key study, the Bogalusa Heart Study (Freedman *et al.* 2000; Freedman *et al*, 2002) published data examining 3,000–3,500 children's growth over the period 1973–92. The 2000 paper showed that the 1992 children were almost an inch taller than their 1973 counterparts at age 12, but that this height advantage was not sustained in early adulthood. The 2002 paper demonstrated that white girls began their periods two months earlier in the 1990s than the 1970s, whilst black girls started nine months earlier. Although a much more geographically limited study (covering one state only), these results also supported the contention that puberty was starting earlier in the United States.

[6] Diagnoses included insulin resistance/hyperinsulinism, congenital adrenal hyperplasia, neurofibromatosis, growth hormone deficiency, hypothyroidism and McCune-Albright Syndrome (Midyett *et al.* 2003: 49–50).

miss out on treatment.[7] In their conclusion, these authors state their intention to ignore the new guidelines and to continue to recommend the referral of all children under age 8 with one or two signs of early puberty (Midyett *et al.* 2003: 51).

In 2004, Herman-Giddens, Kaplowitz and Wasserman published a commentary responding to the spate of articles published in *Pediatrics* following their 1997 contribution. Defending their study against its critics and picking apart their rivals' work, they argued again that the norms of puberty had changed and reasserted the need for revised clinical guidelines defining early onset puberty (although also advising that 'Primary care physicians should not blindly use the age of the child as a rote guide for referral' for treatment) (Herman-Giddens, Kaplowitz and Wasserman 2004: 915). In the United States, they suggested, the increasing numbers of children experiencing early onset puberty meant that physicians would soon not be able to provide clinical assessments to those who under earlier clinical regimes would have been offered them. Arguing against Midyett *et al.*'s (2003) reinterpretation of their original data, they calculated the number of girls going through early puberty if it were defined as development under 8 years of age:

> This totals 195 400 girls <8 years old with at least Tanner 2 pubic hair. There are ~650 pediatric endocrinologists in the United States. If all these girls truly need an evaluation, then each endocrinologist would have to see, on average, 300 of these girls. If we estimate the cost for a basic evaluation as proposed by the authors of an examination and bone age films (including radiologist interpretation) at $250, the cost to evaluate these girls would be $48 850 000. (Herman-Giddens *et al.* 2004: 915)

In contrast, reducing the lower age of 'normal' puberty as they suggested in their earlier work ('black girls <6 years old and white girls <7 years old'), 'the number of girls needing an evaluations for pubic hair drops to 63 000, a still-large but more manageable number' (2004: 915).

In their conclusion, however, Herman-Giddens *et al.* also stated that the increased numbers of girls going through early onset puberty was not in itself evidence that nothing was wrong or that this was a harmless shift. Increasing rates of early onset puberty may well, they

[7] This definition is contentious and was later contested by Hermann-Giddens and her team (2004: 915).

write, constitute a '"canary in the mine" for environmental problems' (2004: 925). They rather bluntly outlined this dilemma in two summary statements:

1. Data show that girls are maturing earlier than they did several decades ago and that there are substantial racial differences between white and black girls.
2. These 'norms' are not the same as the condition of being 'normal' in the sense of indicating optimal health (2004: 925–6).

The debates around historical population (or 'secular') changes in onset of puberty continue to the time of writing. In 2008 a group of ten experts, led by a scientist working at the US Environmental Protection Agency, Susan Euling, came together to perform 'a thorough weight-of-the-evidence evaluation of the data' (Euling *et al.* 2008: S172). Asked to 'resolve the debate' (2008: S172), their work was oriented around the misleadingly simple question: 'Are data sufficient to suggest or establish a secular trend in the timing of puberty onset and/or progression (as measured by puberty markers) in both boys and girls from US data over the time period 1940–1994?' (2008: S173). The majority of the group agreed that the data were sufficient to suggest a trend towards earlier breast development onset and menarche in girls (a minority of this group argued that the evidence was enough to 'establish' both of these), but not for other pubertal markers (e.g. pubic hair onset or growth, i.e. Tanner PH1–5, or later breast development, i.e. Tanner B3–B5). Almost all the panellists agreed that the data were not sufficient to evaluate secular trends in male populations, for either pubic hair or genital development. Importantly, the panel also agreed that 'altered pubertal timing should be considered an adverse event' (2008: S172) but did not elaborate questions of cause, effect or treatments. The consequent question of where to set the outer limits for 'normal' puberty was not addressed.

Responding in part to Euling *et al.*'s report, an American consortium called the Breast Cancer and Environment Research Center (BCERC) set up a longitudinal, prospective study to follow a cohort of girls through puberty into adulthood. In 2010 they reported on the pubertal development stages of their baseline cohort of 1,239 girls, who were divided into three groups: white non-Hispanic, black non-Hispanic and Hispanic. In this paper Biro *et al.* (2010) report a further increase in numbers of girls going through early puberty: almost twice as many white non-Hispanic girls were going through puberty at ages 7 and 8 than reported in the PROS study thirteen years earlier (10.4 per cent at age 7 for BCERC versus 5 per cent in PROS; 17.9 per cent at age 8 for BCERC versus 10.5 per cent in PROS). For black non-Hispanic girls the change was less significant at age 7 (23.4 per cent versus 14.4 per cent in PROS) and insignificant at age 8 (37.0 per cent versus 36.6 per cent in PROS). Hispanic girls were also increasingly likely to go through early puberty: 14.9 per cent at age 7 and 30.9 per cent at age 8 were at Tanner breast stage 2 or more. The authors conclude, then, that 'it seems that age in onset of puberty is continuing to fall in white but not black girls. Black girls continue to mature at younger ages than white girls' (Biro *et al.* 2010: 583).

The publication of these data led to a new spate of media articles in which the late 1990s sense of crisis is reaffirmed. In an article entitled 'Early Puberty in Girls Doubles in a Decade', *New Scientist* journalist Andy Coghlan quotes Marcia Herman-Giddens expressing shock and concern:

> Marcia Herman-Giddens of the University of North Carolina at Chapel Hill, who led the 1997 study, expressed shock at the increases. 'To find the girls are starting breast development earlier and earlier is extremely concerning,' she says. 'To have that much change in such a short time, it has to be the environment.' (Coghlan 2010)

Articles about recent research indicating earlier puberty in boys are more equivocal. In an article entitled 'Boys Now Enter Puberty Younger, Study Suggests, but It's Unclear Why', *New York Times* journalist Pam Belluck (2012) cites scientists trying to damp down public concerns: 'Several experts said the study should not be seized upon as cause for alarm.' Discussion of both cause and consequences of early development in boys is also much more tempered. In relation to cause, Belluck writes, 'the study ... did not try to determine what might be causing earlier puberty, although it mentioned changes in diet, less physical activity and other environmental factors as possibilities'. Regarding consequences, gendered distinctions are clearly made: 'Some experts said that while earlier development in girls can be worrisome because girls may be treated as more socially mature than they are, implications for boys are uncertain' (2012). These debates are explored in Chapters 5 and 6.

Global flows

The studies discussed so far refer to North American populations, but what is the story in the rest of the world? In a 2003 review article collating data from around the world entitled 'The Timing of Normal Puberty and the Age Limits of Sexual Precocity: Variations around the World, Secular Trends, and Changes after Migration', Anne-Simone Parent *et al.* (2003: 674) review studies of normal and precocious puberty. Distinguishing between children living in 'well-off' and 'underprivileged conditions' (both within countries and across them), Parent *et al.* note an overall decline in age of menarche historically, a decline that seems, they argue, to be coming to an end in 'well-off' populations but continues to decline in 'underprivileged' ones (those living in India, China and Eastern Europe, for example). They put this change down to 'current changes in living standards' and note that their 'data highlight the crucial role of socioeconomic and nutritional conditions in the timing of puberty' (2003: 673). Analysing the results of the smaller number of studies focusing on breast development, Parent *et al.* come to the puzzling conclusion that 'In Europe there is no evidence of the marked secular reduction in average age at B2 [Tanner breast stage 2] such as shown in the United States' (2003: 675). This difference, they conclude, remains to be explained (2003: 687). Parent *et al.* (2003: 675) are cautious about the American proposal to reduce the age limit for precocious puberty, noting the internal disputes amongst American endocrinologists: '[T]he question of age limit for sexual precocity does not have any definitive and unequivocal answer' (2003: 675).

A more recent study, published in *Pediatrics* in 2009, came to a different conclusion. Studying 2,095 Danish girls from the Copenhagen area and using palpation to assess breast development, the researchers excluded girls who were not 'European' (i.e. who had one parent 'originating from a non-European country') (Aksglaede *et al.* 2009: 933). This sampling strategy, they argue, meant excluding 'confounding resulting from ethnic differences' (2009: 937). The girls also came from a limited number of schools and were thus deliberately homogenous in terms of social and economic backgrounds (these are not specified).

Aksglaede *et al.* (2009) found that girls' breast development in 2006 started on average at 9.86 as compared to 10.88 in 1991, and that age of menarche had also slightly decreased (from 13.42 in 1991 to 13.13 in 2006) (see also Aksglaede *et al.* 2008). The researchers took blood samples to assess pubertal stage and found to their surprise that earlier breast development was not associated with higher levels of gonadotropins (indeed, 8–10 year olds in the 2006 group had a slight but significant decrease in estradiol levels compared to the 1991 cohort). The authors note: 'This result suggests that our observations may not reflect earlier activation of the pituitary-gonadal axis but, rather, gonadotropin-independent estrogenic actions at the level of the breast' (Aksglaede *et al.* 2009: 935). The change in breast development age found was greater than that of age of menarche onset: the authors thus conclude: 'As a result of the uneven changes in early and late markers of puberty, the length of puberty seemed to have increased' (2009: 935).

A recent UK study found similar results in relation to breast development and pubic hair growth, but no evidence of a secular decline in age of menarche (although at 12.93, this was lower than the Danish median, it remained the same as that of the mothers of the girls in the study). Recruiting from a large cohort of mothers and children enrolled in the Avon Longitudinal Study of Parents and Children (ALSPAC), Rubin *et al.* (2009) asked the girls in the study (or their parents) to fill out questionnaires about their sexual development from the age of 8 to 13. Using this rather weak form of data collection, the authors lost quite a lot of data: forms were not filled in, errors were made and data were not coherent. Despite these difficulties, Rubin *et al.* managed to obtain usable results for 3,995 girls in relation to breast development, 4,102 for pubic hair growth and 4,212 for menarche. Based on these numbers, Rubin *et al.* found that 12 per cent of girls reported having exceeded Tanner breast stage 1 (B1) by age 8. The median age of exceeding B1 was 10.14 years. By age 8, only 5 per cent of the sample had exceeded PH1, although the median age of this stage was 10.92. Rubin *et al.* (2009: 499) write: 'The median ages of breast development identified in our analysis (10.14 [for >BS1] and 11.61 [for >BS2]) were also slightly younger than those reported in studies from other European countries, where the age for transition into stage 2 ranged from 10.32 to 10.90 years and for stage 3 from 11.70 to 12.40 years.' Making comparisons to Marshall and Tanner's 1969 results, they cautiously suggest that these findings are not as notable as they might first appear:

> Our results suggest that girls in the ALSPAC cohort are maturing at younger ages than those in the few published studies that report progression through Tanner stages in British girls. However, more than 25 years have passed between the publication of those results and ours. The secular trends in pubertal development that have been reported elsewhere may, in part, explain our finding of younger ages at breast and pubic hair Tanner stages. (Rubin *et al.* 2009: 499)

The findings about age at menarche were similar to other UK and European studies (e.g. Whincup *et al.* 2001): only one girl (out of 2,953) had started menstruating by age 8, whilst 60 per cent had attained menarche by age 13. The median age of menarche, as stated above, was 12.93 years. Interestingly, Rubin *et al.* state that the strongest predictor of early menarche, above social class, body mass index (BMI) and mother's smoking habits when pregnant, was race (2009: 498). Children in their study were divided into 'non-white' and 'white' categories: only those with two white parents were included in the latter group. I will return to questions of racial and ethnic differences shortly.

In 2011, however, another large-scale British study (the Breakthrough Generations Study, a cohort study of breast cancer aetiology) reported different results on menstruation in 94,170 British women, finding that age of menarche had declined in cohorts born in the early 1990s compared to earlier ones (Morris *et al.* 2011a and 2011b). The mean age for menarche in the contemporary cohort was 12.3, with three girls menstruating before age 7. Unusually, as discussed below, this study focused on socio-economic status rather than race or ethnicity, finding that women from lower socio-economic groups were significantly (although only slightly) more likely to start menstruating earlier than those from higher socio-economic groups (mean age was 12.1 compared to 12.5) (see Figure 5).

Studies in China have also found a declining age of breast development and pubic hair growth and menarche. In a paper published in *Pediatrics* in 2009, Ma *et al.* report on a study of 20,654 healthy urban girls, finding that the median age for Tanner breast stage 2 (B2) was 9.20 years and for Tanner pubic hair stage 2 was 11.16 years. At age 8, 19.57 per cent of girls were at B2. By age 12, 40.14 per cent of the

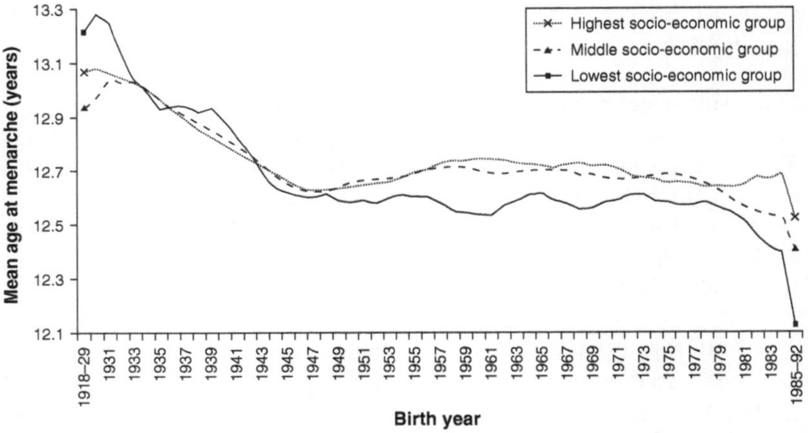

Figure 5 Social class and pubertal timing: Morris *et al.*'s (2001a) findings. Moving average of age at menarche across three socio-economic groups in 93,362 women born 1918–92 (without adjustment for known determinants of age at menarche). Lines represent 7-year weighted moving averages and points represent the mean of the average ages at menarche in each of the birth years 1918–29 and 1985–92. Women born 1908–17 or in 1993 were excluded because not all socio-economic groups included a participant with these birth years.

sample had started menstruating. The authors concluded that Chinese girls are experiencing breast development at ages younger than current norms and that they had one of the earliest onsets of breast development globally. Age of menarche had also decreased by 1.23 years since 1979. Although the time between Tanner B2 and menarche for Chinese girls, the authors report, are today longer than those of girls in most countries, excluding black American and Chilean girls, age of menarche is comparable to many other Asian cohorts (Ma *et al.* 2009: 273). The authors note the consequences of these findings for Chinese paediatrics:

It was noted that >10% of urban Chinese girls had stage 2 breast development before the age of 8 years (3rd and 10th percentile ages were 7.11 and 7.72 years, respectively). So the definition of precocious puberty adopted for white girls, that is, onset of puberty (breast stage 2) before the age of 8 years may lead to overestimation in 10% of urban Chinese girls. However, normal reference data from longitudinal data are necessary for the girls to evaluate whether the age limit of 8 years for defining female precocious puberty is relevant to girls in China. (2009: 273).

Scientists all over the world are currently studying national cohorts of girls to try to answer this question: are the standards developed from a mid twentieth-century population of children living in the English care system relevant for early twenty-first-century populations? That this question is being asked reflects much broader changes in the production and circulation of scientific knowledges globally and, as I argue below, a shift within biomedical research towards an emphasis on differences within and across populations (differences of age, race, ethnicity and nationality as well as historical or 'secular' differences). In the early twenty-first century it is no longer taken for granted that a small population of mostly white, underprivileged children can 'stand in for' children all over the world. Today, differences matter.

The tools and methods of measuring sexual development

One of the great difficulties in comparing international studies, as my story starts to show, is that measuring pubertal timing is not a straightforward task. Indeed, it is not clear what should be measured. As Tanner and Whitehouse's chronologically sequential photographs portray, puberty is a fluid process characterised by initially barely perceptible changes that gradually compound into significant physiological changes. Assessing pubertal stage either requires observing, touching, removing fluids from and describing bodies in flow and measuring them against arbitrary staging points, or using later recall. As described in Chapter 3, these encounters are affective engagements between at least two human actors and an array of machines and devices, involving intimate knowledges and disclosures: mothers describe their children's development at particular ages; boys mark pictures depicting testicles that match their own in size; girls permit physicians to touch their budding breasts. Findings, feelings and figurations entangle as these encounters enact bodies.

In their 2008 review of the field, Euling *et al.* describe the difficulty in comparing findings across studies of pubertal onset: 'Differences in methods to measure puberty markers can affect findings and, thus, comparability of findings between studies' (2008: 175). Different assessors are also likely to produce different results when studying breast development or pubic hair growth. Children's self-assessments (marking their own development stage compared to a drawing or photograph) have been shown to generate different results from those produced by a clinician. Young people tend to overestimate in the early stages and underestimate in the later stages compared to professionals' views (2008: 175). Age at menarche is usually measured by asking the girl or her parents if she has had her first period or asking when it happened. As Euling *et al.* argue (2008: 173), such approaches are not accurate and indeed become more inaccurate as greater time elapses between menarche and the posing of the question. In studies of boys, testicular volume is usually assessed using visual staging rather than palpation or ultrasound: other male pubertal events (voice breaking, first ejaculation, acne, underarm hair development) all occur later in puberty and are subject to greater individual variability.[8] Additionally, the relationship between all these events and the physiological processes constituting the onset of puberty are not well understood (2008: 173). The moment of onset of puberty, then, is difficult to define and challenging to measure.

More technical markers – e.g. measurements of hormones in the blood – are expensive and produce technical problems around 'detection limits and interindividual hormone level variability' (2008: 174). Hormone levels change over the course of hours and days and do not necessarily correlate directly with a particular stage of development. Euling *et al.* (2008: 188) explain: 'For example, in prepubertal boys and girls, gonadotropins in serum exhibit large diurnal [day/night] variations as a result of their pulsatile secretion; therefore any single measurement is unreliable.' Taking blood samples is also invasive and unpleasant for participants. Assessing bone age similarly requires invasive procedures (X-rays) that are, as described in Chapter 3, potentially harmful and sometimes unpleasant. Reading X-rays is not straightforward: as in other fields such as mammography, research groups debate whether computers could provide more accurate data than human technicians (Albanese, Hall and Stanhope 1995).

In their review, Euling *et al.* rather optimistically affirm the need for better measures: 'Puberty markers that are easier to measure, less invasive, less expensive, and more sensitive and reliable need to be explored, developed, and validated' (2008: 187). They recognise the potential stress to the participant in undergoing Tanner staging and

[8] As discussed in Chapter 1, particular cultural sensitivities and assumptions – that it is acceptable to touch girls' breasts but not boys' testicles, for example – are at play in methodological decisions.

suggest several alternative physical markers of puberty that could be developed and validated, including: behavioural markers; muscle mass increases in boys, spermache and voice break. They also suggest using infrared photographs for Tanner staging so children do not have to remove their clothes (2008: 188). Euling *et al.* make a stronger plea for better hormonal tests, stating that 'The development of reliable biochemical markers would represent a major step forward for puberty-timing studies in that biochemical changes may identify precursor events and provide validation of later phenotypic [bodily] puberty changes' (2008: 188). Improved reliability and reduced costs are needed, they argue, for saliva, urine and blood hormone level assays so that they can be used in large-scale studies. In future studies, they suggest, these physiologic markers (hormone and hormone receptor levels) should be measured alongside the traditional Tanner staging assessments so new data can always be compared to existing data.

In addition to these technical questions of the data retrieved from bodies, Euling *et al.* raise important concerns about how to measure 'age'. Like puberty, age is a fluid process. Citing children's ages in whole years can produce misleading results: a child who is 7 and 11 months will be described as '7' although chronologically she is almost 8. Relatedly, reporting the age of first observation of a stage tends to overestimate the age of attainment of that stage: the stage was actually reached at some point before the observation. Euling *et al.* suggest that:

> It is important to cope with these problems by applying statistical tools that account for the structure of the data ... Such tools are available ... and models that incorporate continuous traits that vary over time may be applied. Rather than simply estimating possibly biased observed mean ages, such analyses may provide age distributions and allow for estimation of median or quartiles of ages. (2008: 175)

Statistical techniques, in other words, can be used to guess the 'real' age of the child at the attainment of pubertal stages. These problems were also of great interest to Tanner: his collaborations with statisticians were intended to design solutions to them. Their continued relevance today, however, indicates the ongoing nature of definitional debates in this field.

Debates about how to define and measure puberty demonstrate the inseparability of apparatuses from scientific accounts of bodies or worlds. As discussed in Chapters 2 and 3, many science studies theorists argue that technical devices and practices are central elements of assemblages or networks that literally make or 'enact' (to use Mol's term) bodies and worlds. Even 'facts' as simple as age or physical growth come into existence in the material-semiotic encounters constituting research and clinical practices. As I will go on to demonstrate, particular articulations of 'race', social class and sex similarly animate scientific accounts of sexually developing bodies. Neither pre-existing facts nor only-social constructions, 'race', social class and sex emerge in research on early onset puberty in troubling – and yet contestable – configurations.

Measuring and materialising race

Race is immensely important to the prevalence studies of early onset puberty. Each of the studies cited above articulates racial and/or ethnic categories of research subjects. This is standard practice in contemporary medical research in the United States, which is, as sociologist Steven Epstein (2007) has shown, framed by what he calls the 'difference-inclusion paradigm'. In this policy and scientific paradigm, researchers are expected to pay attention to racial/ethnic differences, to recruit research participants from a range of groups and to report on findings along racial/ethnic lines.[9] Indeed, some journals refuse to publish work that does not 'spell out both gender and ethnic breakdowns and subgroup analysis findings' (Epstein 2007: 169).[10] Epstein argues that this paradigm is a response to critiques of earlier research protocols in which young white men (often college students) were assumed to represent or stand-in for all humans. Although outlining the limitations of such critiques (they usually overlook the fact that African-American and other ethnic minority groups have long been used as research subjects – both alive and dead – with any differences between them and white populations conveniently ignored), Epstein acknowledges the significance of the demand to be included in research. Some bodies are, it seems, more likely than others to be affected by various diseases and do react differently to some

[9] In the UK, researchers are not obliged to use these categories, but many do (Ellison *et al.* 2007).

[10] The website for *Pediatrics* does not contain any guidance on this issue.

medications. These issues notwithstanding, Epstein argues that the difference-inclusion paradigm tends to produce both racial/ethnic and sex/gender differences (and others, such as those relating to age and even sexual orientation) as inherently biological, that is, as stemming from genetic and related physiological differences rather than as differences that are a result of socially differentiated existence (Epstein 2007: 228–31). Quoting Braun (2002) he writes:

> Biologically reductionist explanations, as Lundy Braun has noted 'naturalize racial and ethnic difference and create a conceptual barrier to developing a research program that explores the complex ways in which social inequality and experiences of racial discrimination interact with human biology to influence patterns of disease'. (Epstein 2007: 230–1)

As described above, much research into early onset puberty makes strong claims for racial differences, arguing that African-American and/or black girls are more likely to mature earlier. In all of these studies race and/or ethnicity are treated as obvious or self-evident: authors rarely describe how classifications of individuals were made. Were participants asked to self-identify, were parents asked to categorise themselves and/or their children, or did clinicians make their own assessments (and if so, based on what)? Epstein retells a story reported in the *Washington Post* that highlights the difference such practices might make. The story concerns a woman, Elyse Frazier, who was invited to enrol in a clinical trial of the first drug ever approved only for use in black people, BiDil:

> When research coordinator Jackie Rayford asked her if she might be interested in the study for African Americans, she was puzzled. She considered herself black in matters of politics, but it was not a question she had ever been asked before in a health context. Frazier's mother is half black, half Cherokee Indian. Her father is half black, half Blackfoot Indian. To resolve the dilemma, Rayford asked Frazier: 'Do you consider yourself African American?' When she replied in the affirmative, Frazier was enrolled in the BiDil trial. Needless to say, the findings from the trial were not taken to represent the effects of the medication in people who might be a bit of this and a bit of that, still less in people who consider themselves black in matters of politics. (Epstein 2007: 228).

In Herman-Giddens' 1997 paper the process of ascertaining participants' race or ethnicity is not discussed beyond the statement that 'age, height, weight, race, ethnicity, payment status, reasons for visit, chronic illness and medication history, presence or absence of menses, and stages of development of breast, pubic hair and axillary [under-arm] hair' were all 'collected using a one-page, two-sided standardised form' (Herman-Giddens *et al.* 1997: 507). It is not clear what the difference between 'race' and 'ethnicity' might be; but both are figured as straightforwardly factual (like height and weight). This is in great contrast, it should be noted, to the final items on the list: the stages of breast development and public and axillary hair growth. For these, the authors detail a set of data collection practices in which clinicians were tested before they were allowed to participate in the study (clinicians had to gain an 87.5 per cent score or higher in this test of their ability to accurately rate Tanner stage development from photographs) (1997: 506). Describing breast and pubic hair growth, in other words, is acknowledged to be complex; articulating race or ethnicity is not.[11]

The terms used to describe racial categories in studies of puberty are various. In their 1997 paper, Herman-Giddens *et al.* divide girls into three categories: white, African-American and 'other' ('mixed race' girls and girls from other ethnic groups). Data pertaining to the third category were not analysed. In their 2004 paper, 'Navigating the Recent Articles on Girls' Puberty in *Pediatrics*: What Do We Know and Where Do We Go from Here?', Herman-Giddens, Kaplowitz and Wasserman write instead of 'black' girls in referring to the PROS study data. Similarly, in their re-analysis of the PROS data in 'Earlier Onset of Puberty in Girls: Relation to Increased Body Mass Index and Race' (2001) Kaplowitz and a related group of authors, including Herman-Giddens, write of 'white' and 'black' girls, arguing (as will be discussed in greater detail in Chapter 5) that something other than obesity is needed to explain the racial differences in timing of puberty (their initial assumption was that black girls go through puberty earlier because they are more likely to be obese) (2001: 351). Here 'black' and 'white' are racial groups that are meant to be self-evident: Kaplowitz *et al.* (2001: 350) name the statistical work of this paper 'race-specific analyses'. They describe their results in the following way: 'Although obesity may contribute to the earlier onset of puberty in black girls, genetic and/or environmental factors specific to the black

[11] See Braun *et al.* (2007) for a critical analysis of the role of the 'rapid racial assessment' in everyday clinical encounter: guessing a person's race based on appearance, they argue, is not a good shortcut in medical consultations; for an alternative approach, see Montoya (2007).

population seem to be important in determining how early puberty starts' (2001: 351). Noting other research that comes to a similar conclusion, they add 'Thus, genetic factors within the black population may account for their higher leptin levels for a given level of fatness, which could contribute to their observed earlier onset of puberty' (2001: 351). In both cases, they refer to 'the black population' as a group of people broader than the sample so named in the study. In their conclusion, they write: 'It may be speculated that genetic factors and/or environmental factors specific to this ethnic group also may help to account for the earlier maturation of black girls' (2001: 352). Here population differences can be either genetic or environmental.

Apart from the difficulties of ascertaining race (who decides which race an individual belongs to, and on what basis) and choosing which words to use to describe these classifications, there are also complex problems relating to so-called 'mixed' heritage (see Braun *et al.* 2007). Working in diverse national contexts, researchers approach this question in different ways. In the PROS study, for example, to be 'black', a girl had to have two African-American parents. In Rubin *et al.*'s UK study by contrast, girls only required one non-white parent to be classified as 'non-white'. In Denmark, only 'European' girls were included in the study; those from other backgrounds were excluded (Aksglaede *et al.* 2009). In the 2010 BCERC study, parents were asked to identify the race and/or ethnicity of the child: girls were then 'assigned race/ethnicity by using the criteria that black race superseded other race/ethnicity designations and Hispanic superseded all others' (Biro *et al.* 2010: 584). In comparing their findings to the PROS study (which is one of its main purposes), Biro *et al.* do not comment on the differences in classification of black participants: in PROS a girl needed two African-American parents; in the BCERC study only to be identified as black by a parent.

In their critical examination of the data from 1940 to 1994, Euling *et al.* also refer to problems around classifying the 'racial/ethnic' identity of the participants: 'Racial/ethnic distinctions may reflect genetic or environmental factors or a combination of both. For example, an individual identified as "non-Hispanic black" in NHANES III might have more in common, genetically and environmentally, with others identified differently' (Euling *et al.* 2008: 183). Despite this 'fact', all the panel members 'preferred and recommended that studies present results by race/ethnic group' (2008: 183). Later in the paper, when making recommendations about the physical measurements taken, Euling *et al.* return to this issue, advising the development of 'race/ethnic-specific Tanner staging'. They explain this in brackets: '(e.g. pubic hair staging in Peruvian Indians is not accurate for estimating sexual maturation; it was noted that PH4 for Asians is typically the last, adult-type stage' (2008: 188). The reference to Peruvian Indians is a citation of a paper on ethnic differences and Tanner's pubic hair staging published in the *Journal of Adolescent Health* (Freyre *et al.* 2002). The mention of this rather small and relatively specific group 'Peruvian Indians' in this sentence rather undermines the more complex point Euling *et al.* make earlier, that most American studies (in contrast to Tanner's original English study and, more recently, the Danish study described above, both of which try to minimise racial diversity in their samples) place strong emphasis on what they alternately call racial or ethnic differences in their samples. As noted above, findings of the two key American studies centre around the different experiences of white, African-American and, additionally in the NHANES III case, Hispanic girls. The BCERC study (Biro *et al.* 2010) also analyses differences between 'black' and 'white' girls.

Despite all these difficulties, race is repeatedly identified as significant in pubertal timing. As mentioned above, in their landmark study of early sexual development in the USA, Herman-Giddens *et al.* focused only on children who were 'white' or 'African-American'. Analysing their findings, the authors make a strong claim about 'racial differences' but, importantly, decline to provide an explanation of them:

> Our study found African-American girls entering puberty approximately 1 to 1.5 years earlier than white girls and beginning menses approximately 8.5 months earlier. *We have no explanation* for the discrepancy in timing sequence between the African-American and white girls for either the onset of puberty and subsequent menses of appearance and spacing of the secondary sexual characteristics. Neither can we explain the earlier development in African-American girls in general. (Herman-Giddens *et al.* 1997: 510, emphasis added)

Similarly, although Rubin *et al.* in their UK study describe 'non-white race' as the strongest predictor of early onset puberty, no explanation of this is provided.

Race, then, in scientific studies of puberty is both taken for granted (as something that can and should be studied) and a source of great uncertainty. What is missing in scientific attempts to address this paradox by producing more and more data on differences is an understanding of the ways in which scientific work on children's development in part enacts the categories it claims to find 'in the world'. Attempting to measure racial differences always produces such differences: children become 'black', 'white' or 'non-white', some even 'Peruvian Indian'; those who do not fit clear categories are excluded in order not to produce 'confound'. Thus scientists end up measuring something partially of their own devising; a phenomenon that of course relates, as Epstein shows, to cultural and political categories (such relation is in part dependent on who gets to make the choices about how to describe a particular individual) but which nonetheless is a more or less useful scientific tool. As much research in science studies demonstrates,[12] after having developed classificatory categories, scientists often then make claims as if these relate to a previously existing world: finding, in this case, that black girls are more likely to have early onset puberty. But if many children whose parents might describe them as black have been excluded, what might this result mean?

In thinking critically about pubertal science, it seems essential to open up questions about the psycho-social lived experience of race and racialisation and to refuse to accept scientific racial categories as in any way straightforwardly biological. I will return to these questions in Chapter 5, when analysing claims about the causes of early onset puberty. At this point, however, I want to agree with science studies theorist Amade M'charek (2010: 318) who writes that 'differences, such as race, sex or sexual differences, are neither stable nor given. Rather, they are enacted in specific practices as effects of interferences. Differences materialize in the form of relations between various interfering entities.' The significance differences in pubertal development are material and enacted: they need to be taken seriously but also troubled (Butler 1990).

Enacting social class

Research into early onset puberty is rather less directly structured through enactments of social class differences. Although, as discussed

[12] See for example, Bruno Latour's (1988) classic account of microbial science.

in Chapter 3, most of the children in the Harpenden Study were from lower socio-economic backgrounds, class plays no role in Tanner and Whitehouse's analysis; indeed, these differences are actively denied, as argued earlier. In the contemporary studies described above, social class again is usually absent: the studies either aim for homogenous samples (as in Aksglaede *et al.*'s Danish study) or varied ones (as in Rubin *et al.*'s UK study) but do not generally make hypotheses or produce findings about class differences. Given the emphasis placed on the role of obesity in early puberty, this is surprising: many studies of childhood obesity argue that overweight is linked to socio-economic deprivation (materialised through poor diet, lack of exercise opportunities and/or low parental educational levels) (see, for example, Butland et al. 2007; Health Survey for England 2012).[13]

Morris *et al.*'s cohort study of breast cancer aetiology is one exception here. As described above, their 2011 paper reports that girls from lower socio-economic backgrounds are more likely to begin menstruating earlier than their wealthier peers. In their discussion, Morris *et al.* link this finding to increased risks of obesity in poorer children (2011b: 399). Notably, they describe the limitations in their ascription of socio-economic status, pointing out that their methods assume a correlation between current and childhood status:

> Socio-economic status was based on the participant's current postcode as a proxy for childhood socio-economic status, which might have reduced any true association between age at menarche and childhood socio-economic status if current and childhood socio-economic status differed. The assumption that childhood and adult socio-economic status were similar is, however, plausible because social mobility is low in the UK. (2011b: 399)

This question of variation over time has great significance for the collection of data on social class. Unlike racial differences, economic disparities (and the classed distinctions closely intertwined with these) are widely understood to be socially produced and as such potentially non-permanent factors in an individual's life (see also Krieger and Fee 1994). Although classed experiences may have persistent biological effects – the work of Hilary Graham (2009) and many others on health inequalities in the UK shows that an individual's class has an enormous impact on their health across the life course – these are not biologically

[13] For a critical analysis of these claims, see Herndon (2005).

derived and seem to lie outside the purview of the scientific and biomedical literature on the physiological causes of early development described above. But this does not explain why social class is not well studied in the epidemiological literature on secular trends in puberty. As will be discussed in detail in Chapter 5, some psychologists argue for a 'social stress' theory of early onset puberty, claiming that stressful early childhood experiences are linked to early sexual development (see, for example, Belsky, Steinberg and Draper 1991). Here again, social class could be seen to play an obvious role – poverty and associated social discrimination are highly stressful experiences – but these differences are not addressed in the large incidence studies.[14]

Social class does play a more prominent role in literatures comparing puberty across countries. In these, as described above, attempts are made to compare sexual development timing across wealthy and developing countries, with a historically robust finding emerging that girls in wealthy countries are more likely to develop earlier than their more deprived counterparts. Such comparisons build on early auxological work comparing 'peasants' and wealthy children and are shot through with figurations of ethnicity and race. In these large inter-country comparisons, intra-country socio-economic differences can fade from view: 'China', for example, becomes homogenised (see, for example, the comparative bar graph in Parent *et al.* 2003: 671). In their review Parent *et al.* (2003) try to address this issue by distinguishing national studies of children living in 'well-off' and 'underprivileged' conditions, arguing that 'taken together, these data highlight the crucial role of socioeconomic and nutritional conditions in the timing of puberty' (2003: 673). It is very difficult to ascertain much about social class from these inter-country comparisons, however. Much more fine-grained elaboration of categories and careful selection of subjects to represent these would need to be undertaken. There is apparently little appetite for such work in the puberty field.

Why is race so much more important than class in the epidemiological literature on early onset puberty? Is this in part an artefact of Tanner's refusal to note the significance of social class, or of the

[14] One questionnaire-based British study of the effect of pubertal timing on risk-taking behaviour, discussed in more detail in Chapter 5, found that both boys and girls from poorer socio-economic groups were more likely to experience puberty earlier (Downing and Bellis 2009). The authors argue that connections between poverty, obesity and sexual development require further research.

longstanding interest amongst US scientists in questions of race and fascination with the sexuality of black girls and women (Harding 1993; 2006; Braun *et al.* 2007)? Discussion of race and class in the social science literature on the 'sexualisation' of girls may be instructive here. American sociologist Danielle Egan argues that both public and feminist academic debates around sexualisation focus on white girls, paying only scanty attention to African-American girls and ignoring Latina, Asian, South Asian and Indigenous girls. Sexualisation, in her analysis is 'a racially specific threat to white, middle-class heterosexual girls' (Egan 2013: 68). As I also discussed in Chapter 2, cultural notions of childhood innocence are entwined with whiteness and particular forms of economic and social privilege: 'proper' children, as Erica Burman (1994) notes, do not work, for example. Egan (2013: 74) claims that this historical connection underpins horrified responses to claims about sexualisation. Australian feminist Anita Harris makes a similar point. Citing critical psychologist Valerie Walkerdine (1988) in a discussion of public concerns about the sexualisation of pre-teens or 'tweenies', she writes,

> [T]he tweenie phenomenon may be an extension of the sexualisation of working-class girls – itself a project with a long history – to all preteens. In other words, the positioning of young girls as sexual, as consumers of popular culture and as knowledgeable actors in an adult world of sex and money has perhaps only become problematic now because it has reached out in a process of upscaling to the white and middle class. (Harris 2004: 215)

The concern with race in the epidemiological literature, then, might indicate a worry about early development in white middle-class girls specifically; a desire to 'document' (that is, to articulate) differences as a kind of defensive strategy. Such articulations figure 'black girls' as much more likely to become sexually mature at an early age but also enact concerns about white girls following along this path, a trajectory similar to Harris' 'upscaling' of sexualisation.

In the sexualisation discourses discussed by Walkerdine and Harris, sex, class, race and sexual orientation are inextricably mixed. Egan similarly suggests that 'the endangered girl in the discourse on sexualisation is a white, middle-class, female, and heterosexual subject, whose subjectivity and behaviour are defined through and against the sexualized' (Egan 2013: 102). Public discourses around sexualisation, she shows, replay 'historically trenchant fears of class contagion'

(2013: 83). Observing girls' investments in adult sexuality, popular writers such as Tanith Carey (2011) and Jean Kilbourne and Diane Levin (2008), Egan claims, worry about 'the erosion of middle-class respectability and the transformation of good middle-class girls into their working-class counterparts' (2013: 83). Again citing Walkerdine, Egan argues that the childhood innocence requiring protection from adult sexuality is a specifically middle-class one. The desire to protect this version of childhood may reflect broader anxieties about the fragility of the middle class as a socio-economic possibility (2013: 103; see also Tyler 2013). Here, the sexualised child becomes the object of displaced fears, a useful object for her middle-class parents, teachers, writers and bureaucrats worried about their own potential loss of status and security to try to control.

Social class plays an important role in the academic literature and public debate on sexualisation (see also Renold and Ringrose 2013). In contrast, it is surprisingly absent in the epidemiological literature on early sexual development. This disparity highlights the significant differences between the debates on 'sexualisation' and early onset puberty. Whilst I argue in this book that the two areas need to be brought into dialogue, they are not the same (see also Roberts 2013). The early puberty debate has its roots in technical scientific and biomedical domains, whilst the sexualisation debates are largely cultural and political in orientation. The lack of attention to social class in the early puberty literature highlights the biological orientation of epidemiological articulations of early sexual development: unlike obesity or diabetes, for example, early puberty for most scientists and clinicians is understood as a biological problem concerning genes, hormones, weight (and sometimes individualised experiences of stress in less mainstream arguments) rather than as a materialisation of socio-economic status. As I discuss in Chapter 6, however, concerns about the negative effects of early development are strongly classed, reflecting more directly the worries described in the feminist literature on sexualisation. It is in this part of the puberty debates, then, that class is articulated in more detail.

Making sex and sexed bodies

Studies of early onset puberty are all about sex: puberty is said to be the attainment of the 'secondary sexual characteristics' that in part constitute adult maleness or femaleness. As in the literature on 'normal' sexual development, early puberty research routinely classifies boys and girls into two groups: there is no discussion of children who go through this process in atypical ways or who have atypically sexed bodies (either from birth or at puberty). Although given the relative rarity of atypical sexual development, this might be expected, in other ways it is surprising. Pubertal processes are of great significance to debates around intersexuality or disorders of sexual development: puberty is figured as a period in which sexed identity can radically change and in which surgery and hormonal treatments are frequently used to configure bodily characteristics that 'match' the person's psycho-social sex (Spurgas 2009). In both scientific publications and feminist debates around biology and the body, atypically sexed children are used to articulate the nature of sexual development and gender attainment.[15]

One of the most important population case studies in sex endocrinology, for example, describes a group of children living in three villages in the Dominican Republic who, although raised as girls from birth, became young men at puberty when they grew penises (Imperato-McGinley *et al.* 1979). In sex endocrinology, this story underpins claims about the power of biology to determine sex and (consequently) gender: the children, we learn, shared a genetic difference that suppressed the hormonally stimulated growth of 'normal' masculine genitalia in utero, a development that nonetheless occurred at puberty. According to Julianne Imperato-McGinley and colleagues, 'These subjects demonstrate that in the absence of sociocultural factors that could interrupt the natural sequence of events, the effect of testosterone predominates, over-riding the effect of rearing as girls' (1979: 1233).

Viewed differently, as feminist biologist Anne Fausto-Sterling points out, this case study indicates the complexity of socialisation in the production of sexed embodiments. In her critical engagement with Imperato-McGinley's work, Fausto-Sterling stresses the fact that these children were not raised as girls but were nominated as an unusual group, described as *guevedoche*, *guevote* or 'penis-at-twelve' (Imperato-McGinley *et al.* 1979: 1235). They were very unlikely, she

[15] For an excellent set of articles on this, including debate on terminology, see Holmes (2009). For a detailed ethnographic analysis of the medicalisation of intersexuality, see Karkazis (2008).

argues, to have been raised in the same way as 'genitally normal girls': the decision to become boys at puberty also seems to her to be a reasonable one, as the life of teenage boys was freer than those of girls in that society (Fausto-Sterling 1992: 86–7). Feminist theorist Lena Eckert argues that this categorisation arose from the villagers' encounter with Imperato-McGinley and her team: 'There is no indication', she writes, 'that people were in earlier times distressed by "the phenomenon" or even aware of it ... Through their investigations, Western researchers created a social category of "sexual deviation" that had not previously existed in the community. Local understandings of materiality were overwritten and extinguished' (Eckert 2009: 65). Again, this argument highlights the material-semiotic significance of scientific framings of differences in practice. The entanglements of the Dominican Republic villagers, the scientists, their tools and discourses, and the children's bodies enacted puberty and sexual difference in particular, powerful ways. Although intending, in the face of strong arguments about the social nature of gender, to demonstrate the importance of hormones to sexual development, Imperato-McGinley *et al.*'s research ultimately articulates the material-semiotic nature of embodied sex.

Epidemiological and clinical research on early puberty from Tanner until the present assumes normative sex: puberty is figured as a complex physiological process by which young female bodies develop into adult women and young males become men. In narratives about atypical children, like those in the Imperato-McGinley study, lies a counter-narrative about the entanglements of social, psychological and biological forces in producing sexed bodies at puberty. The 'penis-at-twelve' children's development demonstrates that the attainment of secondary sexual characteristics is not a natural unfolding of a biological truth but a complex bio-psycho-social encounter between bodies, genes, hormones, language, naming and social life (including scientific practices); that is, an entanglement of findings, feelings and figurations. The extensive body of critical literature on atypical sexual development, I suggest, has much to offer analyses of puberty through its highlighting of the implosion of biological, scientific, psychological, social, political and other actors in producing sexed bodies. I return to this literature and particularly to Fausto-Sterling's arguments in more detail in later chapters.

Feminism and science: experimental engagements

The literatures on rising incidence of early onset puberty are complex, contentious and contested. They provide substantial data based on technically highly elaborated and well-debated research but also make claims about processes that are hard to define and challenging to measure. I have argued that they rely on uncritical assumptions about important analytic categories (race, ethnicity and sex) and often fail to take into account the differentiating effects of social class. When these differences are attended to, they are figured as pre-existing; the ways in which scientific work enacts them as categories is ignored. Despite this, the epidemiological research on pubertal timing articulates a problem that is compelling and that resonates with a broader set of social observations and concerns about serious changes to contemporary childhood. How then might we make sense of this literature? How might feminists engage with and learn from these scientific debates?

In Chapter 2 I introduced several arguments from feminist science studies about the ways in which science and medicine perform or enact bodies. In these arguments, the practices and discourses constituting science and medicine are strands in a tangled ball or complex web of forces through which and in which bodies come, temporarily but sometimes solidly, to be a certain way. Haraway uses the term 'congeal' to describe these processes of 'corporealization', emphasising the complex material-semiotic networks that come together as bodies are made. In the quote below she uses the term 'interaction' rather than Barad's later 'intra-action'. This difference is not philosophically significant here: writing of bodies and indeed the world 'taking shape' through contingent activity, Haraway, like Barad, articulates an active, relational ontology:

> Technoscientific bodies, such as the biomedical organism, are the nodes that congeal from interactions where all the actors are not human, not self-identical, not 'us'. The world takes shape in specific ways and cannot take shape just any way; corporealization is deeply contingent, physical, semiotic, tropic, historical, international. Corporealization involves institutions, narratives, legal structures, power-differentiated human labor, technical practice, analytic apparatus, and much more. (Haraway 1997: 142)

Importantly for this book and particularly for my argument as it continues in the next chapter, Haraway includes the biological processes of bodies as active in corporealisations: 'The processes "inside" bodies – such as the cascades of action that constitute an organism or that constitute the play of genes and other entities that go to make up a cell – are interactions, not frozen things' (Haraway 1997: 142). Agreeing with Haraway about the significance of these interactions, I argue that it is important to learn about the 'cascades of actions' within cells and bodies – in the case of sexual development, those pertaining to hormones in particular – in trying to understand puberty. Scientific and biomedical research articulates these cascades but cannot be understood as providing merely factual accounts. Throughout this book, I use the word 'findings' rather than 'facts' or 'data' to highlight the ongoing and contested nature of technical discourses and arguments. Scientific and medical findings are articulated with particular networks of expertise and interests: viewed as a group, they are frequently contradictory, revealing complex patterns of relation amongst diverse actors.

As is evident in this chapter's discussion of the epidemiology of early onset puberty, medicine and science are rarely, if ever, coherent in their enacting of bodies; and they can never be totalising. Carrying personal and social histories, bodies are lived; they are not blank slates awaiting medical or scientific 'inscription' or ghostly forms shaped by social construction (see also Grosz 1994). Bodies and bodily entities (hormones, genes, cells, organs) (intra-)act: the processes of puberty involve material forces of cellular movements and change, hormonal messaging and neuroendocrine events. Scientific and medical discourses and practices describe and analyse these materialities in ways that also carry and articulate material-semiotic histories: scientists and clinicians are embodied actors working in complex and situated fields of social practice.

Feminists and others interested in bodies, then, should not *uncritically* turn to science or medicine to learn about bodies. Science and medicine cannot provide data or facts for the social sciences or humanities in a straightforward way; instead they provide findings. Our engagements with these findings are themselves located practices of body-making and world-making. Engaging with scientific and medical ways of enacting puberty for me involves respecting other intellectual traditions but also insisting that my own (inter)disciplines (namely feminist theory and science studies) have much to offer in theorising bodies.

As mentioned in the two previous chapters, taking this approach means distancing myself from some contemporary feminist theorists who argue for a non-critical approach to science and scientific data. Following Haraway, I think it is important to engage with technoscience and biomedicine as forms of practice entangled with many other economic, political and cultural practices, networks, actors and entities. Neither data nor bodies are extricable from such entanglements. As a feminist theorist, then, I engage with scientific findings as a form of experimentation and learning. I want to listen carefully to what scientists and clinicians have to say about early sexual development but also to bring my own expertise in reading and critical thought to bear on what I hear. In so doing I want to facilitate new articulations of early puberty: articulations that open space for children and young people to live in more diverse, less restrictive ways.

This chapter focused on epidemiological papers and their numerical and graphical findings: percentages of populations; average ages when particular events occur; and numerical comparisons across place and time. Such findings are always-already social: they are produced through practices of collecting, organising, analysing and presenting that are discursive and historically specific. In intra-action with particular feelings and figurations, these findings enact bodies and biological processes (the budding of breasts, the growth of pubic hair) and articulate categories of difference (early/late; normal/abnormal; black/Hispanic/white/European; girls/boys). Biological entities are implicated actors here, not passive recipients of social inscription. Of course I cannot know their actions in any direct way: scientists articulate their activities through practices of touching, visualising, measuring, writing and calculating and I engage with their reports of these activities.

Outlining the research on global change in incidence of early onset puberty, I attempted to grasp and articulate the scale of the purported 'crisis'. Following Kelty and Landecker, I have used 'The Literature' as an informant, reading for practice and plot and attending to problematisation. Although not highly technical (I have not analysed the mathematical processes used, for example), my engagements have cast a critical gaze over the formation of categories used in the statistical work undertaken in these papers. I have traced 'plots' of race/ethnicity, class and sexuality, finding that taken as a group these papers articulate mixed, even confused, understanding of important social differences. Articulating a more complex social scientific version of these differences, I suggest, produces a valuable shift in the making of pubertal bodies, allowing us better to understand where and what the contemporary changes in sexual development might be. My approach also opens up problematisation. If early development is not occurring for all girls, then it becomes a different kind of problem; possibly not even a crisis. Articulating social scientific expertise with epidemiological knowledge, then, remakes the problem of early development, challenging existing notions of 'what should be done'.

Epidemiological literatures on early onset puberty articulate global changes of potentially profound proportions. These claims need both to be taken seriously and to be carefully worked through. It is important to think critically about the enactments of difference that are involved in such claim-making: differences of sex/gender, 'race'/ethnicity and social class amongst others. I have shown here that these literatures articulate particular groups of girls as developing 'out of time' with worrying and as yet inexplicable frequency. These figurations, articulated as findings, underpin contemporary accounts of a crisis in girls' sexual development that resonates with wider concerns about 'sexualisation' and facilitates social, political and medical interventions. Engaging with the literature in an ethnographic mode renders the epidemiological science of early onset puberty as an event open to collaborative, iterative sense-making rather than a set of statements of fact. In the chapters that follow, I move into other scientific and medical debates around sexual development, exploring the explanations given for the rise in rates of early onset puberty described here, the debates around the effects of early sexual development on young people and the clinical discourses that attempt to manage these.

5 *Causes and explanations: genes, fat, toxins and families*

It is useless to proceed by trying to separate nature from nurture and looking at how they interact. The causal effects of nature and nurture on development are simply not separable.

(Keller 2010: 81)

Scientists and clinicians across the world claim that more and more girls are entering into puberty early. Although epidemiological evidence remains contested, there is general agreement that these are notable secular trends. But what is causing these changes?

In her 2000 *New York Times* article, 'The Making of an Eight-Year-Old Woman'. journalist Lisa Belkin reminds us of the social embedding of research questions, noting how cultural concerns shape scientific enquiry. In the quote below, Belkin reports an encounter in which scientist Marcia Herman-Giddens, lead author of the Pediatric Research in Office Settings (PROS) study described in Chapter 3, talks her through a set of powerpoint slides about early onset puberty:

> [W]hat we know is limited by what we think to ask. Scientific hypotheses necessarily reflect a moment in time. The parade of possible triggers that Herman-Giddens clicks onto her wall is also a list of society's front-and-center concerns. Obesity. Pollution. Food additives. Divorce. Soft porn. If we weren't worried about these things, we wouldn't think to investigate them. Puberty research, like so much scientific research, is a mirror onto our fears. (Belkin 2000)

Acknowledging and exploring these fears, this chapter analyses an astonishingly diverse range of explanations of contemporary changes in sexual development: from theories that emphasise the role of genes and obesity to arguments focusing on environmental toxins and familial and psychological patterns of relating. In this, I continue to theorise pubescent bodies as bio-psycho-social; as enacted through a plethora of experiences and discourses that emphasise 'micro' and 'macro' processes and relations at different times and in different places. Early developing pubertal bodies, I argue, demonstrate the intra-actions of biological actors such as hormones, genes, hair or fat with psychosocial encounters and discursive formulations and practices in the naming and living of any particular body in space and time. Pubertal bodies are responsive, changing and stubborn: both flexible and resistant, they speak and refuse to converse. Might feminist science studies help us to listen more carefully to them?

Initially engaging with the physically smallest and most technically elaborated actors implicated in early puberty, the chapter then moves into wider and less scientifically manageable contexts and situations. Starting with genes and hormonal pathways, I discuss obesity and metabolic processes and then engage with debates around the impact of toxic chemicals on growth. The final section deals with psychosocial accounts of early onset puberty, focusing on stress, early attachment patterns and parenting, and describing the effects of contemporary mediatised cultures on sexual development.

The chapter explores claims from a broad range of scientific disciplines and approaches. It tells stories about multiple enactments of early developing bodies, exploring findings, feelings and figurations to highlight the rich and fractured nature of contemporary attempts to understand what is going on in girls' sexual development. Feminist theory and social science more broadly, I suggest, have much to learn from engaging with the range of explanations enacting bodies in this area. Encountered as a diverse collection, these explanations move us away from viewing scientific and biomedical explanations as monolithic or biologically/genetically determinist, demonstrating the multiple and contested ways in which science and medicine 'do' or enact bodies (Mol 2002).

Exploring the diverse explanations of the 'causes' of early puberty enacts scientific and biomedical discourses as something to engage in rather than reject. In my view, feminist theory and politics would do well to be experimental in its approach to science and medicine – we need to listen and come to know, and learn to speak across discursive 'divides' (Roberts and Mackenzie 2006). Importantly, this also means insisting on the value of other knowledge histories and practices, from the social sciences and humanities for example. One of my aims here is to explore how this open-yet-critical engagement might be done, moving across a range of disciplines involved in making claims around early puberty.

From a science studies perspective that might advocate a more situated, ethnographic approach (studying a particular group of scientists in one laboratory for example), the range of sciences I engage with here might seem unwise. I certainly sacrifice depth for breadth. Rather than providing an in-depth account of the workings of any particular scientific or medical tradition, my goal is to map out and explore the diversity of fields enacting early onset puberty. Claiming an ethnographic approach to texts, then, I align myself with contemporary multi-sited ethnography (Marcus 1995) rather than with traditional anthropology.

Direct physical causes of precocious puberty

It is important to note at the outset that some forms of early onset puberty have clear physical causes. Sometimes tumours in the brain near the pituitary or the hypothalamus interfere with the neural pathways that regulate hormonally stimulating messages to the ovaries or testes. Whilst accounting for only a small number of cases, such serious pathologies require urgent medical attention involving surgery and/or chemotherapy or radiation. More commonly, some children have a non-tumoral brain defect known as a haratoma near the pituitary that can press on normal brain tissue and cause early sexual development (Kaplowitz 2004: 37–8). Other children with early onset puberty suffer from pathologies of the ovaries or testes: tumours or large cysts affecting normal function. Some rare genetic conditions, including congenital adrenal hyperplasia and McCune-Albright Syndrome, are also associated with early sexual development. Although these cases are unrelated to the general population trends described in this book they do, as noted in Chapter 4, play a significant role in the politics of classification of early onset puberty. Some clinicians fear that reducing the age for 'normal' puberty onset increases the risk of children with tumours being classified as developing normally (if early) and the tumour being missed (see, for example, Rosenfield *et al.* 2000; Midyett *et al.* 2003). The remainder of this chapter, however, focuses on early onset puberty that has no obvious physical cause.

Biological actors: calculating genetic influence

Understanding the action of genes and DNA in the production of bodily differences has been of immense interest to science and biomedicine since the 1970s. Adele Clarke and colleagues (2003; 2009; 2010) argue that after 1985 this interest was part of a broader shift towards 'biomedicalisation' in which technoscience and biomedicine made significant new inroads into explaining and managing biological processes. Processes of biomedicalisation, they argue, focus not just on cure, but on optimisation and enhancement. Building on elaborations of Foucault's (1978 [1990]) ground-breaking argument in *The History of Sexuality* Volume 1 by Paul Rabinow and Nikolas Rose and others, they suggest that contemporary bodies have become projects for both professional and lay actors (Novas and Rose 2000; Rabinow and Rose 2006; Rose 2007a, 2007b). Bodies today form the basis for subjective identifications – we classify ourselves in terms of kinds of bodies – but these are neither stabile nor fixed. Bodies are figured in terms of risks rather than absolutes – one may have a propensity towards a certain medical condition – but action can be taken to ameliorate such risk. Indeed, as many scholars have argued, biomedicalisation also produces new responsibilities for body-related activity, responsibilities that are notably gendered, racialised and classed (Shim 2000; Roberts 2006; Clarke *et al.* 2010; Raman and Tutton 2010). The genomic sciences have played a significant role in these changes, providing new articulations of the 'interior' processes of bodies, their development from conception, and processes of cell regeneration and death. Although, as I argue below in the case of early onset puberty, genomics has provided little useful knowledge in terms of treatment, it has reshaped what contemporary bodies are and, in some cases, provided new avenues for action (the possibility of using preimplantation genetic diagnosis and IVF to avoid having a child with a serious genetic disease, for example) (Franklin and Roberts 2006).

Attempts to map the complex processes involved in cancer aetiology in order better to predict, diagnose and treat cancers form a central core of contemporary genomic science, providing rich resources to study the contribution of DNA or genes to physiological development more generally. The Breakthrough Generations Study of Breast Cancer Aetiology, for example, has traced the pubertal histories of over 90,000 British women volunteers in order to study links between age of sexual development and later breast cancer. Such work attempts to quantify the contribution of genetic factors to physiological events. In one paper from this study, Danielle H. Morris *et al.* (2011b) analyse the age of menarche of 25,970 women, finding that 57 per cent of the variation in age of first menstruation is 'genetically affected'. Members of families were more likely to go through puberty (measured by menarche) at a similar time. The other half of the variation, Morris *et al.* argue, was due to 'non-shared' environmental factors. This is quite a high figure: other studies allot a much greater proportion of effect to genetic factors. Using the growth spurt as an indicator of puberty (as opposed to menarche or breast development) and studying a cohort of 922 Finnish twin pairs, Wehkalampi *et al.* (2008) for example concluded that 86 per cent of variance in female puberty timing was explained by genetic factors.

The Breakthough Generation study makes no attempt to determine the genes involved in pubertal timing. Indeed, as I will explain shortly, it is important to note that the question of genetic cause ('Do genes cause X condition?' or 'Which genes cause X'?) is not the same as that of genetic contribution to difference ('How much of Y difference is determined by genetic differences?') (Keller 2010). Citing key studies attempting to 'find the genes for pubertal development', Morris *et al.* state that the genetic loci remain undetermined: those currently identified account for less than 2 per cent of variation in age of menarche:

> In recent years, several loci that are associated with age at menarche have been identified, but these explain at most ~2% of the variation in menarcheal age (assuming they act additively). This means that the vast majority of the heritability of age at menarche is not because of the identified loci. Previous genome-wide association studies have included tens of thousands of women and so it seems likely that the remaining loci are either rare or explain a very small amount of variation. (Morris *et al.* 2011b: 310)

According to Morris *et al.*, then, genes account for half the variation in age of pubertal onset but cannot necessarily be located or offered as causes of development. In a recent meta-analysis genome-wide study of data on 87,000 women, described in a paper with 174 authors, the international Reprogen Consortium found thirty new genetic loci related to menarcheal age (Elks *et al.*, 2010). Some of these were related to genes involved in energy homeostasis, thus articulating links between puberty and (over)weight. Despite the wealth of new loci presented here, however, the authors write that 'these together explained between 3.6%–6.1% of the variance in age at menarche, equivalent to 7.2%–12.2% of its heritability' (2010: 1082). This research is also limited by its inability to ascribe cause:

> Although our pathway analyses strongly identified potential new biological pathways involved in pubertal timing, we acknowledge that the ability to assign putative functions to these menarche loci is substantially limited by the lack of identification of the causal variant at each locus. (2010: 1081)

Despite this lack of clarity, the study received significant media attention in the UK, with headlines claiming in *BBC News Online* that 'Genes give clue to early puberty' (Anon. 2010) and in *The Telegraph* that 'Early puberty and obesity are linked in young girls, genetic research finds' (Smith 2010). Alongside the long list of funders of the consortium and the lengthy author list, this attention gives some indication of the scientific value attributed to such research, despite its relatively useless outputs. Such high-cost, low-yield technoscientific investment is typical of the genomics field and speaks to a complex social-technical formation of hope that has been widely analysed in social science (Franklin and Lock 2003; Reardon 2004; Rajan 2006; Helmreich 2008).

Historian of science Evelyn Fox Keller (2010: 5) is deeply critical of such studies, arguing that they posit impossible questions: 'The casting of the debate as an effort to determine "how much of our behaviour is driven by our genes versus the environments in which we grow up and live" poses a question that is not only unanswerable but . . . is actually meaningless.' This kind of research, she argues, produces genes as actors that can cause outcomes, when it is commonly understood in the relevant fields of science that in fact genes (or pieces of DNA) can do nothing of the sort:

> DNA doesn't *do* anything. It does not *make* a trait; it does not even encode a program for development. Rather, it is more accurate to think of DNA as a standing resource on which a cell can draw for survival and reproduction, a resource it can deploy in many different ways, a resource so rich as to enable the cell to respond to its changing environment with immense subtlety and variety. As a resource, DNA is indispensable; it can even be said to be a primary resource. (Keller 2010: 51, emphasis in original)

As a resource, Keller argues, DNA should always be understood as part of a complex network of interacting resources. The language Keller uses – 'entangled', 'interacting', 'unfolds' – resonates with both Haraway's and

Barad's writings. Like Haraway (2003: 9), Keller describes actors and forces relating in all manner of directions to 'give rise to' bodies:

> But a cell's DNA is always and necessarily embedded in an immensely complex and entangled system of interacting resources that are, collectively, what give rise to the development of traits. Not surprisingly, the causal dynamics of the process by which development unfolds are also complex and entangled, involving causal influences that extend upward, downward, and sideways. (Keller 2010: 51)

Mainstream genomic studies, Keller argues, also conflate generational transmission (or 'heritability') of traits – the idea that people in the same family are more likely to share characteristics – with genetic action. Traits can be technically heritable without being genetically transmitted: they might be epigenetically, socially, linguistically or environmentally passed down (Keller 2010: 62, 80). So age of menarche may be heritable but this may relate to nutrition, shared environments or similar modes of physiological processing (epigenetic factors). The search for genetic markers of pubertal onset, in other words, will not establish cause.

Needless to say, such studies also provide little traction for paediatricians working with children experiencing early onset puberty. Despite this, some papers argue the case for potential early identification of patients. Philip and Lazar (2005: 56) for example assert that 'detection of these genes will provide a tool for identification of children at risk of developing CPP [central precocious puberty], enabling early intervention with the aim of preventing its distressing outcomes'. Here genes become markers indicating future risk. Falling into the trap of enacting genes as causal agents, this claim also provokes more practical questions: How would parents know to subject their child to genetic testing on the off-chance that they might have a gene for early onset puberty? And would it ever be worth the risk associated with treatment to treat girls only on the basis of genetic prediction? (The risks of treating early onset puberty are discussed in detail in Chapter 7.) Genetic research, then, has little to offer clinicians and is driven by more distant agendas relating to genomic science more broadly.

Fat: troubling the biological/social divide

Of much more interest and potential use in clinical practice is research connecting early onset puberty to childhood overweight and obesity.

Here two contemporary discourses of great public concern coincide and inform each other (Throsby and Roberts 2010). Indeed, increases in childhood obesity are, like increases in children going through early puberty, often described as a 'crisis' (see, for example, Ebbeling, Pawlak and Ludwig 2002). Biological links between childhood obesity and early onset puberty are figured as obvious: rising rates of obesity coincide historically with changes in pubertal timing. The US-based Bogalusa Heart Study introduced in Chapter 4, for example, found in examining 3,000–3,500 children's growth over the period 1973–92 that girls born in 1992–4 were more overweight and were twice as likely to reach menarche by age 12 than girls of similar ages born 1978–9 (Freedman *et al.* 2000; Freedman *et al.* 2002). But the connecting mechanisms are less than clear: genetic factors, as described above, may indicate a link but these describe only a very small proportion of pubertal timing. Hormonal pathways are more likely candidates but again are non-obvious. Children who are overweight may have higher levels of estrogen in their bodies (fat produces estrogens), which may cause earlier development. Overweight bodies also produce more leptin, a fat cell derived hormone which is thought to be involved in early pubertal development (Jasik and Lustig 2008). But heavy girls may also be misrecognised as developing earlier: as described in Chapter 4, fat can look a lot like breast tissue. Thus, the perceived connection between early puberty and obesity may in part be driven by clinical and social error.

Numerous studies attempt to articulate the relationship between weight and puberty onset. In 2001, Paul Kaplowitz undertook a secondary analysis of the Pediatric Research in Office Settings (PROS) data (Herman-Giddens *et al.* 1997) with two key PROS authors Marcia Herman-Giddens and Eric Slora (Kaplowitz *et al.* 2001). This analysis attempted to determine whether the girls who started breast development earlier had a higher body mass index (BMI). The key findings were that 6–9-year-old girls with early breast development did have a significantly higher BMI compared to girls of the 'same' 'race' and age (readers will remember my concerns about how 'race' and age are articulated in this project). What was surprising to the authors, as Kaplowitz (2004: 96) later wrote, was 'that this difference was more impressive for white girls than for black girls'. They also found that girls with early pubic hair growth (but no breast development) had higher BMIs than their peers. Pubic hair development is regulated by a different set of hormonal processes than breast development and thus a similar outcome was not expected.

As Kaplowitz (2004: 98) points out, the PROS study is cross-sectional and thus cannot establish cause: BMI may be correlated with early puberty rather than a cause of it. In a longitudinal study however, Davison *et al.* (2003) found that higher percentage of body fat at age 5 and at age 7 predicted more advanced puberty at age 9 in 183 white American girls (measured by Tanner breast stage and estradiol levels). In this cohort, 59 per cent of early developers were overweight and 30 per cent were obese (compared to 21 per cent and 8 per cent in later developing girls) (2003: 818). The Breakthrough Generations breast cancer aetiology study also found that girls who were heavier or exercised less were more likely than their lighter or more active peers to go through menarche early (Morris *et al.* 2010). In 2008, Kaplowitz wrote a review of this field, pointing out that although the question of whether earlier puberty is the cause or the result of increased body fat remained unresolved, at least two longitudinal studies suggest that rapid increases in BMI or body fat predicts earlier onset of puberty (Kaplowitz 2008: 214). For him, then, 'it is increasingly clear that leptin has direct effects on gonadotropin secretion and provides the link between body fat stores and the timing of puberty' (2008: 214). An increase in leptin, he states, 'does seem to be the triggering event in the onset of puberty' (2008: 215). Because leptin increase is produced by weight increase, then, the decreasing age of both pubertal onset and menarche in American girls 'could well be explained by the higher prevalence of obesity' (2008: 215). Importantly, Kaplowitz notes that this relationship is not evident in boys and affirms the need for more longitudinal research that uses reliable methods of pubertal assessment and body fat measures (skinfold tests and bioelectrical impedance) rather than BMI.

Somewhat surprisingly in the face of Kaplowitz's assessment of the field, in 2009 the Danish study discussed in Chapter 4 (Aksglaede *et al.* 2009) comparing the pubertal timing of girls aged 5–20 in 1991–3 and in 2006–8 found no correlation between early onset puberty and BMI. Additionally, they found *lower* estradiol levels in the 2006 population despites the generally earlier development of this group. This study was exacting in its assessment of pubertal development, using palpation to assess Tanner breast stages (Davison *et al.* were restricted to visual assessment). Aksglaede *et al.* (2009: 938) conclude that rather than weight, 'factors yet to be identified are involved' in early development. Reporting findings from 'fifty year trends' in sexual development of American children, the Fels Longitudinal Study (Demerath *et al.* 2004a; 2004b), similarly concluded that 'increases in relative weight are a consequence, rather than a determinant, of the age of menarche, and that secular changes in BMI and in the mean age at menarche could be independent phenomena' (Styne 2004: 475). A German longitudinal study of 215 children, on the other hand, found that prepubertal body composition affected the pace of pubertal progression, rather than its onset (Buyken, Karaolis-Danckert and Remer 2009).

Debates around connections between early puberty and weight have been rearticulated in news media. In 2007, a flurry of newspaper and web-based articles reported on a study published in *Pediatrics* by Lee *et al.* (2007) that found that girls with higher BMI well before puberty (at 36 and 54 months) were more likely to go through early puberty than their leaner peers. The young age of the 354 participants facilitated the authors' argument that BMI has causal (rather than correlative) connections to early sexual development (preceding it in time): they argued that 'Our finding that increased body fatness is associated with earlier pubertal development lends support for the hypothesis that increased rates of obesity among children in the United States may be contributing to a possible secular trend of early maturation in US girls' (Lee *et al.* 2007: e629). Reported on BBC News online under the title 'Fat Toddlers "Risk Early Puberty"' the study was said to 'add ... to mounting evidence suggesting childhood obesity is causing the trend of earlier puberty in girls'.[1] Using a photograph of rolls of chubby skin to illustrate its point, the article quotes Helen Crocker, research dietician at University College London, to drive home its key message: 'In our clinics we are seeing girls of seven, eight and nine who are starting their periods and going through puberty. It can be pretty distressing for them. It's another good reason for tackling the wider issue of childhood obesity' http://news.bbc.co.uk/1/hi/health/6410961.stm). Media reports of this study created interest in online parenting forums such as myoverweightchild.com. Here, the parents of overweight children are informed of scientific studies about early puberty through quoted press releases and given the standard advice to ensure healthy eating and adequate exercise (albeit through rather drastic means – enrolment in a

[1] http://news.bbc.co.uk/1/hi/health/6410961.stm.

residential dieting programme or therapeutic boarding school). In a section entitled 'Overcoming the Challenges,' parents read:

> Ensuring that a child follows a healthy diet plan and gets an adequate amount of exercise is the ideal manner of avoiding obesity-related early puberty. Some children who struggle with weight from a young age may need professional intervention, which may include enrolment in a residential weight loss program or therapeutic boarding school for students with weight challenges.
>
> If a child who has entered early puberty responds to the resultant stresses and pressures by engaging in substance abuse, developing depression or impaired self-esteem, or experiencing academic frustration, residential therapeutic intervention – which may include a boarding school or wilderness program – may also be beneficial. (www.myoverweightchild.com/childhood-obesity-articles/childhood-obesity-identified-as-risk-factor-for-early-puberty.html)

Here, early puberty becomes just one symptom of obesity that creates suffering for heavy children.

Attempts to make causal links between early puberty and obesity are seriously weakened by the complexity of obesity itself. Like puberty, obesity remains a rather poorly understood phenomenon, despite huge investments in scientific research on this topic. As critics of obesity discourses point out, explanations of adiposity or fatness are often deeply flawed and contested. Evidence about the causes of fatness and the metabolic processes of weight gain and retention shows that multiple factors are at play: childhood (bio-psycho-social) experiences and contemporary environmental conditions have as significant, if not a far greater role to play than genes, over-eating or lack of exercise and, of course, also contribute in complex ways to the latter two factors (Aphramor 2005; Gard and Wright 2005; Throsby 2007; 2008; Murray 2008; Rich, Monaghan and Aphramor 2010). As I argued in an article co-written with Karen Throsby (Throsby and Roberts 2010), critical studies of obesity have much to offer an analysis of early puberty: highlighting the intertwined actions of biological, psychological and social factors in the production of fat bodies, they resist contemporary scientific and public health attempts to find simple causes and responses/treatments for obesity, arguing that moral beliefs continually inflect all aspects of debate about the health effects of overweight (Gard and Wright 2005; Throsby 2007; 2008). Whilst children's weight may in some way be linked with earlier sexual development, there can be no simple connection made between the two 'crises' of early puberty and childhood obesity. In both cases, bodily changes articulate complex bio-psycho-social intra-actions, moments of what Haraway (2003: 9) would call congealment in ongoing 'multidirectional flows of bodies and values'.

Toxins: the costs of living in a dirty world

'To find the girls are starting breast development earlier and earlier is extremely concerning,' she says. 'To have that much change in such a short time, it has to be the environment.' (Marcia Herman-Giddens, cited in Coghlin 2010)

In Chapter 1, I described environmentalists' concerns about the impact of endocrine-disrupting chemicals on human and non-human animal sexual development. Acting like hormones in the body or affecting endogenous hormonal circuits, endocrine disruptors are part of an ubiquitous chemical saturation of contemporary environments, found in air and water, in food chains, in objects and in human and non-human animal bodies. Examples include pesticides such as DDT, dieldrin and chlordane; heavy metals like lead, arsenic, cadmium and mercury; plastics and phthalates (used to make plastics flexible); perfumes and musks; flame retardants; organochlorines, industrial chemicals and by-products such as PCBs and dioxins; and phytoestrogens such as soy. For leading environmentalist groups such as Greenpeace, Friends of the Earth and the World Wildlife Fund (WWF), connections between the ever-increasing ubiquity of such chemicals and rising rates of early puberty seem obvious: they are chronologically synchronous and are both of an alarming scale.

Scientific and political debates around the impact of endocrine disruptors are fierce. It is often extremely difficult to measure the effects of toxins: they can be active in miniscule amounts and are both additive and cumulative over time, making proof of their effects hard to establish. Endocrine disruptors can also be effective in counter-intuitive ways, with lower doses sometimes having larger effects than higher ones (Langston 2010). The mechanisms of their effects are also complex. Some scientists and environmentalists argue that children exposed to endocrine disruptors, either in utero or in early life, experience atypical development via direct actions of chemicals in pubertal processes; others argue that these chemicals disrupt existing bodily processes such as appetite systems.[2] Many suggest that as a time of great physiological change, puberty constitutes a 'window of susceptibility' to toxins: Garry and Truran (2012: 357), for example, describe the 'interplay of pituitary, adrenal, thyroid and sex hormones' constituting puberty as 'a fertile soil for . . . disruption . . . by environmental chemicals.' Most studies of this interplay use animal models or in vitro experimental design; research on humans tends to follow the outcomes of industrial and medical accidents or focus on particular environments in which people are exposed to abnormal levels of endocrine disruptors (Diamanti-Kandarakis and Gore 2012). The findings of such studies are mixed and cannot decisively point to cause but are consistent enough to claim that 'in general, EDC exposure is associated with earlier onset of puberty or pubertal milestones in girls, whilst delayed puberty is the predominant finding in males' (Wu *et al.* 2012: 349; see also Aksglaede *et al.* 2006).

Sociologist Sara Shostak (2010) argues that claims about environmental toxins are increasingly linked to research into molecular biomarkers of exposure and the genetic susceptibilities thought to mitigate individuals' responses to the chemicals to which they are exposed.[3] These links allow scientists to make more precise claims about levels of exposure (which chemicals can be found in any particular body) and to begin to elaborate different biological pathways of action within exposed bodies. As Shostak argues, following Rose and Foucault, such research also articulates new forms of responsible subjectivity in which individuals should seek to maximize their life chances: 'By opening possible futures to the strategic consideration, choice, and action of individuals, molecular biomarker technologies further contribute to this mode of subjectivity' (Shostak 2010: 245). These kinds of arguments are evident in some work on early puberty. A paper from a

[2] For reviews of this literature, see Cesario and Hughes 2007; Louis *et al.* 2008; Mouritsen *et al.* 2010; Jurewicz and Hanke 2011; Diamanti-Kandarakis and Gore 2012.

[3] According to a recent article in *Nature*, 'A biomarker can be anything that is reliably indicative of a biological state. This can include everything from a gene variant to a behaviour, but the term is generally used to refer to proteins or other molecules found in fluids such as blood or the CSF, or to physiological or anatomical changes that can be observed with techniques such as functional magnetic resonance imaging or positron-emission tomography' (Katsnelson 2011: 139).

leading group in the field, based in Denmark, argues for example that 'There may be a wide range of genetic susceptibility to EDCs' (Mouritsen *et al.* 2010: 354). Connected to such distinctions, as Shostak also points out, are possibilities that such differences reflect social experience rather than 'genes'. She continues,

> At the same time, attending to such possibilities in the context of environmental health and illness, especially given the extensive evidence that people of color and with fewer resources are more likely to be exposed to environmental hazards (Brulle and Pellow 2006), highlights the possibility that such forms of subjectivity may be highly stratified. (Shostak 2010: 245)

Research on endocrine disruptors and pubertal timing speaks to such stratification. Mantovani (2012: 133) suggests, for example, that 'ethnic disparities, such as health behaviors associated with poverty, could ... result in difference in exposure to particular ED [endocrine disruptors]'. These debates point to the entanglements of race, class and health, and remind us (as discussed in Chapter 4) that genetic accounts of racial differences make little sense and should be avoided. Social stratifications such as race and class are lived, felt and embodied.

In news media reports, journalists draw on the scientific literature on endocrine disruptors to articulate individualised risks, producing new responsibilities for particular persons and subpopulations. Although foetuses, babies and children are exposed to endocrine disruptors through countless environmental routes from their mother's bloodstream to furniture, toys and food, mothers are often figured as accountable for such flows and are advised in environmentalist campaigns and mass media articles on ways to reduce their children's exposure (Roberts 2006; 2007: ch. 7). Frequent consumption of particular foods containing sex hormones such as soy, dairy and meat is linked to early sexual development (see for example Karlberg 2002; Rogers *et al.* 2010; Kim *et al.* 2011; Kim and Park 2012) and mothers, as in obesity discourses, are frequently called on to control their children's eating (see for example Gray 2013). In a 2012 article in *The New York Times* that led to numerous television talk show discussions in the United States,[4] journalist Elizabeth Weil describes mothers' shocked responses to Herman-Giddens' initial findings about

[4] This is described in Belkin (2012). For an example of such discussions, see http://loop21.com/black-girls-early-puberty-breast-development-young-age.

early puberty rates and the suggestion that 'ordinary' objects such as processed foods and plastics might be implicated:

> When Herman-Giddens published these numbers, in 1997 in *Pediatrics*, she set off a social and endocrinological firestorm. 'I had no idea it would be so huge,' Herman-Giddens told me recently. 'The Lolita syndrome' – the prurient fascination with the sexuality of young girls — 'created a lot of emotional interest. As a feminist, I wish it didn't.' Along with medical professionals, mothers, worried about their daughters, flocked to Herman-Giddens's slide shows, gasping as she flashed images of possible culprits: obesity, processed foods, plastics. (Weil 2012)

Such shock leads mothers into labyrinthine avenues of action designed to protect their children. For some it also produces business and publicity opportunities. Weil quotes Tracee, the mother of the article's case study (9-year-old Ainsley who started developing at age 6), describing her attempts to 'do something' to help her daughter:

> Over the past three years, Tracee . . . had taken Ainsley to see several doctors. They ordered blood tests and bone-age X-rays and turned up nothing unusual. 'The doctors always come back with these blank looks on their faces, and then they start redefining what normal is,' Tracee said . . . . 'And I always just sit there thinking, what are you talking about, normal? Who gets pubic hair in first grade?' (Weil 2012)

Resisting clinicians' attempts to persuade her that no action was needed, Tracee both pursued alternative therapies and set up a business selling 'sunscreens and lotions marketed to tweens and described by Tracee as "natural, organic, craptastic-free products" containing "no estrogens, phytoestrogens, endocrine disrupters"' (Weil 2012). Enterprisingly, Tracee also established a blog with a mission to 'revolutionize the way we think about, treat and raise girls'. Here mothers are offered the kind of advice Ainsley's doctors and alternative therapists refused to give: '"You can't be more specific?" Tracee asked, pleading. "Like tell me what crap in my house I can get rid of?"' (Weil 2012). Weil reports that for most mothers the attempt to control the effects of endocrine disrupting chemicals ultimately feels futile:

> Over the past year, I talked to mothers who tried to forestall their daughters' puberty in many different ways. Some trained with them for 5K runs (exercise is one of the few interventions known to help prevent early puberty); others trimmed milk and meat containing hormones from their daughters'

diets; some purged from their homes plastics, pesticides and soy. Yet sooner rather than later, most threw up their hands. (Weil 2012)

These dilemmas speak to the impossibilities of the contemporary forms of subjectivity described by Shostak. Although we are encouraged by public health campaigns and corporate advertising to control our bodies, manage our weight, exercise properly, eat well, be mindful, our attempts to negotiate 'health' are constantly thwarted by actors (human and non-human) that elude us. Toxic chemicals are a perfect example: whilst mothers may be able to reduce their children's exposure to particular kinds of food, toys or furnishings, they cannot contain the flow of chemicals in and out of their homes, lives and bodies. Children move through the world and are constituted in and through their relation to it: they cannot be kept apart and are never 'pure' in chemical terms.

I have argued elsewhere that injunctions to protect children from toxic chemicals are gendered: it is mothers specifically who are advised to engage in this labour (Roberts 2006; 2007: ch. 7). Additionally, the literature on early puberty highlights the gendering of concerns about children: it is girls' bodies rather than boys' that mothers should worry most about (see also Roberts 2013; Adams, Murphy and Clarke 2009). In contrast to the discourses above, for example, the 2012 *New York Times* article describing Herman-Giddens *et al.*'s findings about early puberty in boys assures readers that the notable difference between white and black boys in relation to pubertal timing 'is most likely driven by the role of genes' (Belluck 2012). As mentioned in Chapter 4, journalist Pam Belluck also insists that 'several experts said the study should not be seized upon as cause for alarm, but rather as a way to help parents and doctors gauge what to be aware of in boys' development and whether to start conversations about social issues sooner'. Quoting Laura Bachrach, a professor of pediatric endocrinology at Stanford University, she adds,

But the study should not prompt a magazine 'cover article that shows a 9-year-old boy shaving,' Dr. Bachrach said. And because some parents fear that early puberty is related to more hormones in milk – speculation that is unproven – 'I don't want people to get up in arms and rush out and buy organic milk,' she said. 'When patients ask me, I say, "Do that for political reasons or because you like the taste, but don't do it because you think it's going to influence puberty."' (Belluck 2012)

The tone here is such a long way from the panicked response and sense of crisis around girls' development, showing both a relatively relaxed attitude towards early development in boys and a potentially naïve relation to environmental health issues: some recent research does describe the impact of endocrine disruptors on male development (see, for example, Fernandez and Olea 2012; Wu *et al.* 2012).

According to epidemiological studies, early development is much more frequent in girls; boys are more likely than girls to develop late. Mouritsen *et al.* suggest that some of these differences may stem from differentiated responses to environmental toxins: because of girls' higher pre-pubertal estradiol levels, 'additional environmentally derived oestrogen may have more pronounced effect at the hormone-sensitive organs than in boys' (Mouritsen *et al.* 2010: 350). I suggest that it is impossible to separate out cultural figurations of masculinity and femininity from these more technical explanations: every time 'girls' and 'boys' are figured as groups, scientists and journalists inevitably draw on a range of historically and geographically specific sets of expectations, worries and understandings about strength, vulnerability, relationality and health.

Despite the global ubiquity of endocrine disruptors, and although concerns about girls are usually non-specific (all mothers of all girls should be concerned), in some scientific discourses particular populations of girls are articulated as being at heightened risk of exposure to chemicals affecting pubertal timing. Trying to understand the racialised distribution of early onset puberty, for example, scientists have studied the potential effects of shampoos designed and marketed for 'black hair' (Tiwary 1998; Westphal 2002). Containing hormonally active human or non-human placental extracts, these shampoos may be absorbed into children's skin, sending signals to their brains to begin developing. This research is linked to studies finding that parents wearing medical hormone patches or using hormonal sprays may pass hormonal messages to their children through skin contact (Yu *et al.* 1999; Felner and White 2000; Kunz *et al.* 2004; Cesario and Hughes 2007; Gupta *et al.* 2010).

Questions of responsibility are raised here: partly because of their apparent simplicity, these studies are well reported in the news media (see for example Sanghavi 2006; Jamieson 2010: Ebony 2012; Evans 2012) and are linked on medical, parenting and environmentalist websites and blogs to exhortations to change family practices. In the face of great uncertainty, mothers are advised to do what they can to 'help . . . the situation' through consumption choices. As one US-based clinician writes in her blog post on 'precocious puberty', 'Certainly avoid environmental estrogens, eat organic, don't shampoo with estrogen, but make sure you are doing that while waiting for your appointment. That way, when you are told it's idiopathic (i.e. "unknown cause") you'll be well on your way to helping the situation.'[5]

Exhortations to consume wisely and to control children's exposure to endocrine-disruptors assume that early puberty is undesirable. They also sit in tension with other less widely publicised stories about some groups of young women, notably in Jamaica and the Jamaican diaspora, using hormonally active products – colloquially known as 'chicken pills' – to achieve desirable bodies (in this case to stimulate buttock growth) (The Kitchen Sisters 2010; Opelka 2011). These tensions raise important questions about the significance of sexual development and its associated physical changes for young people and their families: should puberty be allowed to unfold without chemical assistance; what kinds of risks should be avoided; and is early puberty always experienced as a problem? I return to these questions in Chapter 6.

In environmentalist discourses, as discussed in Chapter 1, early puberty is but one of a long list of negative consequences of exposure to environmental endocrine disruption. Lists of potential consequences place a diverse range of outcomes in proximity, eliding differences between them: non gender-typical behaviour (such as girls climbing trees or play-fighting) is listed alongside an increased risk of breast or ovarian cancer as if these are comparable in significance. Whilst the rhetorical weight of such lists may be valuable – they do figure the impacts of environmental toxins as widespread and profound – the political implications are alarming (see also Roberts 2003; 2007). Does campaigning against environmental toxins require conviction that mainstream gender norms are natural or right? For me, early onset puberty sits somewhat uneasily and ambiguously in such lists: concerns about early development could be tied to worries about gendered behaviour but also to an emphasis on increased cancer risk. The following chapter turns to questions of risk, exploring biomedical and scientific, environmentalist and news media accounts of the dangers of early development.

[5] http://zrtdocsblog.blogspot.co.uk/2011/08/precocious-puberty.html.

Psycho-social explanations: stress, attachment and parenting

Early onset puberty is explained in other settings in notably different ways. Rather than focusing on the role of biological or other physical actors (genes, hormones, endocrine disruptors) these explanations attend to the social environments and psycho-social histories of early developing girls, claiming sexual development as the consequence of a set of bio-social encounters between parents/caregivers and children. These explanations hold substantial weight in some fields but also give rise to significant controversy: wider claims about the biological effects of parenting practices are both increasingly ubiquitous[6] and deeply challenging to more traditional models of sex and sexual development that position psychological relations and orientations as separate from and/or consequential to biological processes and physiological changes. For me, these debates highlight the impossibilities of drawing clear distinctions between biological, psychological and social forces when articulating sexed bodies.

Literatures on the biological effects of parenting and life histories are daunting terrain for a feminist brought up on critiques of biological essentialisms, most notably those found in socio-biological accounts of human relationships. When I first encountered the argument that early puberty was associated with or even caused by 'absent fathers', for example, I felt dismissive. Mentioning these arguments in academic feminist settings often triggered laughter. Such arguments carry normative freight about the rightness of particular family formations, modes of parental attention and even the biological nature of heterosexuality. Historically, such arguments have been associated with reductive accounts of sex/gender and thus with oppressive sexual politics, so this is a field that feminists have thoroughly critiqued (for an overview, see Fausto-Sterling 2000). Yet such research continues to develop, even thrive. Might there be any value to feminism in engaging again with this work, particularly insofar as it articulates early sexual development? Might taking a new look at its details open up questions around biology and sex that are promising? In the following section I explore the two key areas of debate – the role of international

[6] This is evidenced in the UK, for example, by the popularity of Susan Gerhardt's *Why Love Matters* (2004), a book that provides biological (neurological) accounts of children's behaviour and the effect of parenting practices.

adoption and of early life circumstances in producing early puberty – in order to address these questions.

International adoption

Precocious puberty is a frequent and unnatural event in these girls. (Virdis *et al.* 1998: 152)

One of the most intriguing findings of the epidemiological literature on early puberty is that girls adopted internationally tend to go through puberty earlier than their peers in either their country of origin or their adoptive country. Since the 1990s many parents of girls adopted from developing countries (India, Romania or China, for example) have reported that these children go through puberty notably earlier than their peers in their adopted countries (often in Europe or the USA) and in their home countries (Virdis *et al.* 1998; Mul, Oostdijk and Drop 2002; Parent *et al.* 2003; Teilmann *et al.* 2009). In their study of nineteen girls adopted from India by Italian parents, for example, Virdis *et al.* (1998) found that breast development started on average at 6.9 years. In Belgium one third of girls referred to clinicians for early onset puberty are internationally adopted (Bourguignon *et al.* 1992), whilst in one medical centre in the Netherlands about 20 per cent of children treated for early puberty have these backgrounds (Kempers and Otten 2002). A recent Spanish study came to a similar conclusion, but found also that domestically adopted children were at substantially increased risk of early sexual development (Soriano-Guillén *et al.* 2010). In Denmark too, internationally adopted children were found to have a fifteen- to twentyfold increased risk of early onset puberty compared to non-adopted Danish children (Teilmann *et al.* 2006). This risk was increased for children adopted when they were older than 2 years (uncertainty about the exact ages of adopted children was statistically taken into account) and differed according to birth country. The latter point holds significance in relation to forms of early care: Teilmann *et al.* (2006: 392) found that children from South Korea who had lived in foster homes rather than orphanages were not more likely to experience early puberty. In a later longitudinal study following 276 randomly selected internationally adopted girls, Teilmann *et al.* (2009) found that 16 per cent of the girls had reached Tanner breast stage 2 by age 8 and that on average they both grew breasts and menstruated 1.3 years earlier than their Danish non-adopted peers.

All of these papers report uncertainty about the causes of early puberty in this group of children. Nutritional changes are often discussed: adopted children are commonly underweight when they migrate and many show fast 'catch-up' growth in their new homes (Parent *et al.* 2003: 682). Correlations between early onset puberty and BMI in this group are unclear: Teilmann *et al.* (2009: 244), for example, found that internationally adopted girls had lower BMI than their Danish peers but were nevertheless more likely to develop earlier. Authors also refer to changes in physical environment: increased or decreased exposure to endocrine disrupting chemicals in particular. Change in chemical environment (even for the 'better') might, Parent *et al.* suggest, provoke a pathological response:

> [M]igration may interrupt exposure of foreign children to some EDCs. In such conditions, it is unknown whether central precocious puberty could result indirectly from withdrawal of the negative feedback effects of the sex steroids or their environmental analogs and/or directly from accelerated hypothalamic maturation caused by sex steroids. (Parent *et al.* 2003: 685; see also Krstevska-Konstantinova *et al.* 2001)

These arguments are troubled by the lack of parity between adopted children and those migrating with their parents: whilst some studies show that the children of migrating families moving from underdeveloped to developed countries may also be at increased risk of early puberty (Parent *et al.* 2003: 683), others find this is not the case (Soriano-Guillén *et al.* 2010) or is only marginally so (Teilmann *et al.* 2006). Although exposed to similar changes in physical environment, non-adopted migrating children may not experience significant changes in diet (because they are being cared for by the same people, who are better placed to maintain dietary continuity). More importantly, however, they remain with their birth families and may never have experienced the 'affective deprivation' that usually precedes adoption (Parent *et al.* 2003: 683). Claims about the significance of such deprivation lead us into a connected literature on the relationship between suffering in early childhood and the timing of sexual development.

Embodied histories of suffering: 'uncanny' connections

It is time that developmentalists interested in adolescence begin to systematically examine pubertal timing as *an outcome of social experience*, rather than presuming the reverse causality. (Belsky, Steinberg and Draper 1991: 664, emphasis in original)

Internationally adopted children by definition share two powerful experiences: the loss of birth family and foster or institutional carers and transition to new parents; and (usually if not always) some trauma associated with early abandonment and/or institutionalisation. Contemporary psychological literatures on child development and adoption argue that such experiences are costly, potentially having long-lasting physical and psychological effects. Much of this research focuses on brain development, arguing that early experiences of care-related trauma (neglect, abuse, separation, institutionalisation) forms neuroendocrinological pathways and habits that are difficult to change: babies who are regularly exposed to danger or whose basic needs are not met can become highly sensitive to arousal, exhibiting strong reactions to small threats for many years even when in a relatively safe situation (Hughes 2006; Hughes and Baylin 2012; Schofield and Beek 2006). Such difficulties are often framed through attachment theory, a set of ideas originally proposed by John Bowlby (1969) and revised by Mary Ainsworth *et al.* (1978) that characterise a child's habits in forming relationships with caregivers (for an overview see Fonagy 2001).

Children exposed to early trauma and encountering changes in caregivers at early stages are, it is argued, likely to develop 'insecure' or 'disorganised' attachment patterns that presume that caregivers are unreliable, dangerous and/or unavailable. These patterns are said to correlate with particular brain states in which, for example, high levels of cortisol (the so-called 'flight or fight hormone') become relatively constant. Many children with insecure or disorganised attachments thus experience the world and caregivers as dangerous or unreliable, their bodies biochemically feeding this back to them as a 'truth' after they have been removed to what others would perceive as 'safety'. These brain states, it is argued, also provoke particular reactions and behaviours in children to match their internal 'danger mode' states: reacting strongly to relatively small threats (the loss of a toy, a change in routine, new foods), they will fight, argue or cry as if the danger is life threatening. Such behaviour can provoke strong reactions from well-intentioned carers, thus affirming a view of the world as dangerous ('this carer is so angry, they might leave me') and of the self as unlovable ('people always get angry with me, I must be a bad person'). Thus rather than returning to a calm, regulated state, the insecurely attached child gradually becomes more and more intensely dysregulated, often resulting in extreme rage or despair and/or physical exhaustion (Schofield and Beek 2006; Hughes 2009; Hughes and Baylin 2012).

Some scientists writing from a 'life history perspective' argue that children's development and reproductive futures are affected by inter-uterine experience, largely determined by maternal nutrition but also taking into account exposure to estrogens and other chemicals, such as those in cigarette smoke (for a review, see Sloboda, Hickey and Hart 2011). This view suggests that early sexual development may be a self-protective and 'strategic' biological response initiated by the foetus' 'use of maternal cues to anticipate its future environment': it is better for the individual to develop early, so she or he does not die before reproducing (2011: 221). For these scholars, pre-birth life would be as important as post-birth experience.

The physical effects of pre- and post-birth experiences are not thought to be limited to the brain: some researchers and therapists claim that children exposed to loss, neglect and/or trauma in their early lives are more likely to experience sensory difficulties (hypersensitivities of the skin and problems in temperature regulation for example) and physical complaints such as skin conditions, stomach pains, anxiety and sleep difficulties. Early traumatic experiences are also thought to affect physical growth and development: such children are sometimes slow to grow and fail to meet 'normal' developmental goals related to physical skills such as walking and talking (Schofield and Beek 2006). Such findings take us back to Tanner and Whitehouse's research subjects living in the Harpenden branch of the National Children's Home. In the *Atlas of Children's Development*, Tanner and Whitehouse (1982) asserted that delay in growth could be 'psycho-social' in nature: caused by neglect, poverty and family difficulties. As discussed in Chapter 3, however, Tanner and Whitehouse also argued that moving out of difficult families into care institutions like Harpenden would lead to 'catch-up' growth (1982: 170). In Tanner's view, such growth was positive. In contrast, as I show in Chapter 6, contemporary discourses of early onset puberty figure such growth as having potentially negative outcomes for the children concerned (initiating premature sexual development and therefore long-term height loss).

More controversially, some scholars suggest that the timing of puberty may be affected by early childhood experience of parenting. In 1991, developmental psychologists Jay Belksy and Laurence Steinberg and anthropologist Patricia Draper published a ground-breaking paper in which they proposed 'an evolutionary theory of socialization' (Belsky *et al.* 1991: 647).[7] Combining the concept of 'reproductive strategy' taken from behavioural ecology with contemporary attachment theory, they argued that children generally follow one of two pathways through development. The first, characterised by 'good enough' parenting building secure attachment patterns, leads to 'normal' timing of sexual development, the formation of healthy pair bonds in adult life, and a long-term risk-avoidant investment in raising a small number of children. The second strategy, founded on inadequate parenting that builds insecure attachment patterns and often involves trauma and/or loss, leads to early puberty, poor pair bonds and low or short-term investment in raising children (and often more children).

Although arguing that this bi-partite classification is not a moral one (the second strategy, they suggest, is a reasonable response to some individuals' life circumstances), 'good' and 'poor' outcomes are certainly at stake here. Early puberty is figured in these arguments as one of a consequential string of negative outcomes: associated with early sexual experiences, increased risk-taking and future poor parenting. Such strings of consequences, as I will argue in Chapter 6, are continuously rearticulated in the literature on early puberty: what is unique to Belsky, Steinberg and Draper's theory is the causal linking of early onset puberty to infantile or early childhood experience of care. The core of this argument is that individuals have a biological (evolutionary) orientation towards reproduction: a harsh early environment speeds up childhood in order that the individual might reproduce before dying. As many have pointed out, this argument is potentially counter-intuitive: one could imagine that in a dangerous or stressful environment it might be better for the individual not to reproduce but to wait for better times. For Belsky *et al.*, the drive to reproduction takes precedence over care, either for the self or for others. An

[7] Ellis claims that this paper stimulated a major body of research and theory in the puberty field and that prior to its publication it would not have been possible to seriously argue that 'social experiences influence something as biological and presumably genetic as pubertal timing' (Ellis 2004: 948).

individual will reproduce at significant cost to oneself and even when the world is perceived as dangerous – the new child will have to make the best of a bad lot. For Belsky *et al.* this means continuing in the same vein – a child raised in difficult circumstances would be likely to reproduce a similar pattern of development and reproductive behaviours.[8] Although predictable, then, Belsky *et al.* (1991: 662) describe the relationship between early experience and pubertal timing as 'uncanny'.

The dynamic and complex interplay between biology and the social posited here is unusual in the puberty field. Belsky *et al.* (1991: 658) 'suggest that early stress may affect pubertal timing by making the individual more biologically reactive to social conditions as she approaches the age of pubertal onset'. Here stress (a socially caused yet undefined condition) produces a biological state that renders an individual biologically more likely to react to social situations as she ages. For Belsky *et al.* (1991: 658), this is an argument against those positing a genetic causation of pubertal timing – for them puberty is characterised by changes in an individual's neuroendocrine system, a biological system that is seen to be much more amenable to social influence than genes (see also Roberts 2007: ch. 1). In one part of the paper they postulate a mechanism in which particular styles of thought (described as 'internalizing') connected to sadness, social withdrawal and depression changes produce metabolic effects that provoke hormonal changes:

> In the case of females, we suspect that 'internalizing' problems serve to lower metabolism, store fat, and thereby stimulate menarche. Such experientially and behaviourally induced maturation sets the stage for sexual activity, and thereby, procreation. Early maturation, then, is part of a constellation of biological and behavioural processes that facilitate a quantity-oriented reproductive strategy. (Belsky *et al.* 1991: 652)

Despite their underlying evolutionary emphasis on reproductive drive, then, Belsky *et al.* describe their theory as non-biologically determinist;

[8] For a detailed discussion of this debate, see Chisholm 1999. Belksy, Steinberg and Draper's theory also stands in a somewhat counter-intuitive relation to existing research showing that high levels of stress in adults can suppress reproductive processes: in times of war or starvation, for example, many women stop menstruating. Ellis and Boyce propose an additional theory to address this difference (see Ellis 2004: 936).

as articulating 'an evolved flexibility of organismic response to variations in context, in the service of biological goals (i.e., reproductive fitness)' (1991: 648).

The literature on international adoption cited above did not exist when Belsky *et al.* posited their theory of early development. This literature, as I suggest below, does arguably lend support to their claims about early attachment experiences and sexual development. In Belsky *et al.*'s paper, however, adoption appears in a rather more traditional role, one that sheds some light on the underlying orientation of this work. Near the end of the paper, in a section entitled 'Strong inference tests of the theory', adopted children appear in the generic role assigned to them in 'nature–nurture' debates: that of useful research subjects whose lack of biological connection to their (adopting) parents can be academically exploited. In proposing two research designs to test their theory, Belsky, Steinberg and Draper write:

> The correlational design would involve identical and fraternal twins reared apart and/or adopted and biological children. The central goal of the research would be to test the effect of the hypothesized antecedent conditions (contextual stress, problematic parenting, and child behaviour problems), after controlling for the heritability of pubertal timing and, ideally, of problematic parenting and behaviour problems as well. If the hypothesized antecedents of early puberty did not emerge once behaviour genetic variance was statistically controlled, then a critical theoretical proposition would have been disconfirmed. (1991: 662)

Here, then, adopted children are figured as 'different' only in so far as they do not have a biological relation to their parents: the fact that they are also much more likely to have encountered 'problematic parenting' before being adopted than non-adopted peers remains unacknowledged (although a statement is made that 'problematic parenting and behaviour problems' could be controlled for). In proposing such traditional research paradigms and figuring adoption as something separable from 'problematic parenting and behaviour problems', Belsky *et al.*'s (at least partial) commitment to a rather conventional biological–social distinction becomes apparent. In my view, the paper displays significant tensions in shifting between more and less conventional framings of this relation. In the paragraph above, the biological and the social become 'factors' that can be separated and 'statistically controlled for' in a way that the proposed theory problematises. If stress, endocrinology, social existence and behaviour are all interimplicated, how can such clear lines be drawn? 'Causal influences', as Fox Keller (2010: 51) reminds us, 'extend upward, downward, and sideways.'

Belsky, Steinberg and Draper's theory has been subjected to argument and to empirical testing since publication in 1991. Inevitable criticisms have come from geneticists, who argue that the theory underestimates the power of genetic factors in determining pubertal timing. They suggest that the similarities within families theorised by Belsky *et al.* as evidence of the repetition of particular strategies are more likely to have a genetic basis (for a review of these critiques, see Ellis 2004: 944–5). In a friendlier vein, some developmental psychologists (often collaborating with Belsky or his associates) have tried to test the theory empirically (see, for example, Mofitt *et al.* 1992). In reviewing this work, both Belsky and others suggest that whilst correlative evidence exists (linking, for example, 'warm, cohesive family environments' with later puberty), proving causality remains challenging due to the diverse factors possibly influencing pubertal timing (Ellis 2004: 935–6).

Belsky *et al.*'s research builds on a longer tradition of work on the importance of early childhood experience on adolescent and adult sexual and parenting behaviour. Underpinned by evolutionary and genetic theory on sexual difference in reproductive 'investment' (Bateman 1948; Williams 1966; Trivers 1972; Dawkins 1976), this work deploys anthropological evidence from many countries.[9] Draper comes from the anthropological wing of this tradition and, long before her association with Belsky and Steinberg, had worked on the importance of 'father absence' on adolescent sexuality and later parenting (see, for example, Draper and Harpending 1982; 1988). In contrast to the biological focus of her more recent work, Draper's earlier theories rely on social learning (Draper and Harpending 1982: 265). These 'paternal investment theories' were developed by Bruce J. Ellis and colleagues and empirically tested in several countries: Ellis (2004: 943) claims that this research demonstrates that 'in well-nourished populations, girls from father-absent homes tend to experience earlier pubertal development than do girls from father-present homes, and the earlier the father

[9] For feminist analyses of this field see Fausto-Sterling (2000) and Gowaty (2003).

absence occurs, the greater the effect'. In his review of this field, Ellis (2004: 938–44) outlines a series of possible mechanisms for such effects. Citing animal studies, he mentions the possible role of pheromones (airborne chemical signals passed between individuals that effect internal hormonal processes, including the HPG axis triggering puberty) and of tactile, olfactory and auditory cues.[10] Research on social influences on human ovulation cycles also provides some grist to his mill, as does research indicating correlations between sexual abuse and earlier puberty.[11] 'In sum', Ellis (2004: 944) concludes, 'the direction of causation remains an open question … Further research is needed.'

The notable shift over the last thirty years in this field from an emphasis on social learning to attempts to theorise the neuroendocrine pathways of sexual abuse and 'family ecology' (Ellis 2004: 943) replicates the ever-increasing emphasis on biological factors such as genes and hormones in theorising behaviour, which Clarke *et al.* (2010) argue is part of wider processes of biomedicalisation. Although such models are not simply biologically determinist – both Ellis and Belsky *et al.* specifically argue *against* the claim that puberty is biologically caused – they demonstrate significant investment in theorising the biological routes through which social experience 'gets into' the body.

In his review, Ellis summarises the theoretical approaches to early puberty coming from developmental fields. Addressing critiques of Belsky, Steinberg and Draper's theory (which Ellis names 'psychosocial acceleration theory'; 2004: 921), he suggests that both Belsky, Steinberg and Draper and he himself in earlier work have 'reached too far in conceptualizing pubertal timing as a link in the causal chain connecting childhood experiences, not only to age at onset of sex and reproduction, but also to qualitative differences in reproductive strategies such as pair bond stability and parental investment' (2004: 921). His paper offers a new, less far-reaching framework he calls 'child development theory'. This account 'reconceptualizes pubertal timing as the endpoint of a developmental strategy that conditionally alters the length of childhood in response to the composition and quality of family

[10] For feminist readings of scientific work on pheromones see Brennan (2004) and Sieben (2011).

[11] Fascinatingly, this work takes us back to the PROS study of early puberty, which was inspired by Hermann-Giddens' earlier findings about earlier puberty amongst girls who had been sexually abused (Hermann-Giddens *et al.* 1997).

environments (capitalizing on the benefits of high-quality family environments and mitigating the costs of low-quality ones)' (2004: 921) but declines to make claims about later reproductive life.

In a 2010 paper, Belsky outlined responses to the 'BSD' (Belsky, Steinberg and Draper) theory since its publication. Responding to Ellis' criticism that the theory had been 'too far-reaching', he agrees that more empirical evidence is needed to establish the proposed connections between early experience, puberty and later sexual and reproductive behaviours (pair bonding and parenting). Rather approvingly, he discusses Ellis' reframing of the issue in terms of 'length of childhood', arguing that both approaches signal the importance of early experience in determining pubertal onset:

> Irrespective of whether one embraces Ellis' (2004) reconceptualization of BSD's uncanny prediction linking social-developmental experiences in the family to pubertal timing (i.e. as just terminating childhood rather than facilitating mating, pair bonding and parenting), the fact remains that he, just like D&H [Draper and Harpending] (1982), BSD and Chisholm (1996), regards early experience in the family as playing an influential role in shaping human reproductive strategy. This remains an all too uncommon way of thinking about development within the field of developmental psychology. (Belsky 2010: 32; abbreviations in original)

As Belsky indicates, despite the detailed debate constituting this field, his and his colleagues' ideas have received relatively little attention in wider scientific and clinical literature on early onset puberty.[12] Most of the literature discussed in earlier chapters of this book pays no heed to Belsky *et al.*'s calls for an evolutionary approach. Although Kaplowitz writes in his parental guide to early puberty that it is 'entirely possible that Belsky's theory of psychological stress triggering puberty in young girls has some merit' (Kaplowitz, 2004: 91), for example, the relevant arguments seem poorly understood. Kaplowitz conflates Belsky, Steinberg and Draper's (1991) argument and Draper and Harpending's views, suggesting that the stressors involved in early puberty are reducible to 'absent fathers' and 'divorce' (he argues that the divorce rate

[12] In other work Belsky takes a different tack, arguing more broadly for a view of both foetal and child development as flexible and plastic, arguing that some foetuses/children are genetically and/or temperamentally more susceptible to both negative and positive influences on their development (see, for example Belsky 1997; 2005; Belsky, Bakermans-Kranenburg and van Ijzendoorn 2007; Belsky and Pluess 2009).

has decreased over the time period in which early puberty has become more common) (Kaplowitz 2004: 92). As noted above, Belsky, Steinberg and Draper's argument is more encompassing than that of Draper and Harpending, suggesting a range of stressors including inadequate parenting, poverty, exposure to danger, and abuse and neglect (rather than just 'absent fathers').[13]

News media articles also focus on the 'absent father' element of this research, often wrongly attributing this sole emphasis to Belsky. In her *New York Times* piece quoted at the beginning of this chapter, for example, Lisa Belkin cites Belsky's work to suggest that girls raised in households where biological fathers were not present were more likely to mature earlier. Here too, Belkin notes the striking silence with which Belsky and others' work has been greeted, both scientifically and culturally. She describes these scientists' concerns that their work would disturb others:

> The outrage these researchers fear, however, has not materialized. So far, their work has been met mostly with silence. Belsky and Ellis each published their results in respected peer-reviewed journals, and yet it has not made a huge splash in the academic world. 'Ours is not a popular theory,' Belsky says. 'It is treated like a biological determinism theory, and that gives it a bad name among some people. They think we're saying biology is destiny here, but this is a theory of nurture not nature.' (Belkin 2000)

Quoting her conversation with Herman-Giddens, Belkin continues on this theme of the cultural discomfort triggered by Belsky's and Ellis' research:

[13] Other research focuses on the effects of childhood abuse and neglect. Brown *et al.* (2004), for example, studied 816 American young people who had been in care, finding that those who had experienced more than two incidents of officially documented sexual abuse were more likely than others to go through puberty early. This research reminds us of the origins of Hermann-Giddens' interest in early onset puberty (described in Chapter 3): a correlation between incidence of sexual abuse and earlier onset puberty. In related research in which Ellis is one author, Deardorff *et al.* try to disentangle the effects of father absence, body mass index, family income and ethnicity on pubertal timing. Although hypothesising that girls from lower-income father-absent families would develop earlier because of compounded stress, their results indicated the opposite: that 'father absence predicted earlier onset of breast development only in higher-income families and onset of pubic hair development only in higher-income African-American families' (Deardorff *et al.* 2011: 441). Unsurprisingly the authors were unable to identify 'social and biophysiological mechanisms' through which these effects occurred (2010: 441).

Whatever they are saying, it is not taking hold on the playgrounds or at P.T.A. meetings or in the research papers of other developmental scholars. The fact remains that while research tends to mirror our fears, we can't always handle what is learned. The absent-father hypothesis is 'a theory that makes us look inward, and we don't tend to like to do that,' Herman-Giddens says. 'We like to point fingers at something simple, but we don't like to make complicated changes in our lives.' (Belkin 2000)

I agree with Herman-Giddens that there is much potential discomfort here: such claims raise difficult questions of responsibility for physiological and social events. Belsky and colleagues' recent repositioning of their work within epigenetics, a field focusing on the interactions of genes, proteins, bodily systems and social experience, only intensifies these dilemmas (see, for example Belsky and Beaver 2011).

Theorising about the biological significance of present fathers runs serious risk of affirming a heterosexual, two-parent model of the family that is neither desirable nor possible for many people.[14] Sociological studies in the UK and the USA report increasing numbers of (both lesbian and heterosexual) women choosing to have and rear children without men's active involvement (Pringle 2004; Bradshaw and Richardson 2009; Bradshaw 2011), with notably higher rates of single-female headed households in the USA than in Europe and, in the USA most notably, within black and working-class communities (Ellwood and Jencks 2004).[15] Importantly in relation to discourses about the biological effects of absent fathers, both American and British studies have shown that these single-parent living arrangements do not necessarily mean that fathers are not involved in their daughters' lives: many fathers live nearby and children often have meaningful

[14] It is important to note that some scientists working in this field are aware of such potential: as early as 1982, Draper and Harpending noted that research in the area had been undertaken by people who were 'products of Western culture and upper socioeconomic class' who assumed that their own ideal family forms led to the highest reproductive 'fitness' (Draper and Harpending, 1982: 256). Their attempt to outline the role of social learning, like Belsky *et al.*'s (1991) later focus on the effects of stress and attachment formation, tries to distance itself from moral presumptions about the most appropriate family forms. Indeed, Draper and Harpending (1982: 270) note that, despite massive social disapproval, working-class teenage mothers in the 1980s show more 'reproductive fitness' than their college-educated middle-class comparators.

[15] See Hancock (2004) for a detailed analysis of the 'public identity' of black single mothers in the United States.

and regular contact with them (Bradshaw and Richardson 2009; Bradshaw 2011; Way and Stauber 1996).

Arguments suggesting that certain kinds of familial structures may have negative biological effects are potentially inflammatory. Commentaries on this research slip easily into reproducing oppressive social norms: Kaplowitz, for example, moves seamlessly from his discussion of research on absent fathers to noting rates of 'out-of-wedlock' births, mentioning that black girls have higher rates of such births than white girls: 'Many girls born out of wedlock are raised in homes without their fathers, so this is another area that needs further investigation' (Kaplowitz 2004: 92). This shift from absent fathers to out of wedlock births is problematic: one does not need to be married to be present in a parenting or partnering capacity. As noted above, this section also seems to misunderstand Belsky *et al.*'s point about stress that it takes more than having an absent father for an individual to be led down the path of early development.

Developmental psychologists are on dangerous territory when making claims about the likely effects of early childhood experiences on sexual development: cultural beliefs about 'inadequate' or 'poor' parenting are always based on historically and geographically specific norms and cannot be easily measured or assessed. Much social scientific scholarship seriously criticises contemporary attempts to delineate 'positive' parenting strategies, noting that the attempt to do so is often linked to conservative social policies in which poverty and related forms of suffering are blamed on 'bad parenting' rather than on economic and cultural deprivation, thus creating an oppressive and unjust culture of blame in which necessary services such as affordable childcare, adult education and healthcare are withdrawn and replaced with parenting classes (Hancock 2004; Furedi 2008; Jensen 2010; 2012). Restrictive focus on the family in theorising children's 'socialisation' is also conceptually unconvincing. Family forms are but one element constituting children's social worlds: childcare, schooling, economic and social structures (including racism and heterosexism), friendships, communities and cultural activities all play important roles.[16]

[16] Belsky also has a substantial and controversial track record in research on childcare in which he argues that poor-quality childcare can have serious long-term effects on children's development (Belsky 1990; 2001; Belsky *et al.* 2007).

Finally, early stress (whether caused by neglect, poverty or racism) is not straightforwardly transformed into biological or behavioural 'outcomes'. Current literatures on the effects of early trauma emphasise significant individual differences (often conceptualised as 'resilience') resulting in various outcomes, even for children coming from the same families (Agaibi and Wilson 2005). Although difficult early experiences may well have biological and/or behavioural echoes, these are neither inevitable nor straightforward: the biological, social and psychological are in on-going interplay over an individual's life, and perhaps particularly in early childhood (Rutter 2006).

Given all these concerns, feminists might be tempted simply to dismiss developmentalist arguments about pubertal timing. What remains potentially important for feminist theorising, however, is their focus on the productive interplay between social, psychological and biological forces. Is there any way in which these arguments might help tell a more complex and less politically regressive story about sexual development?

Bio-psycho-social entanglements: emergent ecologies

During her interview with Belkin for *The New York Times*, Herman-Giddens presents a PowerPoint slide show on the possible causes of early puberty. After slides on genes, obesity and absent fathers, she introduces a new topic. Belkin writes:

> Click. The last slide is of a jeans ad from a magazine. The female reproductive system is exquisitely sensitive to external influence, she says – as college women who room together know well, because their cycles often mysteriously fall into sync. 'Can visual images also have a biological effect?' Herman-Giddens asks. 'Does constant exposure to this sort of thing act as a premature trigger? I certainly think we need to find out.' (Belkin 2000)

Belkin describes Herman-Giddens' approach to this issue, suggesting that Herman-Giddens believes that the 'outside' or social world can produce biological effects:

> Marcia Herman-Giddens's view of the world is a constant back-and-forth between how things are and how they used to be. She describes standing in line recently with her 12-year-old granddaughter when 'I happened to notice that her eye level is exactly on the level with Cosmopolitan magazine. The headlines were "10 Ways to Drive Your Man Wild in Bed," and my

granddaughter was standing there, reading, looking at this half-naked woman. I'm thinking to myself, I wonder what in God's name is going through this child's mind. It's in their face, all the time, literally.'

Considering the various theories has led her to develop a hypothesis of her own. 'If you watch somebody cut a grapefruit from across the room, you're going to salivate,' she says, 'which is just one example of how what you see can have a biological effect on your body. We worry about what all the violence is doing to children. Well, what about all the sex? While we're doing all this research, we ought to be researching that.' (Belkin 2000)

This suggestion returns us to my introductory chapter, in which I described intense contemporary concerns about the 'sexualising' effects of contemporary cultures in which children are said to be constantly exposed to adult sexual desire and representations. Most existing research examining the link between television-watching and early puberty, however, does not study the content of programmes but rather the sheer volume of time spent watching, arguing that children who watched a lot of television had disturbed melatonin levels, which affected sleep patterns and thus pubertal development (Hooper 2004). Other research, building on work arguing that watching 'sexy media' is likely to lead to sexual activity, claims that early puberty creates interest in sexual media which then leads young people into sexual activities (Brown, Halpern and L'Engle 2005). Such studies run the risk of making overly simple, causal connections between images, bodies and practices/behaviours. What counts as 'cause' in this work is messy: is television-watching a cause of sexual interest or a symptom of it? Are early sexual practices a result of biological changes or a reflection of encultured interests? How might we theorise these connections in ways that articulate more dynamic flows?

Much cutting-edge developmental science tries to move away from simple determinist accounts, arguing instead for dynamic models of cumulative change (see, for example, Fausto-Sterling, Coll and Lamarre 2011a; 2011b). It is to this field, in my view, that the literature on adoption and early parenting might make a useful contribution by highlighting the complex intertwining of bio-psycho-social factors in sexual development. Ellis, interestingly, cites dynamic change models when he writes, 'Genotypes are capable of producing a range of phenotypic expressions, and actual timing of puberty is an emergent property of the genotype and the environment in which it occurs'

(Ellis 2004: 924). The term 'emergent', I suggest, does a lot of relatively undescribed but potentially important work here. Figured in opposition to claims of biological determination, cause or programming, the term signals both that causes are multiple and that outcomes are not fixed.

Feminist biologists Anne Fausto-Sterling and colleagues also use 'emergence' to describe processes of sexing that occur from birth to age 3 in humans, arguing that models from dynamic systems theory can illuminate that fact that 'experience changes the body and is not merely driven by events internal to the individual' (Fausto-Sterling, Coll and Lamarre 2011b: 1700). In distinction to Ellis, however, Fausto-Sterling and colleagues lean heavily on the term 'embodiment' in theorising the development of sex differences in early childhood, arguing that 'embodiment is a social process' in which social interactions affect neural development via hormonal signalling (2011b: 1697). This term forges a connection to more philosophical feminist work on bodies, including that of Elizabeth Grosz, Rosi Braidotti and Elizabeth A. Wilson, which, as I described in Chapter 2, argues that bodies are inextricably part of physical, cultural and psychical environments or worlds.

Haraway (2008: 135–6) is more cautious in her embracing of the term emergence, writing in a footnote to her own use of the word that 'I would now demote the language of emergence in favour of reciprocal inductions in order to stress that there is no emergence from a thing in itself, but always a relational knot of intra- and interactions' (2008: 356). Although fine, this distinction is significant: like Mol's argument against new materialist accounts of ontology (described in Chapter 4), Haraway's note marks the intrinsic relationality of worlds as temporary congealments of actors and forces. Nothing in such ontologies is fixed or certain. Morphing a well-known Hindu cosmological myth in which an elephant holds up the world, Haraway writes: 'Historical specificity and contingent mutability rule all the way down, into nature and culture, into naturecultures. There is no foundation; there are only elephants supporting elephants all the way down' (Haraway 2003: 10).

If emergence runs the risk of misrepresenting ontologies as foundational, what other language might capture what is valuable in the mixing of findings, feelings and figurations that are latent in the literatures on adoption, early stress and sexual development? In a report on early onset puberty published by the US-based National Breast Cancer Fund (which I will discuss in detail in the next chapter), ecologist Sandra Steingraber (2007: 59) suggests that 'Early puberty is a phenomenon best understood as an ecological disorder.' Whilst wanting to refuse the naming of early puberty as a disorder, I want to suggest that the term 'ecological' might do some useful work in describing the enactment of bodies-in-worlds. As in science studies theorist Susan Leigh Star's (1995: 2) phrase 'ecologies of practice', this term signals a refusal of social/nature and social/technical dichotomies and a desire to 'invent' new modes of analysis.

Christine Hughes and Celia Lury (2013: 786) also propose an 'ecological methodology' for thinking about how 'we live in relation to, and are of, a more-and-other-than-human world'. Borrowed in their case from Isabelle Stengers (2000; 2010), the term 'ecological' signals the multiple, dynamic and entangled nature of entities and causalities and, indeed, creations of meaning. For Stengers (2000: 86), and thus for Hughes and Lury, an ecological methodology requires us to '"dream along with" other disciplines in constructive, rather than deconstructive or destructive practices' (Hughes and Lury 2010: 792).

Thinking of early puberty as part of a sexual bio-psycho-social ecology opens up space not just for thinking about how the social produces embodied differences, but how such processes or 'systems' evolve within and through wider worlds. Early puberty not only emerges through the social but makes it in a particular way: sexual development is thus always political, as is any ecology. Early sexual development matters because it changes our sexual landscapes and alters the potentialities of girls' bodies and actions. As in environmentalist and scientific accounts of physical ecologies, changes in one area are important partly because of their effects on others: what matters about girls going through puberty earlier is whether this produces new bio-psycho-social sexual worlds that may reduce rather than expand girls' potential becomings.

Campaigners organising against the 'sexualisation' of girls argue that contemporary media and popular toys and clothes are stripping children of their inherent sexual innocence, forcing them to engage with modes of 'adult sexuality' before they are ready to do so (Rush and LaNauze 2006; Andrusiak 2009; Reist 2009). Feminist critics of such claims argue that appeals to childhood innocence are both historically and geographically specific and themselves limiting for children and that their descriptions of sexualising effects of mass media representations figure girls as passive and naive consumers. Sociologists Danielle Egan and Gail Hawkes (2008a: 293–4) write, for example, that 'The discourse of sexualization promotes a mechanistic and passive construction of the child. As a result, the discourse on sexualization fails to acknowledge the complexity and multiplicity of reader response and ignores how children might submit to as well as subvert particular cultural messages as well as forms of fashion and commodification' (see also Harris 2004 and 2005; Bray 2008; Egan and Hawkes 2008; Hawkes and Egan 2008; Egan 2013; Attwood and Smith 2011).

Empirical studies in various countries have shown that girls do actively engage in and sometimes resist 'sexualizing' discourses: drawing on ethnographic data about three British girls, for example, Emma Renold and Jessica Ringrose argue for a Deleuzian theorization of their relation to contemporary sexual cultures. Troubling binary logics of passivity versus empowerment, they suggest that these girls navigate and perform 'new schizoid formations of subjectivity,' both expressing 'female desire' and being 'caught up in' limiting models of it: embracing the term 'slut' to avoid sexual regulation, for example (Renold and Ringrose, 2011: 403–4). Rebecca Coleman (2008) makes a related argument, using Deleuze's theory of becoming to explore the ways in which teen girls' bodies come into being through engagement with media images. Although diverse, all of this work refuses to figure girls as pure, arguing instead for recognition of their affective and effective activity.

In collating explanations of the causes of early puberty in this chapter, I run the risk of positing a potentially 'pure' space or time of sexual development in which girls are subject to none of these factors and are hence 'free' to develop as they somehow should, thereby becoming happy and healthy. Within such a framing, if we deal with obesity, reduce exposure to environmental toxins and parent our children well, sexual development will return to normal; the crisis will be resolved. Worryingly, such an orientation chimes rather tunefully with problematic elements of anti-sexualisation politics, reproducing a sense of a desirably innocent and 'healthy' form of childhood sexuality in which children's sexual interests and desires are almost inevitably pathologised and/or constrained.

Resisting such a move, my framing of puberty as 'ecology' aims to stay with the problem. Whilst I agree that claims about childhood innocence tend to figure girls as passive, our engagement cannot end there. Sexual development happens: over time children turn into adults and begin to enact 'adult' sexualities. Sometimes this is not a pleasant, exciting or welcomed process; sometimes it is. In either case, puberty is a bio-psycho-social flow of situated bodies; the result of intra-actions of a wide range of actors, an entanglement of findings, feelings, and figurations. Studying this process, I suggest, we would do well to listen to Haraway's assertion that 'Nothing is passive to the action of another, but all the infoldings can occur only in the fleshly detail of situated, material-semiotic beings' (Haraway 2008: 263).

Like Fausto-Sterling *et al.*, I find the term 'embodiment' helpful in thinking these intra-actions. As a form of embodiment, puberty is perhaps best thought of as:

> syntactically and materially . . . always a verb, or at least a gerund. Always in formation, embodiment is ongoing, dynamic, situated, and historical. No matter what the chemical score for the dance – carbon, silicon, or something else – the partners in infoldings of the flesh are heterogeneous. That is, the infolding of others to one another is what makes up the knots we call beings or, perhaps better, following Bruno Latour, things. Things are material, specific, non-self-identical, and semiotically active. (Haraway 2008: 249–50)

The range of explanations of early onset puberty discussed in this chapter highlights the complexity both of contemporary scientific knowledge production and of pubertal bodies themselves. Enacted in these discourses, pubertal bodies are indeed 'material, specific, non-self-identical, and semiotically active'. Sometimes overweight and/or poorly cared for, sometimes shaped by childhood stress and/or exposure to endocrine-disrupting chemicals, pubertal bodies are always in-the-making in particular flows or folds of time and space. In my view, none of these 'factors' will ever provide an explanation of early development on its own; we need instead to keep exploring early maturing bodies as dynamic multiples. On-going research in all these areas will doubtless continue to provide overlapping, contradictory and contested theories of sexual maturation: our role as feminists and social scientists, I suggest, is to work across these fields, exploring the ways in which their findings intra-act with feelings and figurations.

I have argued throughout this book that early developing bodies provoke widespread concern, from parents, clinicians, policymakers and journalists. But what is the specific nature of these concerns? And what scientific and biomedical evidence underpins them? The next chapter addresses these questions, picking up and working with Haraway's language of 'infolding' to explore the dynamic intra-actions of biological, social and psychological forces in enactments of pubescent bodies.

6 *Consequences of early onset puberty: sex, drugs and shortness*

Early development is considered an adverse effect because of its impact on outcomes in adolescence, such as accelerated skeletal maturation and short adult height, unwanted pregnancies, sexually transmitted infections, and psychosocial difficulties, and because of its potential impact on adult diseases such as breast cancer and elements of the metabolic syndrome.

(Hiatt *et al.* 2009: 1815)

Across the global North, sexually developing female bodies are culturally troubling. Adolescent girls' desire for new sexual experiences and potential to become pregnant are framed as problems requiring management through education, regulation and biomedicalisation (most notably via hormonal contraception). The reproductive capacities that are initiated in many – although not all – women at puberty are, like sexual intercourse, widely figured as something that should be 'saved for later', fulfilled only at an appropriate time. In biomedical and popular discourses such concerns also enact particular forms of sex/gender, class and race: different worries become attached to particular kinds of bodies.

Most feminist research in this area addresses public debates around teenage pregnancy, birth and parenting, sometimes undertaking empirical work with young women in order to produce critical counter-narratives in the face of significant misogyny and 'class disgust', to use Imogen Tyler's (2008) term. In her classic book *Feminism and Youth Culture* (1991), for example, Angela McRobbie tells stories about teenage mothers living in a deprived area of south Birmingham. Unlike the selfish or ignorant victims portrayed in news media and reviled in television comedy (Tyler 2013), McRobbie's research participants are resourceful young women trying to get by in the face of severely limited opportunities for employment, education, and physical and social mobility. Spending time with these women and their families, McRobbie notes that 'motherhood had pushed them towards a precocious maturity'; a maturity denied to their male partners who were unable to find paid employment (McRobbie, 1991: 227; see also Sharpe 1984). This experience of achieving maturity through motherhood is highly classed: the bodies of middle-class girls in contrast, as Walkerdine, Lucey and Melody's (2001: 215) interview-based research shows, have 'to be regulated at all costs' in order to avoid pregnancy and birth: indeed, pregnant middle-class teenagers are more likely to have an abortion than their working-class counterparts. The relative freedom of contemporary middle-class girls, McRobbie (2009: 85) later wrote, is contingent on not getting pregnant: 'Delay in age of marriage and also delay in the birth of a first child on the part of young Western women, are directly connected with their being able to come forward into the labour market.'

This enactment of contemporary middle-class femininity leaves working-class women who have children when they are young vulnerable to vilification both directly in social encounters and indirectly in media representations and debates. Building on Castañeda's work on the child (2002), Tyler analyses media representations as world-making figurations, arguing that figurations of working-class white young mothers reveal cultural anxieties about contemporary changes in reproduction. Referring to a Blairite British context, she (2008: 29) writes: 'The figure of chav mum has a particular resonance in terms of anxieties about fertility and motherhood and is used instrumentally to classify bodies according to more or less desirable forms of reproduction' (see also Tyler 2013).

Anxieties about young people's sexually maturing bodies are also expressed in media stories about sexually transmitted infections. Cultural theorist Cindy Patton (1995), for example, shows that North American media coverage of HIV articulates three forms of adolescence: (1) dominant white youth moving 'appropriately' from an innocent childhood through a stage of hormonally driven sexuality through to 'civilised adulthood' (i.e. heterosexual reproductive marriage); (2) gay youth moving from innocence to a male subcultural world that is outside civilised adulthood and (3) 'at risk teens' – young people of colour who are associated neither with innocent childhood nor with civilised adulthood. North American young people of colour, in other words, like young white-working class people in the UK context, are consistently rhetorically connected to risk (see also Hancock 2004;

Mamo, Nelson and Clark 2010: 133; Bute and Russell 2012); indeed Tyler (2013: 188) argues that the racialized figure of the chav 'bodies forth a whiteness polluted by poverty and contaminated by proximity to poor black and migrant populations'.

How does the figuration of black girls as 'at risk teens' illuminate the North American scientific and popular literatures on the effects of early puberty? As discussed in Chapter 4, black girls are said to be more likely to experience early onset puberty; one could imagine, then, that these literatures might highlight black girls as objects of particular concern. Whilst many scientists have explored 'racial' differences in sexual development, I argued in the previous chapter that such explorations are beleaguered by inevitable problems of categorisation: there seems to be little agreement about how to define membership in 'racial' categories. Counting such differences is difficult: accounting for them even harder.

Despite this epidemiological interest in 'racial' differences in pubertal timing, North American news media pay little attention to 'race' in their discussions of the *impact* of early sexual development. In these discourses, the girls figured as at risk represent normative categories: accompanying images commonly depict white, middle-class, able-bodied children (see for example Jamieson 2010; Moorhead 2010; Weil 2012).[1] This signals an important difference between figurations of girls going through early puberty and those of girls said to be at high risk of sexually transmitted infections or teenage pregnancy. Whilst the latter are seen as dangerous (literally contagious in some instances) and as draining of state resources and therefore requiring control and blame, early developers remain blameless. News media articles present early sexual development as a worry for parents, who are encouraged to act to protect their daughters' innocence. As I will argue in Chapter 7, pharmaceutical companies have much to gain from such worries. Girls experiencing early onset puberty are not a potential drain on state resources or source of contamination but instead constitute a growing and potentially lucrative market.

Despite this key difference, feminist research on teenage mothers provides an important methodological and political backdrop to this

[1] Rogers' (2007) *Mail Online* article, featuring a non-white and a white girl, is an exception. The same image was reused in Moorhead's (2010) article in *The Guardian* newspaper but not the online version.

chapter's exploration of gendered, classed and racialised discourses of sexual and reproductive risk. Exploring a range of scientific, biomedical, environmental and media discourses, I argue here that current enactments of the 'problems' posed by early sexual development – increased cancer risk, reduced adult height, and psychological and behavioural 'outcomes' relating to sexuality and risk-taking more broadly – demand critical feminist engagement. Discursive elaboration of these risks, as I will show, overflows the bounds of scientific and biomedical journals, often via health and science journalism, reverberating with wider public debates about the contemporary 'loss of childhood' and concerns about women's sexuality and reproductive capacities. As in earlier chapters, here I simultaneously take seriously the risks described in various scientific and related literatures and explore the logics of, omissions in and feelings associated with such descriptions through a critical feminist lens. Staying open to the possibility that early sexual development is articulated with physical, psychological and behavioural patterns or practices that might limit girls' lives in undesirable ways, I also keep a rather sceptical eye on the way that risks are enacted within particular literatures, contributing to figurations of reproductive and sexual crisis.

As discussed in Chapter 1, articulating a crisis means demanding that something should be done. Worries about the effects of early sexual development are linked to demands for action on both individual/familial and societal levels. In Chapter 7, I explore biomedical treatments of early puberty, asking questions about the physical, psychological and social implications of using hormones to delay sexual development. This chapter explores the justifications for such medications; that is, the effects they are intended to minimise or negate and the dangers thought to lie ahead for untreated girls. Starting with the most weighty, if less often emphasised, risk (cancer), it moves through physical risks (most notably reduced adult height) to psycho-social concerns, arguing that discourses of puberty in crisis intra-act with existing cultural anxieties in rather insidious ways, contributing to problematic figurations of (certain) girls' bodies as risky. Building on this discussion, I develop my alternative approach that explores early puberty and related physical and psycho-social phenomena as ongoing processes or foldings rather than cause and effect (that is, crisis).

Longer-term risks: cancer

In earlier work on sex hormones, biomedicine and feminism (Roberts 2007; chs. 5 and 6), I described debates around the risks of hormone replacement therapy for older women and the potential effects of endocrine disrupting chemicals on sexed bodies and human and non-human animals' health. These debates highlight historical connections between exogenous hormones (or hormonally active chemicals) and increased risk of cancer, particularly of the breast. Such hormones, to put it bluntly, are widely considered dangerous to women's bodies (although, as argued in the earlier book, they are also viewed as essential for health: dosage or amount of exposure is key here). In reading scientific, biomedical, environmentalist and news media discourses around early puberty, then, I expected such concerns to be prominent: as a hormonal process, early sexual development was likely to constitute a cancer risk. Somewhat surprisingly, however, concerns about cancer figure only minimally in the epidemiological and clinical literatures on early puberty. Although there is debate within cancer epidemiology about the effect of pubertal timing on breast cancer risk (see for example Hamilton and Mack 2003; Ahlgren *et al.* 2004) such concerns are not highlighted in most medical and scientific papers on early puberty. As exemplified in the epigraph to this chapter, clinical concerns focus on loss of adult height and the behavioural 'consequences' of early development.

Advocates and researchers interested in the environmental causes of breast cancer, in contrast, describe early puberty as an established risk factor and make connections to claims around exposure to toxins. In August 2007, for example, biologist and environmentalist writer Sandra Steingraber published a report for the American breast cancer prevention organisation, the Breast Cancer Fund, which claimed to be 'the first comprehensive review of the scientific literature on the timing of puberty' (Steingraber 2007: 5). In her executive summary Steingraber outlines 'What we know about the consequences of early puberty':

> Early puberty poses several risks for girls. *It raises the risk for breast cancer* and is associated with many high-risk behaviors in later adolescence –such as smoking, drinking, drugs, crime and unprotected sex – that have potential life-long consequences. Early-maturing girls are also more likely to suffer violent victimization and psychopathologies such as depression and anxiety. It is not clear whether the social or physiological experience of pubertal

change is responsible for these negative outcomes. In either case, interventions that reverse the trend toward ever-earlier puberty in girls are a public health imperative. (2007: 13, emphasis added)

This quote summarises many of the scientific and biomedical concerns about early puberty (although interestingly leaving aside the most straightforwardly medical and most frequently researched issue – that of reduced adult height). It states as 'fact' ('what we know') that early puberty is 'responsible' either directly (physiologically) or indirectly (socially) for a range of serious outcomes that need to be addressed by public health initiatives: using words such as 'risks', 'life-long consequences', 'responsible for' and 'imperative', the text establishes a crisis requiring action.[2] The Breast Cancer Fund's Executive Director Jeanne Rizzo affirms Steingraber's emphasis on breast cancer in her preface: 'The reports and images [of early puberty] are deeply disturbing. *For breast cancer advocates, there is something else that is disturbing*: early puberty increases breast cancer risk' (in Steingraber 2007: 5, emphasis added). Written for clinicians, scientists and members of the public (2007: 8–9), this report uses early puberty to make an argument about breast cancer prevention.

Reviewing the scientific literature, Steingraber uses nine studies to argue that 'early puberty, as measured by onset of menarche, is a well-established risk factor for breast cancer. As age of menarche decreases, overall risk of breast cancer increases' (2007: 24). An additional study, she notes, reports a 'modest' increase in mortality from breast cancer for breast cancer patients who went through early puberty (2007: 24). 'The mechanism' for this connection, Steingraber argues, 'is not entirely clear', but seems to involve two aspects: increased lifetime exposure to estrogens; and the role of early breast growth in creating a 'wide "estrogen window" that is thought to be favourable to the future development of breast cancer' (2007: 25). In both framings, early puberty increases carcinogenic exposure to estrogens, enabling Steingraber to make connections to existing debates about estrogen-disrupting chemicals and to promote messages about organic farming, the regulation of industrial chemicals and environmental justice (2007: 60–3). Although ostensibly about research on early puberty ('What we

[2] Steingraber's text makes a distinction between 'social' and 'physiological' experiences, as if these could be separated. My argument refutes this standard dichotomy.

know, what we need to know'), this report uses 'the falling age of puberty in U.S. girls' to promote the Breast Cancer Fund's core message about complex disease causation and the importance of proactive cancer prevention strategies. In its final sentence, Steingraber writes, 'Known as "bias for action," this early identification and response approach, which is community-based and collaborative, holds much promise for addressing the problem of early puberty in U.S girls' (2007: 63).

In a scientific review article describing their national research programme, the US-based Breast Cancer and the Environment Research Centers [BCERC] network similarly figures puberty as an inherently risky period of hormonal change and 'exposure':

> Two major hypotheses are being investigated by BCERC: First is that puberty is a window of biological susceptibility to carcinogenesis; second is that the advent of puberty initiates a window of hormonal stimulation ending in menopause. (Hiatt *et al.* 2009: 1815)

Early onset puberty, Hiatt *et al.* argue, brings such risk forward, extending its length and therefore the chance of developing cancer in later life; like Steingraber, they claim that the risk for breast cancer among those with an earlier age of menarche is 1.2–2.2 times greater than for those who have later menarche (2009: 1815). Puberty is thus 'a critical period during which to assess the impact of exposures to endocrine disruptors in the environment that interfere with normal hormonal synthesis and metabolic pathways, such as agents in the families of phenols, phthalates, and phytoestrogens' (2009: 1815).

Debates around the role of endocrine disruptors in increasing breast cancer risk are immersed in international breast cancer politics, with some organisations – those more closely aligned with corporate and/or medical and scientific interests – refuting others' claims about environmental toxins.[3] Sometimes, then, as on the website of Breakthrough Breast Cancer (UK), the effect of early puberty on increasing breast cancer risk is presented as only 'small and gradual' (www.breakthrough.org.uk/about-breast-cancer/breast-cancer-risk-factors/our-genes-and-bodies). For this organisation, breast cancer risk is not related to hormonally active chemicals: 'Overall, there is no good

[3] For a critical consumer organisation's view, see http://bcaction.org/our-take-on-breast-cancer/environment/; for academic work, see King (2008) and Klawiter (2008).

evidence that exposure to environmental chemicals increases your risk of breast cancer, based on the levels you would normally be exposed to in the UK' (www.breakthrough.org.uk/about-breast-cancer/breast-cancer-risk-factors/our-surrounding-environment). Significantly, pubertal timing is discussed on the page about 'our genes and bodies' rather than the page entitled 'our environment'.

More critical organisations, like Breast Cancer Action, Breast Cancer UK and the Women's Environmental Network, raise questions both about early puberty as increasing potentially risky exposure of breast tissue to toxins as described above and as itself an outcome of exposure to the endocrine disruptors that may be involved in breast cancer. They engage in political actions around endocrine disruptors (bisphenol A for example), promoting the precautionary principle that chemicals should be regulated and controlled unless there is clear evidence of safety. In contrast, as Samantha King makes clear, pharmaceutically sponsored elements of the movement, such as National Breast Cancer Awareness Month (NBCAM) and the American Cancer Society, 'continue carefully to avoid environmental issues, or indeed reference to prevention in general', preferring to focus on screening (King 2006; xxi).[4]

Despite the concerns of breast cancer activists and the scientific work in this field, the question of increased risk of breast cancer is not covered in Kaplowitz's (2004) otherwise informative and critical book for parents. Like the clinical literatures he cites, he emphasises more immediately significant risks: those occurring in childhood and adolescence such as effects on height and on sexuality-related behaviour. This may be because, as Hiatt *et al.* (2009) stress, understanding early puberty and breast cancer risk requires transdisciplinary approaches that exceed and challenge conventional divisions of scientific labour. Other foci, such as adult height, are far simpler to research and are more easily configured as sites of action in a crisis. As I have suggested, however, environmental arguments about cancer risk are also aligned with left-leaning and anti-establishment politics, and so may be more likely to be seen as somehow tainted or unreliable by some authors.

[4] NBCAM was founded by Zeneca (now AstraZeneca), the manufacturer of tamoxifen, the best-selling breast cancer drug, who were until 2000 'under the auspices of Imperial Chemical, a leading producer of the carcinogenic herbicide acetochlor, as well as numerous chlorine and petroleum-based products that have been linked to breast cancer' (King 2006: xxi).

Longer-term risks: reduced adult height

Significant impairment of final height in untreated CPP has dominated the rationale for intervening with GnRH treatment. (Mul and Hughes 2008: S5)

The most frequently described risk posed by early onset puberty concerns growth: children going through early puberty are at risk of being shorter adults. As Tanner and Whitehouse (1982) confirmed in their ground-breaking longitudinal study (described in Chapter 3), puberty involves a growth spurt initially involving growth in feet and hand bones, then legs, arms and trunk. This growth – its initiation, progression and form – is of great scientific interest and has been much studied. Early growth spurts also finish early and raise concerns that 'full' or 'expected' adult height will not be 'achieved'. The child's young age means that processes of bone lengthening cannot fully unfold; growth is prematurely capped when high levels of estradiol in late puberty lead to the fusing of skeletal growth plates, the zones of soft cartilage from which bones grow.[5]

Systematically analysing international medical research on bone growth, Anne Fausto-Sterling (2004: 1504) points out that 'many studies on children and adolescents address the contribution sociocultural components of bone development [including diet, exercise and body weight] make to male–female differences that emerge just after puberty'. In sharp contrast, these factors are usually ignored in the literature on early onset puberty, which focuses on the physiological aspects of bone growth, articulating development as an intricate biological process involving hormones, hormone receptors and genes. As I will suggest, such an emphasis is closely tied to discourse and practices of using hormonal medications to delay or block puberty.

Early maturing girls are usually tall at diagnosis compared to their peers. Rather than focusing on an absolute measure of shortness, the biomedical literature describes the effect of early development on individuals' 'target heights', calculated by averaging the height of both birth parents and adding 2.5 inches for boys and subtracting 2.5 inches for girls. Girls who develop early are said to be less likely to reach their target height.

[5] A stream of contemporary research focuses on the hormonal processes involved, often using mouse models: see for example Vanderschueren and Bouillon (1995); Biro *et al.* (2001); Chagin and Sävendahl (2007); Börjesson *et al.* (2010).

In making decisions about whether or not to treat early developing girls, 'likely final height' is predicted using hand X-rays to measure 'bone age'. These X-rays are visually compared to images from an atlas of X-rays taken in the 1930s and 40s of 'healthy white children in the Cleveland area' (Kaplowitz 2004: 55) by Greulich and Pyle (1950) that function internationally as normal standards in the same way Tanner's pubertal stages do. These visual comparisons, according to Kaplowitz, are 'somewhat subjective': 'It is not uncommon', he notes in his parental guide, 'for readings to differ by about a year between the endocrinologist and the radiologist' (Kaplowitz 2004: 55). Height predictions are then made using charts developed by Bayley and Pinneau in 1952 based on Greulich and Pyle's (1950) original atlas. Although these charts perform well to analyse the growth of large populations, Kaplowitz writes, they do not work so well in clinical settings to predict height outcomes for specific girls: 'When one looks at *individual* girls, in some cases the height is slightly overpredicted and in other cases it may be slightly underpredicted, so I tell parents that the height prediction I give them is my best guess but could be off by up to two inches in either direction' (Kaplowitz 2004: 60, emphasis in original).

As in Tanner's case, the use of these images as norms or standards is problematic. Some scientists have argued that the Greulich and Pyle's (and therefore Bayley and Pinneau's) norms are historically and racially specific – the children in the original study were 'upper class' and white – and lead to miscalculations of bone age and height, particularly for black girls (Loder *et al.* 1993; see also Mora *et al.* 2001). In 1977 Tanner and Whitehouse developed a more sophisticated method to predict height in normal children but Zachman *et al.* (1978) argued that the increased accuracy of Tanner's method did not hold for those going through early puberty. Despite a further revision, most clinicians still use the Bayley-Pinneau method (Bar *et al.* 1994; Proos *et al.* 2006; 2010; Carel *et al.* 2009). UK clinicians I have spoken to use 'Bone Xpert', software for automated bone age measurement from X-ray that relies on the Greulich and Pyle and Tanner-Whitehouse scales (www.bonexpert.com). As Proos *et al.* (2010: 35) state 'The only drawback of the GP [Greulich and Pyle] method was that it requires an experienced pediatric radiologist. Automated methods are being developed and may soon facilitate the use of the GP method for those less experienced.'

Most recent studies of the effect of early puberty on adult height discuss hormonal treatments, attempting in many instances to establish criteria for medical decision-making: that is, to answer the question: who will benefit from treatment? Of the 1,500 articles in my database of scientific and biomedical articles on early onset puberty, more than 300 concern treatments, focusing mainly on height outcomes.[6] Here it is clear that the articulation of a problem (loss of height) goes hand in hand with a proffered solution and attempts to optimise its use. In his parental guide, Kaplowitz writes: 'In my experience, parents worry most about the behavioural consequences of early puberty, while physicians ... tend to worry more about adult height' (Kaplowitz 2004: 62). Readily measurable and relatively predictable, height-related growth is a process in which intervention is comparatively simple.

But what might it mean to worry about a girl's adult height? Popular scientific literature on the psycho-social effects of shortness on boys argues that low height is linked with lack of academic achievement and economic success (Hall 2006). A similar discourse exists about 'tall girls', whose height has historically been (and is sometimes still) understood as so socially significant as to require treatment (Rayner 2008; Rayner *et al.* 2010). Height – too little or too much – can constitute a (highly gendered and gendering) social problem. (This is discussed in more detail in Chapter 7.) In the early puberty literature, however, this 'problem' is never spelled out: loss of adult height is widely assumed to be bad.[7] The word 'loss' is frequently used to describe height outcomes of early developing girls, as if that which would have been predicted was already theirs; something to be protected before it disappears. In the epigraph to this section, clinicians Mul and Hughes (2008: S5) refer to final height 'impairment', an even stronger term. Stressing the differences between predicted and final height, they emphasise that 'it has been calculated that height loss is of the order of 20 and 12cm in boys and girls respectively' in untreated children rather than outlining what

[6] As described in Chapter 2, this database compiles the results of systematic searches of scientific and medical literature made in 2012, using PubMed and Web of Science.

[7] Typically, Kaplowitz (2004: 58–60) provides an important counter example, pointing out that in at least one study, 90% of untreated girls ended up with a height in the 'normal' adult range, that is, 5 feet or greater and suggesting that height should not be a driving force in decision-making around medication.

might be achieved by treating children (Mul and Hughes 2008: S5). In contrast, Mansfield *et al.* (1983) report a modest increase of 3 cm in girls treated long term, whilst Massart *et al.* (2009) found that effects of treatment on final height were 'doubtful'. Mul *et al.*'s earlier work in The Netherlands reported an average increase of 5 cm in treated children: 'In girls, GnRHa treatment seems to restore FH [final height] into the target range' (Mul *et al.* 2000: 765).

It is hard to avoid the significance of culturally and historically specific aesthetic ideals here. None of this work describes medical or physical consequences of shortness, nor mentions the potential social benefits of not turning out to be 'too tall': girls' 'target' height is assumed to be 'normal' (that is, socially desirable). Cultural differences in valuing height – that shortness might constitute a rather different problem in The Netherlands (Mul *et al.* 2000) than in the United States (Boepple *et al.* 1991) or Thailand (Wacharasindhu *et al.* 2001; 2003; Jaruratanasirikul *et al.* 2011) – remain unexplored. Swedish psychologists Johansson and Ritzén make a similar critique, arguing that:

> It is remarkable that almost all studies have focused on the outcome in centimetres rather than on quality of life. The latter has been the subject of many short adults in general, with or without specific diagnosis, with or without treatment aimed to improve final height. To our knowledge, none of these studies is able to demonstrate that the quality of life is poorer among short adults than among those with average height. Neither has it been shown that adding some centimetres to the final height will significantly increase their quality of life. Therefore other factors other than final height should be considered when the decision to treat or not to treat girls with precocious or early puberty is made. (Johansson and Ritzén 2005: 127)

But what are these other factors? How might pubertal timing affect a girl's quality of life?

Risk-taking: sex, drugs and vulnerability

In the news media, in scientific and biomedical texts, in parental guides and online discussion forums, early puberty evokes concerns about female sexuality and its 'timing'. In Chapter 1, I quoted Lemonick *et al.*'s *Time* magazine article in which 'the potential psychological effect of premature sexual development' is described as 'even more troubling than the physical changes ... The fear, among parents and professionals alike', they argue, 'is that young girls who look like teenagers will be under intense pressure to act like teenagers' (Lemonick *et al.* 2000). In the UK, similarly, journalists depict early maturing girls as becoming emotionally 'teenage'. In the *Mail Online*, for example, Tanith Carey (author of *Where Has My Little Girl Gone?* [2011]) recounts a conversation with a mother of a 10-year-old girl: 'For Emma, the metamorphosis of her daughter Atlanta from a cherubic little girl into an angst-ridden mini-teen seemed to happen almost overnight' (Carey 2012). In the same publication, Tamara Cohen quotes a clinician affirming the 'strong link' between early development, early sexual activity and teen pregnancy:

> Dr Tabitha Randell, of Nottingham University Hospitals NHS Trust . . . said: 'We need to help parents deal with the physical and psychological consequences of early puberty which are very serious and can be very distressing for the child. There is a strong link with early onset of sexual activity when they are not emotionally ready, and with teenage pregnancy for which we already have the highest level in Europe.' (Cohen 2012)

Seen as producing forms of physical sexual maturity that are out of temporal step with individuals' mental states and age-appropriate social norms, early development heralds a disturbing set of psychosocial risks: that girls will become the sexual targets of boys and men who misread their chronological age; engage in inappropriate sexual activities and thus be at risk of pregnancy and sexually transmitted infections; even that they will desire sex before their peers (or before their parents wish them to). Elizabeth Weil from *The New York Times* writes:

> Social problems don't just increase the risk for early puberty; early puberty increases the risk for social problems as well. We know that girls who develop ahead of their peers tend to have lower self-esteem, more depression and more eating disorders. They start drinking and lose their virginity sooner. They have more sexual partners and more sexually transmitted diseases. (Weil 2012)

Psychological research supports and feeds these concerns. Julie Grabner, Jeanne Brooks-Gunn and Michelle Warren (1999: 110), for example, write: 'Early maturing girls are more likely to be unprepared emotionally and cognitively for the changes of puberty itself and the social pressures that they may experience from boys and adults who perceive them to be more mature than their age and experience.' In such discourses, early puberty is seemingly inextricably linked with teenage sexuality and all the dangers and pleasures that that entails. But what evidence underpins these worries?

For many, the effect of early puberty on sexuality seems almost too obvious to be researched. Clinicians and scientists publishing in paediatric endocrinology, and particularly those promoting hormonal treatments, tend to make rather simple statements about the sexual risks of early development, with little reference to research evidence and without any historical or geographic contexting. In their paper on GnRH analogues, for example, Mul and Hughes write:

> Few studies have evaluated psychosocial outcome following early or precocious puberty, but a long-term Swedish study reported more antisocial behaviour in adolescence and lower academic achievement in adulthood. There is evidence that normal, early maturing adolescents are more likely to have sexual intercourse and engage in substance abuse at an earlier age than normal or late maturing adolescents. (Mul and Hughes 2008: 5)

The Swedish study cited here, a paper by Therése Johansson and E. Martin Ritzén (2005) entitled 'Very Long-term Follow-up of Girls with Early and Late Menarche', was published in the journal *Endocrine Development*. The paper analyses findings from a long-term study of 456 girls born in one Swedish town in 1955, who were recruited, interviewed and measured at age 10, and then followed up at 13, 15, 27 and 43 years of age. Participants were asked detailed questions about their physical and psycho-social development. Not from a study of early puberty per se, these findings are used by Johansson and Ritzén to explore the long-term effects of timing of sexual development and particularly to address issues of quality of life.

Although 'in agreement with previous research, the study ... revealed that the mid-adolescent years were problematic in many ways for the early-maturing girls', Johanson and Ritzén found that quality of adult life was not diminished either by early puberty or indeed by height (2005: 130). Their key findings are summarised as follows:

- At age 15–16, girls with menarche before age 11 (early) were more norm-breaking, including being delinquents ... [and] had earlier advanced sexual experiences.
- By adult age, there were no differences in psycho-social adjustment between the early- and late-developed women.
- At ages 27 and 43, early-developed women had lower academic education.

- At 43, women with early menarche were shorter and heavier, had worse physical fitness and dieted more frequently compared to other women. There was no difference in quality of life. (2005: 126, formatting in original)

Although Mul and Hughes and many others cite this paper as evidence of the adverse effects of early development, then, its details indicate that the psycho-social effects of early puberty are short-lived and rather insignificant.[8] Indeed, Johansson and Ritzén (2005: 126) ultimately argue that 'the effects of early pubertal timing for psycho-social problems seem to be adolescent-limited'. Although noting that by age 43 most of the early developers had caught up with their later developing peers in terms of education, at age 27 and 43 the early developers did have lower academic achievements, despite equal IQ levels (2005: 132). Johansson and Ritzén (2005: 132) argue that these lower achievements were most likely due to earlier heterosexual relationships, often with an older partner. Such relations led to earlier childbearing and fewer opportunities to pursue education. This finding was statistically significant. Johansson and Ritzén write: 'Actually, heterosexual relations was the factor that correlated most strongly with social problems behaviors when the influence of pubertal timing and regular heterosexual relations were compared' (2005: 132). Early developing girls who did not become sexually involved with older boys, in other words, did not experience more psycho-social problems at adolescence than their later developing peers and did not have lower educational achievements (2005: 134). Socio-economic status, interestingly, was not technically significant in this.

It is important to note the historical context to which Johansson and Ritzén's research refers. Women born in 1955 went through puberty in the late 1960s, forming sexual relationships in the 1970s. It is unconvincing, to say the least, to draw inferences about contemporary girls from such dated examples. A paper by American public health researcher Carolyn Tucker Halpern and colleagues (2007), however, makes a similar argument based on contemporary young women's

[8] Google Scholar cites forty-five citations for Johansson and Ritzén (2005). Those I checked cited the paper as evidence of negative effects of early development (see for example Ong, Ahmed and Dunger 2006; Walvoord 2010; Berenbaum and Belz 2011).

experiences, comparing the timing of puberty to the importance of sexual relations. Entitled 'Perceived Physical Maturity, Age of Romantic Partner, and Adolescent Risk Behaviour', the article describes a questionnaire-based study of a nationally representative sample of 4,000 adolescents participating in the National Longitudinal Study of Adolescent Health. Questionnaires were completed by the participant on a laptop and pubertal stage was ascertained by self-assessment of 'physical maturity'.[9] Although the study found that advanced physical maturity increased the risk of girls becoming involved in sexual and drug-taking related behaviours, having an older romantic partner had a much stronger effect in this direction (Halpern, Kaestle and Hallfors 2007: 8).

These kinds of arguments are poorly cited by epidemiological and clinical researchers who instead make direct connections between early sexual development and sexual activity. They are also frequently misrepresented in news media reports. In part, this misrepresentation can be attributed to the processes by which scientific results are disseminated to journalists. Researchers are encouraged by their employing institutions to prepare press releases to promote their work, as press-released articles are more likely to be reported in newspapers and other news media (de Semir, Ribas and Revuelta 1998; Healy 2004). In such texts, complex findings are often simplified, with less surprising or culturally challenging findings highlighted (Woloshin and Schwartz 2002).

In March 2007, the University of North Carolina, Chapel Hill issued a press release about Halpern *et al.*'s work entitled 'Girls with Early Puberty, Older Boyfriends at Greater Risk for Drugs, Sex, Alcohol' (News Services 2007). This text emphasised the role of early development more strongly than of older boyfriends, thus misrepresenting Halpern *et al.*'s research. The text of this press release was faithfully reproduced in a range of medical and related websites, usually as if it were an original article. I came across it on public health websites, on websites for general practitioners and on a site for practitioners

[9] Respondents were asked to choose their own racial category and researchers later classified these responses into 'White, Black and Other' (Halpern *et al.* 2007: 3). Like social class (measured by one parent's highest educational achievement), however, race does not figure as an important category of analysis in the paper but rather something to 'be controlled for'.

involved in preventing sexual violence.[10] The story was also picked up by science journalists. Stefan Anitai's (2007) 'Early Puberty Makes Girls Prone to Sex and Drugs. And to Relationships with Much Older Partners', for example, was published on Romanian news aggregator and software download website softpedia.com. Using the text of the press release, Anitai figures early puberty as causal in girls becoming involved in relationships with older men, rather than reporting the finding that relationships with older men had a more significant impact on sexual activities than early development, referring in his only original sentence to early development as something that can 'turn nasty later on'.[11]

In contemporary contexts press releases do not simply provide resources for print journalists but are reproduced across multiple professional and lay websites without investigation, analysis or even comment. In this case, one scientific group's figuration of the connections between early puberty and sexual activity is made available for American doctors and sexual violence prevention practitioners and Eastern European technology geeks (amongst others). Media portrayals of puberty in crisis are strongly dependent on scientists' (re)figurations of their own work in press releases.

Epidemiological and clinical scientists and journalists also make strong claims about the impact of early puberty on drug and alcohol use. Again, these claims tend to simplify the arguments made in the relevant literature, which in some cases provides a more nuanced picture of the ways in which pubertal timing and 'risky behaviours' are connected. UK researchers Jennifer Downing and Mark Bellis (2009), for example, find in their questionnaire-based study of young British people that social class plays an important mediating role between early development and behaviours such as smoking, problematic alcohol use (drunkenness), fighting and risky sexual activity (unprotected intercourse).[12] Young people from poorer backgrounds

[10] See http://news.bio-medicine.org/?q=medicine-news/girls-with-early-puberty-at-greater-risk-for-drugs–sex–alcohol-19274; www.health.state.mn.us/injury/new/svpnnews_pdf.cfm?gcNews=93.

[11] http://news.softpedia.com/newsPDF/Early-Puberty-Makes-Girls-Prone-to-Sex-and-Drug-50131.pdf)

[12] American research by Negriff, Dorn and Huang (2010), in contrast, argues that racial differences do not mediate the impact of early development on smoking initiation.

were more likely to develop early and to engage in all of these behaviours at a relatively early stage (before age 14). Unable to sort out the causal relationships in their correlative data, Downing and Bellis conclude that their results 'suggest occurrence of early puberty should be explored as a potential factor influencing adolescent behaviour especially in deprived communities and as a possible contributor to health inequalities' (Downing and Bellis 2009: 554).

Claims about the role of social disadvantage in mediating the effects of early development sometimes appear in news media articles. Such articles figure poor, racialised young people as subjects in crisis, putting inordinate weight on the causal effects of early sexual development in explaining troubled lives. In her *New York Times* piece, for example, Elizabeth Weil argues for a biologistic causality in which early development itself increases risk-taking. Relying on the literatures on early childhood stress discussed in the previous chapter, she develops the idea that 'social problems' might be both an outcome of and a causal factor in determining pubertal timing. Quoting paediatrician Tonya Chaffee, Weil writes:

> 'You can almost predict it' — that early maturing teenagers will take part in more high-risk behaviors, says Tonya Chaffee, associate clinical professor of pediatrics at University of California, San Francisco, who oversees the Teen and Young Adult Health Center at San Francisco General Hospital. Half of the patients in her clinic are or have been in the foster system. *She sees in the outlines of their early-developing bodies the stresses of their lives – single parent or no parent, little or no money, too much exposure to violence.* Some of this may stem from the same social stresses that contribute to early puberty in the first place, and some of it may stem from other factors, including the common nightmare of adolescence: being different. (Weil 2012, emphasis added)

In confusing contributing factors and outcomes, Weil both evokes troubling figures and exemplifies the conceptual difficulties inherent to this field. As there are no 'pure' children to function as standards, disentangling the biological, the psychological and the social in sexual development is impossible.

It is fascinating to note, reflecting back on Chapter 3's discussion of Tanner's study of sexual development and Chapter 5's account of claims about early childhood stress, that half of the patients in the San Francisco clinic mentioned 'are or have been in the foster system'. Although to my knowledge not reported in the medical or scientific literature or in any other media article, this claim may be significant in conceptualising early onset puberty. Weil's article unfortunately shies away from addressing this issue. Avoiding discussing the possible contribution of early or current stress on early developing girls, she cites psychologist Julia Graber (mentioned above) to argue that early development triggers long-term emotional difficulties (specifically depression) rather than the reverse (although she does not follow through the logic of this to argue that early development leads children into foster care). The difficulties experienced by early developers, which Graber characterises as 'very serious' and 'severe', are represented as produced by a hurried childhood and lack of time for psychological development before encountering the 'challenges' of adolescence:

> Some of this may stem from the same social stresses that contribute to early puberty in the first place, and some of it may stem from other factors, including the common nightmare of adolescence: being different. As Julia Graber, associate chairwoman of psychology at the University of Florida, has shown, all 'off-time' developers – early as well as late – have more depression during puberty than typically-developing girls. But for the late bloomers, the negative effect wears off once puberty ends. For early bloomers, the effect persists, causing higher levels of depression and anxiety through at least age 30, perhaps all through life ... Graber offers a broader hypothesis, perhaps the best understanding of the puberty–depression connection we have for now. '*It may be that early maturers do not have as much time as other girls to accomplish the developmental tasks of childhood. They face new challenges while everybody else is still dealing with the usual development of childhood. This might be causing them to make less successful transitions into adolescence and beyond.*' (Weil 2012, emphasis added)

In retaining a focus on the sexual body as cause, the logic described here fails to consider the possibility that 'risky' adolescent behaviours might arise from subjectivities and circumstances directly associated with childhood stress. Although there may be biological consequences and/or correlates of these stresses (including early development) there is no need to figure these as causal (or even as mediating) in order to make sense of links between childhood deprivation and adolescent difficulties. As the feminist literature on teenage pregnancy cited earlier shows, young people who come from stressful backgrounds often continue to live in very difficult circumstances, engaging in activities described by researchers as 'risky' for complex reasons, both restrained by and resisting historically and geographically specific social norms.

Similarly, as discussed in Chapter 5, children fostered or adopted in order to remove them from physical and/or psychological danger often continue to experience their new (relatively safe) environments as dangerous and to act accordingly.

Claims about the effects of early development on mental health have been contested. In an article in *Social Science and Medicine*, for example, Norwegian psychiatrists Lien *et al.* (2010) argue that any negative effects of early development on mental health are transitory, disappearing as girls move beyond 15 years of age. Relying on survey responses from 1,377 15-year-old girls, and comparing their responses to a follow-up questionnaire completed three years after participating in a survey about sexual development at age 12, they write:

> In the analysis of the follow-up data there was no statistically significant difference in mental distress across age of menarche, even though the differences in body and weight satisfaction and average body mass index remained at the same level between baseline and follow-up. We therefore conclude that the effects of age of menarche on mental health problems are a transitory problem during puberty. (Lien, Haavet and Dalgard 2010: 529)

Similarly, in an earlier paper analysing ethnic differences in experience of distress around early puberty, comparing Eastern European, North African, Middle Eastern, sub-Saharan African and East Asian/Pacific immigrants to Norway with 'Norwegian/Western' girls, Lien *et al.* (2006) found girls' weight (BMI) had a much stronger effect than timing of puberty: 'the association between age of menarche and mental distress might be mediated via differences in current and desired weight', they argue (Lien *et al.* 2006: 285). Unsurprisingly from my perspective, attempts to disentangle distress from more obviously material factors such as weight often falter.

Other research comes to more negative conclusions about the mental distress of early developing girls, both reciting and reproducing the view that early puberty is usually connected to (and indeed causes) psycho-social distress, expressed through depression, poor self-esteem, self-harming behaviours and/or poor relationships with others. Based on quantitative studies of young people's self-reported experiences (published in, for example, the *Journal of Early Adolescence* or the *Journal of Research in Crime and Delinquency*), this work establishes correlations between early puberty and experiences of victimisation. Papers in this field by Nadeem and Graham (2005), Trembly and

Frigon (2005) and Schreck *et al.* (2007), for example, argue that for girls of all ethnicities going through puberty early leads to distress that can consequently lead to victimisation: distressed people, Schreck *et al.* (2007) argue, tend to be victimised more often because they are annoying.

As indicated above, these connections are also articulated by American psychologist Julia Graber and colleagues, who form the most prolific research team in this area. In a 1999 paper, for example, Graber, Jeanne Brooks-Gunn and Michelle Warren (1999: 110) state that early onset puberty is associated with 'poorer adjustment, including poorer body image, greater internalizing behaviors, and increased eating problems than other girls or boys'. Early maturing girls, they argue, 'are more likely to have lifetime history of depression, eating disorders, conduct disorders, and reported suicide attempts' (1999: 110). Although very interested in the role of weight in early development, Graber's group also suggest that conflict within families and peers and lack of approval is correlated with early onset puberty (Graber, Brooks-Gunn and Warren 1995; Graber *et al.* 1997; Graber *et al.* 1999: 111; Graber *et al.* 2004; Sontag and Graber 2010). Pointing out that most research on the effects of early puberty has been undertaken with white, middle- to upper-class girls, they stress that class and race need to be 'unconfounded' in future studies of early puberty and the intersecting roles of biological and social factors in sexual development explored (Graber *et al.* 1999: 112). Despite this, in a later paper they discuss research on non-white girls, arguing that it has 'often replicated and extended findings across ethnic groups ... The trend', they argue, 'has been towards similarity rather than differences in early timing effects' (Graber, Nichols and Brooks-Gunn 2010: 255). As noted above, however, this is not the case for social class: researchers claim that early developing young people from lower socio-economic groups are more likely to engage in risky behaviours than those from more privileged backgrounds (see for example Downing and Bellis 2009).

Psychological research runs into serious difficulties in its attempts to distinguish between the effects of family interactions and physical development. In Graber, Brooks-Gunn and colleagues' work, early sexual development, difficulties in family life and psychological and psycho-social problems during adolescence are causal factors that could and should be disentangled. In their 2010 paper, they approvingly cite a 'weathering' model drawn from Geronimus (1994) and Foster *et al.* (2008) to highlight the physical and subjective ageing effects of factors such as poverty and racism. 'Both physical and subjective weathering [the experience of feeling one is ageing rapidly] may be mechanisms that link childhood stress, maturational timing, and subsequent adult health-related behaviors and outcomes in females over the first decades of life', they suggest (Graber *et al.* 2010: 259). In Foster *et al.*'s study of the development of depressive symptoms across adolescence,

> Childhood trauma predicted earlier maturation in girls; earlier maturation was associated with increased risk for partner violence during adolescence, along with lowered rates of high school graduation; both partner violence and early maturation contributed to accelerated role transitions and subjective and physical weathering by young adulthood; these processes predicted depressive symptoms. Interestingly, as part of subjective weathering, early maturing young women reported feeling like they were older than other young adults – taking on more adult responsibilities, growing up faster. Such perceptions are to some extent accurate in that these young women had experienced more interpersonal traumas and stress resulting in earlier entry into adult roles. Further model testing may extend this model to other outcomes or this may be unique to depressive symptoms in girls and young women. (Graber *et al.* 2010: 259)

Although rhetorically evocative, the concept of weathering does little more than describe a set of possible connections between challenging life experiences and mental distress. The arrows in the diagram presented in Graber *et al.*'s article (see Figure 6) do not convincingly render causal relations: the chronological separations they describe between psychological trauma, physical maturation and psychological experiences of ageing remain arbitrary. It seems to me – as I will argue in the final section of this chapter – that rethinking the presumed separability of biological, social and psychological factors may provide more traction in theorising early development.

Overall, arguments around the connections between early development and sexual behaviour are rather weak. This runs counter to the overwhelming tendency in medical and epidemiological research papers to emphasise the 'obvious' problems of early sexual development. Analysing this field of medical and scientific research, psychologist Rachel Posner (2006: 316) suggests that it is imbued with racialising and classist anxieties about adolescent women's sexuality:

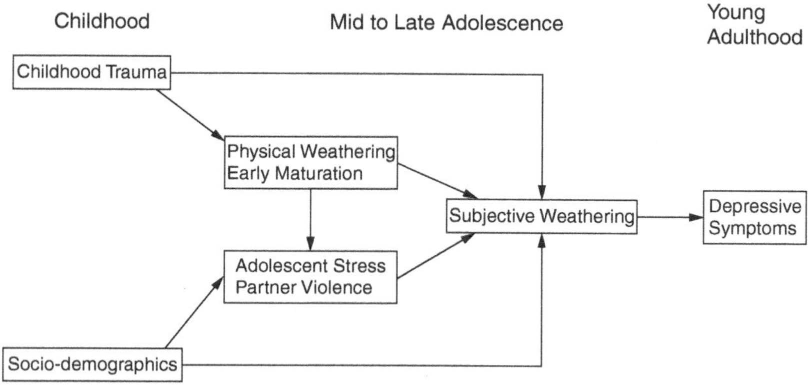

Figure 6 The 'Subjective Weathering' model, linking childhood experiences, maturational timing and depressive symptoms.

When educators, parents, and policy makers have expressed anxiety about 'adolescent sexuality' they have mostly referred to female adolescent sexuality. In many ways, to be an adolescent girl is to be over-identified as a sexualized being. Additionally, implicit in much of the research on teenage sexuality has been the assumption that to be urban, poor, and/or a member of an ethnic minority is to be hypersexual (Tolman, 2002). Accordingly, the focus of research into early puberty has almost exclusively targeted girls. Girls tend to suffer more negative psychosocial consequences related to early puberty than boys do, so this focus makes some sense. *Nevertheless, underlying the agenda of most of the research into the antecedents and consequences of early puberty has been a drive to control and limit adolescent girls' sexuality.* (Posner 2006: 320, emphasis added)

'This line of research', Posner continues, 'has aimed to determine how sexual behaviour among adolescents can be prevented' (2006: 320). Although the language of 'drives' and 'underlying agendas' is not one I find helpful, I have shown above that unexamined concerns about women's sexuality are repetitively enacted in these texts.

In a context of 'crisis', such concerns may have serious consequences, fuelling demands for and justifying potentially harmful actions. When uncritically racialising and classist distinctions between groups enter the frame, as Posner suggests they do, researchers enter even more fraught territory, running the risk of uncritically (re)articulating wider cultural concerns about black and working-class girls' sexual and reproductive behaviours in ways that affirm rather than challenge existing figurations, thus in part enacting the differences they claim to describe. As Patton (1995) and Tyler (2013) suggest, through such figurations black and working-class girls come to inhabit categories of 'at risk teens' which are problematically dissociated from both childhood innocence and civilised adulthood. But how might we think early developing girls' sexuality differently?

Puberty, childhood adversity and survival

Searching for feminist work on early puberty, I came across an article by US-based women's studies academic Kristina Pinto (2007) published in the *Journal of Early Adolescence*. Entitled 'Growing up Young: The Relationship between Childhood Stress and Coping with Early Puberty', the paper reports on a qualitative, interview-based study with sixteen African-American and white girls (she does not describe how racial identifications were made). In this work Pinto listens carefully to the voices of early developing girls: a practice that, as Posner (2006: 320) argues, is rare in the otherwise expansive literatures on the effects of early onset puberty. In doing so, Pinto comes to the stark yet compelling finding that, for girls living very stressful lives, the experience of early puberty is not particularly disturbing. Defining stressful lives as involving, for example, losing parents, being sexually abused or experiencing serious psychiatric problems, Pinto finds that such experiences tend to produce a demand on girls to 'grow up young' in any case. This claim echoes the notion of 'subjective weathering' described above but articulates early development in quite a different, less negative (or crisis-oriented) way.

At young ages, the girls in Pinto's study became aware of cruelty and social suffering, had to take on heavy social responsibilities, and/or were left to fend for themselves in unsafe situations. When puberty came early too, then, it was experienced either as just another issue to deal with (and a relatively minor one at that) or, more positively, as a physical embodiment of a sense of being more grown up than age-peers, a kind of physically recognisable sign of an already burgeoning maturity, brought on by adversity (Pinto 2007: 531). Pinto writes:

> To summarize the experiences of these inspiring girls, their narratives indicate that a history of childhood adversity can mediate the salience and meaning of early puberty for girls when the stressors occur in proximity to

the onset of puberty. Although stress served as a distraction from the significance of puberty or the risks associated with early timing for some girls, other girls noted that the developmental demands of early psychosocial adversity moderated the psychological difficulties often associated with early puberty. This is not to imply prior stress was unequivocally beneficial. (2007: 531)

As I have shown in earlier parts of this book, scientific, news media, environmentalist and public policy debates around early development and sexualisation tend to represent all young girls as sexually innocent and thus requiring protection from their own and others' sexual desires. Pinto directly challenges this representation, arguing: 'The effort to protect the inexperience and naiveté of girls assumes . . . that the young are unknowing of cruelties familiar to adults' (2007: 509). After analysing the narratives of development provided by the girls in her study, she returns to this issue:

[I]f puberty is cast as a crisis, early puberty is popularly considered to be psychologically and behaviourally endangering, akin to the sexualizing of a child. The narratives of the girls in this study suggest, however, that the puberty-as-crisis paradigm might not apply to some early developers who confront childhood developmental demands that accelerate the maturation process, whether socially, behaviourally, or intrapsychically. (2007: 532).

This research, as Pinto briefly points out (2007: 535), also challenges the literature on the psychological and social effects of early puberty at a deeper level. Citing the biomedical claim that childhood stress (such as international adoption) can 'precipitate' early puberty, Pinto asks whether existing studies of the effects of early puberty might not be regularly confounded by not controlling for such stress. That is, if childhood stress is correlated to behaviours such as drug-use and sexual activity *and* early puberty, how can the claim be made that early puberty is the *cause* of these behaviours? It would only be if thoroughly 'innocent' girls going through early puberty engaged in such behaviours that such a claim could be made. Importantly for my argument here, Pinto concludes that 'puberty implicates other narratives and does not operate independently'; there is, she argues, 'reciprocity between physical, emotional and cognitive development' (2007: 535–6). Thus, for her, 'puberty is not a singular and discrete catalyst for maturity and gender identification following the closure of childhood, but rather an outpouring of the past, channelling into womanhood' (2007: 536).

Pinto's research provides excellent direction for feminist work on early puberty. Her refusal to lump all girls into one category and her careful attention to how particular life experiences intersect with sexual development resonate with a feminist science studies approach that highlights the specificities of scientific knowledge production and the careful examination of the ways in which biological bodies are enacted across a range of sites (clinical, scientific and others). It also chimes with Egan and Hawkes' (2008) suggestion that feminist work on 'sexualisation' should pay attention to the specificities of particular groups of girls' experiences (see also Harris 2004; Renold and Ringrose 2013). Pinto's work highlights the importance of resisting overarching discourses of alarm about early sexual development, instead contextualising such development in the life histories of particular girls. Socio-economic deprivation or childhood neglect, for example, may play important roles both in how sexual development is experienced and in when it occurs. Experiences of racism may also have related embodied effects, as Anne Fausto-Sterling's work on hypertension (2004) and bone growth (2008) suggests.[13]

Hints of such connections can be found in existing literatures on early development. Finding an association between early sexual development and mental health problems in adolescence amongst Finnish teenagers, for example, Katiala-Heino *et al.* (2003) concede that 'Some previous research has suggested that psychosocial factors like problems in the family may trigger earlier onset of puberty ... There might be common underlying reasons for both mental health problems and early maturation, or the associations between psychosocial distress, early maturation and mental health problems might be reciprocal' (2003: 1062). This reference to reciprocity resonates both with Pinto's argument and with the core argument of this book: that sexual development is best understood as articulating entangled biological, social and psychological forces.

Theorising bio-psycho-social relations: puberty as folding

As discussed in the previous chapter, Haraway (2008: 263) describes embodiments as 'infoldings of the flesh'. Taken from biology, this term emphasises a movement inwards rather than outwards and fruitfully

[13] I explore this argument in my final chapter.

retains strong focus on the materiality of bodies. In embryological development, infolding refers to the folding in of outer layers to make a pocket in the surface; this is also known as invagination or gastrulation. This embryological simile is also explored by French philosopher Gilles Deleuze in his work on folds as dynamic and non-dichotomous relations. Reading Foucault's (1988) later work on the practices constituting Ancient Greek sexuality, Deleuze (1988) describes subjectivation as a process by which, through marriage and dietetic (pleasure-related) and sexual practices, individuals form a self and a relation to the self; forming an inside from without. Deleuze likens this to the invagination of embryological tissue in which the outside cells of the hollow sphere of cells known as the blastula clump together to form three concentric tubes that are the basis of the embryonic body which has an outside and an inside (Deleuze 1988: 98). In subjectivation, this process articulates a relation to power: 'just as power relations can be affirmed only by being carried out, so the relation to oneself which bends these power relations, can be established only by being carried out. And it is in sexuality that it is established or carried out' (Deleuze 1988: 102).

Thinking of puberty as a form of folding reframes it as a process of becoming involving biological, social and psychological forces. Commenting on the significance of Deleuze's concept, science studies theorist Geoffrey Bowker writes:

> The nature of the fold is to perpetually bring the outside within (folding) and the inside without (unfolding) – the false dichotomy between the two is both politically and philosophically charged: politically because we have a tendency to smuggle our 'inside without' back into our world as transcendent truth about the nature of reality . . .; philosophically, because it breaks up a world that by its very nature should be understood as one. (Bowker 2010: 129)

The language of the fold, then, avoids making non-credible distinctions between self, society and nature or configuring any part of this triumvirate as 'removed from time, flow, the world' (2010: 129). It is this sense of flow in time that resonates, I suggest, with Pinto's empirical findings about early maturing girls. As folding, sexual development remains a temporal process; an 'outpouring' or 'channelling' of the past, to borrow Pinto's words.

Theorising puberty as folding does not mean that all distinctions or categories are rendered useless. In research terms it still matters at some moments and in some ways to think with categories, as I have done in this book by focusing on findings, feelings and figurations. But it is important, Bowker argues, to do this without positing origins (see also Bowker and Star 1999). Thinking through folds 'gives us a way of understanding the world as inherently multiple and porous, without losing the value of categories' (Bowker 2010: 131). Because forces interpenetrate, categories are always approximations: we need then, as science studies theorists Helen Watson-Verran and David Turnbull (1995) argue, to think about both differences and similarities without 'hardening the categories' (in Bowker 2010: 130).

Using the concept of the fold should change research and writing practices. Bowker helpfully notes that it is not enough to proliferate scare quotes (and one could make the same argument about hyphens) to change established patterns of thought. 'If all the fold does it to put scare quotes around insides, outsides, identity and categories without changing practice', he suggests, 'then it is not so interesting. Through their very proliferation, scare quotes slowly fade into the background leaving old habits of thought unchanged' (2010: 131). Instead, Bowker argues for folded readings of science that bring together philosophy, history and science: he wants to recognise that the work of scientists, social scientists and humanities scholars, and the entities enacted therein, are folded into each other, into the socio-political realm and into a dynamic ontology (2010: 131). In this book I have attempted to produce such a reading of pubertal science through taking an ethnographic approach to texts. Throughout the chapters I have explored the ways in which pubertal bodies are enacted across and between scientific, biomedical, environmental, social scientific, news media, educational and feminist texts. In so doing, I have articulated a version of science that interpenetrates with related cultural discourses, parental practices, commercial activities and historical figurations of bodies, sex and sexuality.

Learning from Pinto's study and her articulation of puberty as an 'outpouring of the past, channelling into womanhood' (Pinto, 2007: 536) and from Haraway and Deleuze's use of in/folding, I want to argue that the biological, social and psychological processes that constitute puberty are foldings of personal histories (of care in particular), of material bodily encounters with the world (exposure to chemicals, nutrition and sunlight) and of broader social meanings and histories (what it means to be a girl or a woman). Pubertal bodies express these foldings; indeed *are* these foldings. Thus puberty is an infolding and an unfolding, a living of history in the present and the formation of new ways of being, a framing of potentialities.

In articulating this, divisions between biological, psychological and social causes and effects become decidedly blurry. As noted above, however, this is not to argue distinctions are useless or that puberty should always be studied or considered as an undifferentiated process. It is to suggest, rather, both that none of these elements should be posited as independent origins and that the consequences of studying or highlighting particular aspects of sexual development are serious. Research practices that isolate elements (genes, sexual behaviour, endocrine disruptors, height, for example) are always political interventions (whether intentional or unintentional).

As the psychologists I have cited above found, attempts to distinguish the effects of early sexual development on timing of sexual activity amongst girls is extremely difficult. Early developing girls, it seems, are more likely to have older boyfriends, and those with older boyfriends are more likely to engage in sexual activities. Attributing this directly to pubertal timing seems unnecessary and, as I will argue in the next chapter, potentially harmful. If going out with older boys is risky, might it not be better to help girls make safer decisions about partners or to help young men understand their own desires for relationships with younger (albeit physically developed) girls? Rather than trying to hold off pubertal development with medications, could efforts be focused on understanding the social and psychological dynamics of relationships that span age groups and helping young people to recognise and respect each other's differing needs? Early onset puberty, in my view, should not be figured as a trigger of problematic behaviour but configured as but one element of many girls' situated, embodied sexual lives.

Teenage motherhood could similarly be thought as a folding process in which physical capacities (fertility), desire for maturity and adult status, needs for care and love, and particular socio-material conditions fold together to form a young woman's and her child's life. Addressing any problems arising from such events can never be simple and should not be oriented simply towards biomedical interventions or indeed only towards educational ones focused on individuals (although this is not an argument against either of these in particular circumstances). Strategies for helping teen mothers or helping women avoid becoming mothers in ways that jeopardise their own or their children's happiness or wellbeing must be developed at wider social levels too: fighting poverty; opening up educational, political and cultural possibilities of expression; increasing women's capacities to act in multiple worlds, to express agency, to have effects, to care for themselves and others. Framing women's bodies as problems is utterly unhelpful in any of these endeavours and must be strenuously avoided.

Like Chapter 5, this chapter has discussed a wide range of claims about pubertal bodies concerning cancer, height, depression, risk-taking and sex. The intersections and articulations of scientific, medical, news media and environmentalist debates described here demonstrate the diversity of actors and stories constituting early sexual development as contemporary crisis. This diversity requires new modes of engaged feminist analysis. Interdisciplinary approaches, as suggested by Bowker, offer a form of story (re)telling that explores the links and disjunctures between variant disciplines and discourses and the movement of findings, feelings and figurations across a range of material-semiotic fields. These movements or flows are highly consequential; not only for how we articulate puberty-as-crisis, but also for how early developing girls are treated, both socially and medically. The next chapter, then, turns to issues of treatment.

7 *Treatments: pharmaceuticals, sex and suffering*

If you have a normal girl, a girl who's 8 or 9, there's a big ethical issue of giving them medicine. Giving them medicine says, 'Something is wrong with your body,' as opposed to, 'This is your body, and let's all find a way to accept it.'

(paediatric endocrinologist Louise Greenspan, quoted in Weil 2012)

The pharmaceutical company webpage advertising Lupron Depot injections for 'Central Precocious Puberty (CPP)' depicts a beautiful blonde girl of about 6 or 7 in a hot pink blouse smiling toothily to camera (www.lupron.com/). The medication – leuprolide acetate in depot suspension – was originally manufactured by Illinois-based Abbott Pharmaceuticals, tag line 'A Promise for Life' (www.abbott.com/index.htm) but now belongs to AbbVie, a new company formed when Abbott split in two in 2013. Abbott was formally part of Takeda-Abbott Pharmaceuticals, an American-Japanese group who claimed to 'Turn Science into Caring'. Lupron is used to treat several conditions, all of which are advertised here in a matching style: readers can click on a photo of a handsome man to read about prostate cancer or one of two glamorous women to find out more about endometriosis and fibroids. Clicking through to the pages on early puberty (or CPP), readers access definitions of the condition, information about symptoms and tests, and guidance about the medication and how to talk to children about early development. More spectacularly pretty children are pictured, with and without adoring mothers alongside them. Clicking on a flower icon for girls or a sailing boat icon for boys, parents can enter data to create a monitoring chart on which to track their child's progress once on Lupron and to record visits to clinicians. Clicking on a dollar sign icon, they are offered an 'Instant Savings Card' which will 'Save up to $150 off each LUPRON DEPOT-PED prescription (after a $10 co-pay expense)' for monthly injections or 'up to $1,000 off each LUPRON DEPOT-PED prescription (after a

$10 co-pay expense)' for 3-monthly injections. Such savings, visitors are told, can be of the order of $2,000 per year. Clicking on an icon of a phone, parents can 'talk live to a nurse' by calling a toll-free hotline.

In its mixing of economic, scientific, medical and advertising discourses, this website epitomises contemporary US arrangements for diagnosing and treating bodily conditions. Although accessible internationally, such websites are not part of the UK medical setting: there are no British equivalents for the most commonly prescribed puberty blocking pharmaceuticals, Prostrap and Zolodex (Fry and Stanhope 2004: 13). The National Health Service's website for citizens has a page on 'complications of puberty' but the information on treatment provided here is brief and generic and does not mention any particular medication or brand names. It simply states:

Depending on the cause, there are two ways early puberty can be treated:

- treating the underlying cause, such as a tumour
- lowering the high levels of sex hormones with medication to stop sexual development progressing

Treatment with medication is usually only recommended if it is thought that going through an early puberty would cause you problems later in life, such as having weak bones, or growing up particularly short. If this is not the case, having an early puberty will not usually cause any health problems. (www.nhs.uk/conditions/puberty/pages/complications.aspx, formatting in original)

Of course, parents with internet access in the United Kingdom or elsewhere could access the American website, although the AbbVie webpage may feel alien to British viewers unused to the direct marketing of pharmaceuticals and unfamiliar with private health insurance and talk of the commercial price of drugs.

In contrast to this notable national difference in information intended for parents, the medical literature on early onset puberty treatments addresses an international English-speaking expert audience. Rhetorically (if not materially) separated from the goal of promoting particular treatments, this literature articulates an international child–parent dyadic subject of treatment. Although most frequently coming from US-based research teams, it reports the use of hormonal treatments for early onset puberty across the developed world. Speaking to US and British medical regimes, in this chapter I both note the substantial differences between the two national health-care systems and cultures and refer to a broader set of international shifts – what Clarke *et al.* (2010) refer to as biomedicalisation – affecting them both.

This chapter explores the use of drugs like Lupron to treat early sexual development. Wanting to tread a careful path between critical and more open, even affirmative approaches, I work both with sociological literatures on pharmaceuticalisation and with Elizabeth Wilson's Baradian account of the intra-actions of children's bodies with medications. Engaging also with existing research into young trans people's use of puberty-blocking medications, I make an argument for paying close, sustained attention to the worlds that are made through using pharmaceuticals and for theorising drugs as active in the making of pubertal bodies.

The 'Promise for Life'

Although continually tipping its hat to medical expertise, the AbbVie site firmly encourages parents to access its information directly, representing it as disinterested and simply factual. Reading the website, even speaking live to an AbbVie Pharmaceuticals nurse, is presented as an important part of fully engaging in a child's treatment and ensuring treatment success. In the section 'Treatment Options for Central Precocious Puberty (CPP): Which CPP treatment is best for your child?' such actions become imperatives: something a parent 'should' do, that a child 'needs' and that constitute 'part of successful treatment':

> Your pediatric endocrinologist is the best authority on determining how and when to treat CPP. The medicine he or she prescribes can help slow or even stop the signs and symptoms of puberty until a more appropriate age for puberty to start up again.
>
> However, you *should* also learn as much as possible about the different types of treatments for CPP, because it can help you and your child prepare for the treatment process. After reviewing all of the options, you *should* discuss them with your pediatric endocrinologist. Once your child begins treatment, he or she will *need* to be monitored to make sure the medication is working. *Part of successful treatment* is keeping your child's appointments for medication and monitoring. (www.lupronped.com/central-precocious-puberty/treating-precocious-puberty.aspx; emphasis added)

What is figured here is not only a medical condition and its treatment, but also a contemporary child–parent dyad actively engaging with pharmaceuticals in order to give themselves time to manage puberty well. In the section 'About Central Precocious Puberty (CPP): When are early signs of puberty actually a sign of CPP?' parents read:

> Growth spurts, breast development, pubic hair, first periods . . . puberty is a time of big changes in your child's body. Normally, you have time to prepare for it. But what happens if your child starts showing signs of puberty at an age you think is much too young?
>
> **Central precocious puberty** (sometimes called "CPP" or "precocious puberty") is a condition where puberty starts too soon in children – usually **in girls under 8 years old and boys under 9 years old.** If you start seeing early signs of puberty in your child, you should talk with your child's physician. (www.lupronped.com/central-precocious-puberty/default.aspx, emphasis in original)

Again, parents are clearly told what they should do to manage their child's sexual development; that is, seek medical advice with a view to accessing Lupron.

Abbott's tag line 'A Promise for Life' cleverly condenses the aims of the contemporary pharmaceutical industry. As anthropologist Joseph Dumit (2012) argues, medications are increasingly figured as necessary to achieve a normal or healthy life; something to be taken for years, even permanently (see also Marshall 2009). In the North American context, this approach is intensely promoted through direct-to-consumer (television, radio, print and web) advertising in which both medical conditions and their pharmaceutical 'solutions' are elaborated. Such advertising, Dumit shows, produces consumers as self-monitoring active subjects, who recognise themselves as ill or at risk of becoming so (sometimes without experiencing any symptoms) and demand particular, branded treatments from their doctors.

Morphing Irving Zola's (1972) phrase 'medicalization' – developed notably by Peter Conrad (2007) – sociologists Simon Williams, Jonathon Gabe and Peter Davis (2008) describe this as pharmaceuticalisation: the increasingly ubiquitous use of medications to address bodily conditions that were previously understood as social or moral – children's challenging behaviour, shyness, alcohol addiction, sexual proclivities or inhibitions, for example. For Adele Clarke and colleagues (2010) these changes are part of biomedicalisation, a wider process focused on controlling and manipulating biological life through industrialised science, technology and medicine; what they call 'the Biomedical Technoservice Complex Inc.' (Clarke *et al.* 2010: 22). Biomedicalisation, Clarke *et al.* argue, orients itself towards 'actualizing optimal futures' involving 'engagements with regimes of risk and surveillance, extended responsibility for knowledge accumulation and consumption, and taking up new kinds of biomedically inflected identities' (2010: 23–4). The self in this model (or, in the case of early puberty, the child's body/self) becomes something to bring about, to tailor or transform. 'The Promise of Life' is a project to be achieved through engagement with technologies of reading, injecting, monitoring, attending. The sexually developed child emerging 'out of time' – that is, too early – can be enrolled into interventions that will hold her back. An early slogan for Lupron for central precocious puberty exhorted clinicians and parents to 'Pause the Child Within'; to use medication to return a child to a more 'normal' or desirable timetable.

Hormones, sex and the brain

Lupron is a gonadotropin-releasing hormone analogue: an industrially produced hormone that mimics the actions of gonadotropin-releasing hormone (GnRH) in the brain. As described in Chapter 4, at the onset of puberty this hormone messages the gonads (ovaries or testes) to begin sexual development.[1] Adding more of this hormone as medication paradoxically overrides this response by flooding the hormonal feedback circuits, although initially the treatment will trigger symptoms of sexual development, including menstrual bleeding.[2] Injecting GnRH analogues like Lupron interrupts hormonal messaging, maintaining the gonads in quiescent state until treatment ends, at which point messaging recommences and sexual development occurs. For this reason, GnRH analogues are often colloquially referred to as 'puberty blockers'. For men with prostate cancer or women with endometriosis or fibroids, the effect is similar: taking Lupron shuts down the gonadal secretion of testosterone or estrogen associated with tumour growth and related pathologies. GnRH analogues are also used in IVF

[1] My use of the contemporary verb 'to message' (arising from mobile phone texting practices) nods to the conundrum I discuss in Roberts (2007) that whilst hormones are frequently described as 'messengers of sex' they are also themselves 'the message'.

[2] Another medication can be offered to children at this time to prevent or minimise these effects.

treatments to intervene in ovarian function, and in the treatment of male sex offenders to reduce sexual desire.[3]

As mentioned in Chapter 6, a body of medical research focuses on the use of these drugs to treat early onset puberty: in my database of around 1,500 medical and scientific articles on early puberty, over 300 papers analyse the effectiveness of GnRH analogues in addressing the issue of reduced height. Some studies also focus on the acceptability of different modes of delivery (injections versus implants). Articles report injections to be painful (e.g. Hirsch *et al.* 2005), noting that both children and parents are reluctant to continue interventions over time. Long-lasting depot injections (delivered every three months) or implants (lasting up to twelve months) are described as more attractive alternatives.

It is important to note that such research is often sponsored by the drug's manufacturers. Hirsch *et al.*'s paper, for example, is entitled 'The Histrelin Implant: A Novel Treatment for Central Precocious Puberty' and one of the authors works for the manufacturer who also funded the work. Such 'research', as psychiatrist and social scientist David Healy (2004) argues, is as much a form of marketing as it is scientific work. Pharmaceutical companies pay ghost-writers to prepare papers that contain only positive results about their products obtained through their own clinical trials. Indeed, Healy (2004: 231) claims that 'up to 75 per cent of the papers on randomized controlled trials on therapeutic agents appearing in major journals may now be ghost-written' by authors paid by pharmaceutical companies (see also Dumit 2012).

There is little independent research on parents' and children's experiences of using these medications. An article in *Archives of Disorders of Childhood* written by parents of a 6-year-old girl going through puberty, however, describes intense feelings of 'dismay, anger and frustration' with the UK medical system's procedures around diagnosis, testing and treatment. Describing themselves as 'devastated' by their daughter's early development, O'Sullivan and O'Sullivan

[3] GnRH analogues have also been suggested as a treatment for autism, and for increasing the adult height of children with various other conditions (severe hypothyroidism, growth hormone deficiency, idiopathic short stature, those born small for gestational age and with congenital adrenal hyperplasia). The evidence for use in each of these conditions is weak and such use is not widely officially recommended (Carel *et al.* 2009: 757)

(2002: 320) are very positive about the effects of GnRH analogues once they are prescribed. This medication, they write, returns their daughter to a 'normal' state in which she 'comes back' to them as a child:

Our daughter's periods stop, her skin improves, moodiness reduces, *and our child comes back to us*. She even prefers an injection to a period and her confidence with her peers returns to previous levels. She is normal again! But to what end and at what cost? Our daughter finished her 12 months treatment early this year and her recent final bone age test now confirms that 'too little was done too late'. So what is the net effect after three and a half years? I will leave you to imagine what we think of most of the medical profession we have encountered. (O'Sullivan and O'Sullivan 2002: 320, emphasis added)[4]

This idea that taking medication returns consumers to a former, healthy state is widespread in contemporary direct-to-consumer pharmaceutical advertising, as Dumit shows. Analysing advertisements for 'cholesterol awareness' that encourage viewers to submit to testing (and potentially medication) he writes: 'These commercials . . . aim for a retroactive status change. Rather than illness punctuating ordinary life, the everyday conceals illness. Once this is identified, once you identify with it, then your true, real life can be returned to you' (Dumit 2012: 60). For adults who might have raised cholesterol, this is about self-recognition and coming to understand that 'your body is not what you think it is' (2012: 62). In early onset puberty, it is about parents' recognition of their child's out-of-time development and the consequent organising and monitoring of pharmaceutical interventions. As Dumit writes, 'If one is sick, the promise is that one will then be treated and reunited with one's true self and true community' (2012: 73). For children with early puberty, as O'Sullivan and O'Sullivan articulate,

4 Similar stories of difficulties accessing timely medical treatment are reported by journalists. In an article in the *Daily Mail*, for example, Rogers (2007) writes: 'Debbie Smith, 41, a GP dispenser, from Nottingham, tells a similar story. Her daughter, who is now 12, was just eight when she reached full sexual maturity. "We felt very alone. We weren't even told drugs to stop puberty were an option," says Debbie.' Interestingly, however, this story frames medical treatments as undesirable: 'But neither Miranda nor Debbie would have wanted their daughters to have taken hormone-blocking drugs. "What we really need is for someone to recognise this is a horrible thing for the affected families," says Debbie. "We need more support."'

this is about returning to family ('she came back to us') and friends ('her confidence with her peers returns to normal').

The effectiveness of GnRH analogues is most frequently measured in terms of impact on height. As discussed in the previous chapter, height outcomes are both easily calculated and eminently flexible: children can be measured but their height gain is always set against a calculated target height. Other measures of effectiveness are limited to whether or not puberty is effectively halted. Studies do not measure whether or not children engage in less sexual activity or drug-taking or suffer less teasing from peers: all of this is assumed to happen once physical development is paused and they return to their community of peers.

Somewhat naively stating that he 'often wonders' why clinicians overprescribe, in his parental guide Paul Kaplowitz criticises his fellow paediatric endocrinologists for being over-keen to prescribe GnRH medications:

> I often wonder why some of my colleagues are in such a rush to start girls on treatment before they are even sure what they are treating. It is not as though precocious puberty is like cancer and you have to 'catch it early', or the child cannot be cured. If the signs of puberty are early, as they most often are, *there is no harm whatsoever in waiting four to six months or as long as necessary to accurately access the rate of progression.* (Kaplowitz 2004: 149, emphasis in original)

This statement is in direct opposition to the idea that 'too little was done too late' in O'Sullivan and O'Sullivan's daughter's case. Unlike his unnamed colleagues, Kaplowitz claims to have treated very few children with Lupron. Rather than treating girls aged 7 or 8 (who would be considered to have early or precocious puberty according to the older guidelines), Kaplowitz adheres to the new recommendations (which he was instrumental in establishing) that suggest that 7 and 8 year olds with signs of sexual development could be considered the 'tail end of normal':

> M]any of these girls have been 7 or 8 years old, which is slightly precocious by the old definition and early but not precocious by the new guidelines. In these situations, I have a talk with the parents and the child to find out what potential problems they are most concerned about; if I allay those concerns without drug therapy, they usually opt for no treatment. (2004: 147)

Treatment with Lupron, as Kaplowitz (2004: 147) points out, is expensive in the US system, costing in 2004 at least US$8,000 per year, which may or may not be paid by insurance companies (2004: 151–2). His claim that educating parents leads to less intervention is important, and requires empirical investigation. In the UK, the prescribing situation is entirely different, with children being prescribed GnRH analogues on the National Health Service (NHS) at no cost. Clinicians at a leading English children's hospital stated in conversations with me that they also try to dissuade parents from using medications, only prescribing when levels of distress around menstrual bleeding or behavioural changes seem intolerable.

The act of prescribing any particular drug is the outcome of a complex network of actions and actors. As Dumit, Healy and others have shown, prescribing behaviours are not founded solely on medical research or findings but are driven also by consumer/patient demand and doctors' own brand loyalty. Patient demand is, in North America at least, co-articulated through direct-to-consumer pharmaceutical advertising, which not only teaches consumers to identify their bodies as needing particular medical interventions, but also provides specific modes of speech through which demands can be made of clinicians (Dumit 2012: 77). Articles on this topic published in the *British Medical Journal* similarly acknowledge that 'doctors feel pressurised by direct to consumer advertising' and are strongly influenced by patient demand (Spurgeon 1999: 1321; see also Mintzes *et al.* 2002). Doctor's loyalties are built through drug company incentives such as conference sponsorship, gifts and motivational visits (Braithwaite 1984; Healy 2004; Dumit 2012). Such practices, as described below, have had a notable history in the case of Lupron. Kaplowitz's criticisms of his colleagues fail to acknowledge the complex forces leading to GnRH analogue prescription.

Hormonal histories

Prescribing hormones to intervene in sexual processes has a long and complex history. Early, clear warnings of the physical dangers of hormonal medications came with the terrible intergenerational effects of the widely-prescribed (yet ineffective) anti-miscarriage medication diethystilbestrol (DES), which was a form of synthetic estrogen (Seaman 2003; Bell 2009). In 1971, teenage daughters of women prescribed this medication were found to be at increased risk of rare reproductive cancers and other related illnesses and this risk continues to affect the women's grandchildren (Newbold *et al.* 1998; Newbold 2004). Using hormones in older people to protect against the effects of ageing has also resulted in increased risk of cancer and other serious health conditions, such as heart disease (Rossouw *et al.* 2002). In earlier work, I argued that such use also articulates particular versions of 'healthy' sexed embodiment in racialising and gendering ways (Roberts 2007). Activist author Barbara Seaman (2003) argues that the use of estrogen to medicate various women's conditions (including menopause and fertility) since 1938 has constituted 'the greatest experiment ever performed on women'. 'I call the marketing, prescribing, and sale of these drugs an experiment', Seaman writes, 'because, for all these years, they have been used, in the main, for what doctors and scientists hope or believe they can do, not for what they *know* the products can do' (Seaman 2003: 5, emphasis in original).

Other researchers have focused on the use of hormones to treat children born with indeterminate sex. Feminist psychologist Katrina Roen (2009) explores wider medical programmes of intervention (including surgery and psychological practices as well as hormonal medications) that attempt to eradicate sexual ambiguity and to normalise children into one of two assumed sexes. Such interventions, she argues, involve the projection of parental fantasies and fears about what is 'normal' and 'desirable' in children's sexual futures (Roen 2009: 21). As many scholars and activists working in this field have shown, such practices prioritise normalisation over protecting children from medical trauma and injury (see also Spurgas 2009 and other chapters in Holmes 2009; Karkazis 2008). Roen writes:

> [Parents'] fear and ideas become embodied in the child who wakes up from surgery to find that part of her clitoris is missing, or that his urethral opening has been moved and his penis is scarred, or that she now needs to undergo regular vaginal dilation. The child's scars and lost genital tissue are the physical manifestation of the adults' fear of atypicality. Here the adults are imagining a kind of embodied subject and surgically moulding the children's body in the hope that the child will become that subject; that is, that the child will embody the kind of normativity that the adults imagine. (Roen 2009: 22)

The problem here, Roen contends, is that parents (and clinicians) fail to imagine that the medical procedures designed to create normality often produce suffering: 'The parents' picture of a normal, healthy child probably does not include repeated hospital visits, genital scarring, and profound mistrust of adults in medical contexts' (2009: 22). Such medical interventions, she suggests, may actually produce a different kind of child than that imagined: the difficulties and shame involved in such medical encounters shape subjectivities.

This claim is supported by ethnographic research. In 2008, for example, Katrina Karkazis found that many adults diagnosed with intersexuality as children felt very angry about the medical treatment they had endured and that these feelings had long-lasting resonance:

> These experiences had the unintentional effect of making these girls feel that something about their body was wrong or shameful and of giving them a sense of deep bodily vulnerability and of a loss of control over their bodies. This loss of control can lead to depression, anger, a sense of disconnection from their bodies and a disinterest in taking care of them, and a retreat from family members and friends. (Karkazis 2008: 223)

Women's studies scholar Rebecca M. Jordan-Young makes a related point within a wider argument about girls diagnosed with Congenital Adrenal Hyperplasia (CAH). Conventionally described as having 'masculinised' brains due to exposure to androgens in utero, the behaviour and interests of these girls and women are often used to support theories about the effect of prenatal hormones on sex/gender. Jordan-Young convincingly argues that explanations of such behaviour and interests systematically overlook the potential effects of:

> 1) physiological effects of CAH, including complex disruption of steroid hormones from early development onwards; 2) *intensive medical intervention and surveillance, which many women with CAH describe as traumatic*; 3) direct effects of genital morphology on sexuality (versus indirect effects that 'masculine' genitals may have on gender socialization); and 4) expectations of masculinization that likely affect both the development and evaluation of gender and sexuality in CAH. (Jordan-Young 2012: 1738, emphasis added)

In tune with my own argument about early onset puberty, Jordan-Young suggests that alternative explanations that can take all of these factors into account – encompassing the 'complex and iterative interactions among postnatal biological variables, medical interventions, and social context' – would be far more convincing (Jordan-Young 2012: 1738).

Related research focuses on the use of growth hormones to address issues of height. Here gender plays a highly significant role: in the mid to late twentieth century, hormones were used to treat boys who were 'too short' and girls who were 'too tall' (Pyett *et al.* 2005; Bruinsma *et al.* 2006; Morrison 2008; Rayner 2008; Rayner *et al.* 2010). In both cases, hormones act as agents of hetero-normalisation, helping to produce bodies that fit social norms of appearance and sexual relationality. Counter to medical claims that taking drugs to avoid adult tallness would lessen girls' future suffering, an Australian long-term follow-up study comparing outcomes for women who had and had not taken hormones as children, found that medicated women were more likely to suffer depression and anxiety as adults (Bruinsma *et al.* 2006; Rayner 2008). These women often had traumatic memories of treatment and became upset during interviews about their experiences. Others, who often came from tall families in which tallness was normal and appreciated, showed few signs of having suffered due to their height. These histories raise significant questions around the prescription of GnRH analogues to early developing girls by highlighting the potential physical risks of hormonal interventions and the likely psychological consequences of treating children for an appearance- and sexuality-related phenomenon. As medications, hormones can have powerful effects on situated, lived, sexed bodies; effects that have lifelong consequences.

In 2009, the US-based Lawson Wilkins Pediatric Endocrinology Society and the European Society for Pediatric Endocrinology convened a thirty-member consensus conference to produce an international Consensus Statement on the use of GnRH analogues (Carel *et al.* 2009). Although some of the funding for the conference was provided by pharmaceutical companies that produce and market GnRH analogues (including TAP who made Lupron), representatives from these companies did not participate in deliberations, contribute to the content of the report, or review or comment on the report before it was published (2009: 758). Although the authors agreed that GnRH analogues were effective in increasing the adult height of girls starting puberty before 6 years of age, they found that there was little high-quality evidence about the effectiveness of these drugs on any other parameters (e.g. psycho-social effects) or for older children: 'many conclusions rely in part on collective expert opinion' (2009: 752). The authors also advised that all children diagnosed with early puberty before 6 years should be given a head MRI scan to search for brain tumours, although performing such scans for 6–8 year olds remains 'controversial' (2009: 754). 'Whether delaying puberty with GnRHas may improve social functioning', they conclude, 'is still an open question' (2009: 753). Height gain in girls treated before they turned 6 was substantial: an average gain of 9–10 cm (2009: 753). Importantly, the group also argued that available data on long-term 'undesired' effects of GnRH analogues are limited and that long-term data on the fecundity and ovarian reserve of treated patients are needed (2009: 756). It is important to note that the absence of such data does not prevent prescribing.

In 2004, the British Society for Pediatric Endocrinology and Diabetes commissioned the writing of a 'shared care protocol' for the use of GnRH analogues in central precocious puberty (Kirk 2004). This document suggests that consultants and general practitioners (GPs) should agree an individual treatment plan for each child, with the consultant recommending a programme of injections for the GP to carry out after the initial dose is delivered by a specialist nurse in the endocrinology clinic. The consultant should undertake twelve monthly reviews of the child's development and 'audit patient's response to GnRH analogue therapy compared to nationally agreed criteria' (2004: 7). Like the *International Consensus Statement*, this document states that GnRH analogue therapy does not improve adult height in girls beyond 8 years of age and that only 40 per cent of patients 'reach their individual target height range' (2004: 8) but does not elaborate potential risks beyond listing short-term side effects (2004: 6). One senior clinician I spoke with, in contrast, articulated concerns about the long-term effects of GnRH analogues on bone formation. I return to the complexities of bone growth in the final chapter.

Although noting parents' and patients' concerns with pain or discomfort (and consequent adherence to treatment regimens), papers published by clinicians presume taking GnRH analogues to be a neutral experience. The psychological consequences of becoming involved in such treatment are not explored. Rayner *et al.*'s work on tall girls and the important literature on children with atypical sex show us in contrast that such engagements can be highly consequential. As I argued in Chapter 3 in relation to young people's participation in Tanner and Whitehouse's longitudinal study, becoming an object of medical or scientific investigation shapes subjectivities in particular, often highly durable ways. In these practices, findings, feelings and figurations are always intra-actively at play. Figuring a child's sexual development as a problem requiring observation, measurement and often painful treatment is likely to produce a relation to sexuality that is troubled in some way. Puberty in contemporary western cultures, as described in Chapter 1, is already widely figured as problematic; an embarrassing time of difficulty requiring increased levels of physical and emotional privacy particularly for girls. Although the aim of treatment may be to avoid such difficulties in young children, medically attending to sexual development may have the opposite effect. Evidence from both the atypical sexual development and tall girl fields indicates that supportive acceptance and even celebration of changing bodies would be more likely to facilitate a positive sense of embodied sexual self.

Support for parents

In the area of atypical sexual development, changing attitudes and practices amongst both clinicians and families of children born with atypical sex have been led by political collectives such as the Intersex Society of North America (1993–2008) and the Discord Alliance (2008–present). Organised by adult survivors of childhood medical interventions, these collectives are fuelled by a deep sense of rage about the long-term effects many members have suffered. Treatments of early puberty are not of the same scale: they are non-permanent and do not involve surgery. However, they are far more common and may involve significant numbers of children. Although the potential for future activism is great, current activist groups are constituted by concerned parents rather than adult former patients. In the UK, for example, an independent charity called the Child Growth Foundation works to educate clinicians about the impacts of early sexual development and to support parents and children going through this experience (this is only a small part of its work, which concentrates in the main on children with specific medical conditions that affect growth, such as Turner Syndrome, Prader-Willi Syndrome and Growth Hormone Deficiency).[5]

The Child Growth Foundation publishes a series of booklets for parents, including one on 'premature sexual maturity, including

[5] See www.childgrowthfoundation.org.

precocious puberty'. This series is sponsored by the pharmaceutical company Serono and the British Society for Paediatric Endocrinology and the booklet has a positive orientation towards medical treatment of early development. There is also a strong focus on the psychological effects of early development. Although adult height is offered as the most important reason to use GnRH analogues, the text states:

> As well as growth there may be other reasons to treat early puberty. *It is important to arrest or regress the signs of puberty as the child may be extremely distressed that they are different from their peer group.* There are numerous psychological reasons why therapeutic options should be discussed. Going through puberty is often difficult enough when it occurs during the usual age range (which many of us can remember). However puberty that commences too early ... can be associated with behavioural difficulties in both boys and girls. Problems in the very young children may include masturbation at socially inappropriate times and need to be dealt with sensitively. Concentration in school and social integration is usually affected in precocious puberty and needs careful assessment and management. (Fry and Stanhope 2004: 8, emphasis added)

A section on the 'social concerns' associated with early puberty is explicit about the significance of parents' reactions to the situation. The authors write that parents may feel 'alarm, distress, distaste, guilt and confusion' when witnessing their child's early development (2004: 14). Medicating a child is figured here as not simply for the child's benefit. Although behavioural problems are described as stemming from early development (rather than, for example, parental distress), the authors also state that 'even with successful treatment, behavioural difficulties may remain' (2004: 15). Treatment is 'successful' when it halts puberty, but it cannot necessarily turn children into amenable creatures; the stresses involved in being identified as an early developer and medically treated may not be so easy to reduce.

In his parental guide to early puberty, Kaplowitz (2004) makes a similar point. As noted above, Kaplowitz argues quite forcefully against the use of Lupron and other GnRH analogues in most early maturing children. Stating that little is known about the long-term effects of these medications, he adds:

> parents who have a generally healthy and happy 7-to-9 year old with early puberty should give serious thought to how the child might react to monthly shots and visits to the specialist for a physical exam, including breast

measurement and blood tests, every three to four months. There is to my knowledge no study that has specifically looked at how young girls cope emotionally with the stresses of being treated for precocious puberty, especially those who do not see their early breast development as a big deal (and I have seen many such girls). However, I would not be surprised if the treatment were shown to *cause* as many behaviour problems in young girls as it alleviates. (Kaplowitz 2004: 146–7)

Agreeing with Kaplowitz, it seems to me that having a more positive discourse around sexual development – that resists and alleviates alarmed, distressed or disgusted responses – would be more likely to help children and parents than an approach that promotes medical recognition and treatment. Exploring the psychological risks of treatment should become an important element in politics around the prescription of GnRH analogues to children.

Radical resistance and health activism

In notable contrast to this pro-medical approach, the use of GnRH analogues (specifically Lupron) in other arenas is fiercely contested in the United States. The website www.lupronvictimshub.com was established by a North American registered nurse, Lynne Millican, who underwent treatment with Lupron in 1989 for endometriosis and infertility. This very matter-of-fact site, consisting mostly of detailed lists (Millican states she has no time for formatting), documents a range of claims about serious and long-term side effects of Lupron, including court cases and class actions. Claims about the negative effects of Lupron are strongly worded, with sections of the website compiling examples of risks, deaths, adverse events reporting system data and lawsuits. Lupron is described as an antineoplastic agent (cancer chemotherapy drug): 'Like all antineoplastics', the website text states, 'Lupron is harmful to both cancerous and non-cancerous cells.' Wanting to demonstrate the dangers of the drug, Millican notes that 'The National Institutes of Health (NIH) and the Occupational Safety and Health Administration (OSHA) categorize Lupron as a "hazardous drug" that health care workers should only handle when wearing protective gowns and gloves.' The site states that the American pharmaceutical regulator, the Food and Drug Administration (FDA), had received more than 22,667 reports of adverse events linked to Lupron, including 651 deaths, between 1997 and 2006 (http://lupronvictimshub.com/aers.html).

The Lupron Victims Hub also tells a story about the nefarious practices of Takeda Abbott Pharmaceuticals (TAP):

> Even more startling, the Federal Dept. of Health and Human Services' Office of Research Integrity determined that the lead investigator involved with studies on Lupron's use in treating fibroids and endometriosis committed scientific misconduct, and admitted to falsifying or fabricating 80 percent of the data in two published studies on Lupron. (http://lupronvictimshub.com/index.html)

In 2001, TAP pleaded guilty to civil and criminal misconduct over Lupron and was heavily fined, paying $600 million in restitution to Medicaid and Medicare and a $290 million criminal fine. The US Department of Justice found that TAP bribed doctors to prescribe Lupron, encouraging doctors to bill Medicare or Medicaid at $500 per dose for the samples they were providing for free (www.ca1.uscourts.gov/pdf.opinions/10-2494P-01A.pdf). Numerous individuals and groups have filed related claims around costs, as well as claims around physical damage caused by Lupron (http://lupronvictimshub.com/lawsuits.html). These cases have mostly been settled out of court.

The National Women's Health Network also reports on Lupron on its website, but their documentation is mostly written by Millican, repeating the phrases and points made on the Victim's Hub (nwhn.org/lupron®-what-does-it-do-women's-health). The US-based patient advocacy group Endometriosis Research Center has also undertaken critical work around Lupron, asking women members about their experience of taking it. Contradicting Abbott's claims that any side effects would pass after six months of discontinuing treatment, over half of their respondents (51.67 per cent) experienced side effects lasting for longer than six months; and almost a quarter (23 per cent) of the women experienced side effects lasting longer than five years (Endometriosis Research Center 2003: 2). In the UK, interestingly, the leading endometriosis patient organisation, the Endometriosis Society, provides no information on Lupron or GnRH analogues on its website.

Most of this literature deals with Lupron's effects on women rather than children. In the correspondence section of the Lupron Victims Hub, however, Millican reproduces correspondence between the leading feminist health group Our Bodies Ourselves collective (represented by then editor Judy Norsigan) and the US Department of Health and Human

Services (www.lupronvictimshub.com/documents&correspondences.html).[6] In this correspondence, dating from 1994, Millican asked,

> How can children tolerate 7.5 mg lupron depot injections indefinitely for treatment of precocious puberty, yet adult women are prescribed 3.75 mg. and are not to exceed 6 months of treatment?

The reply from the Department of Health and Human Services Medical Officer Lisa Rarick, MD stresses the differences between children and adults hormonal bodies:

> Concern: Use in children questions
> Comment: The use in treating inappropriate GnRH secretion in children with central precocious puberty is very different than the use in normal adult women. Children with precocious puberty have an abnormally high level (and abnormally timed secretion) of GnRH to be countered. Use in adult women involves countering a normal secretion. Regarding bone loss, it is thought that women lose bone due to estrogen deficiency. Estrogen is not a factor for bone loss in pre-pubertal children (they normally have low levels of estrogen).

This response draws helpful distinctions between women and girls but does not in my view adequately address questions of physical risk. The Lupron Victim's Hub describes a range of long-term negative outcomes of using Lupron in relatively small amounts: does children's higher secretion of GnRH protect them against these?

The politics of patient activism around Lupron are highly complex. On the Victim's Hub, and via associated feminist organisations like the National Women's Health Network and the Our Bodies Ourselves collective, Millican and her peers (it is unclear how many women she speaks for) agitate strongly against the misuse of pharmacological agents in treating serious conditions, conditions that in many ways women have had to fight to have medically recognised. This is not a politics oriented around leaving women's bodies alone (as is often the case in activism around disorders of sexual development or intersexuality) but is fuelled by a sense of outrage that treatments ultimately cause more harm and suffering to women who have already endured a

6 For a sociological analysis of the global significance of the Our Bodies Ourselves collective, see Davis (2007).

lot.[7] The demand here is for better science and more caring medicine. The Lupron Victims Hub hosts and promotes, for example, a petition to Congress demanding that patients be given complete information about the risks of any drug before accepting it and that they must sign a document each time they receive an injection to say they have been so informed (www.petition2congress.com/4340/doctorsnurses-heath care-professionals-should-have-to-have-consent/). Although arguing that Lupron should be taken off the market until such protection is in place, this approach ultimately leaves decisions about taking Lupron to individuals, relying on a model of risk education and choice rather than refusal or banning. Although not openly espousing feminist politics, this approach builds on a long history of feminist agitation around medical treatments, particularly in relation to breast cancer and reproductive health (fertility and infertility) and resonating with safe (rather than anti-) vaccination politics (see Murphy 2012).

Making differences with pharmaceuticals

In an editorial of a special issue of the journal *Science as Culture* entitled 'Living Drugs', Suzanne Fraser, kylie valentine and I (2009) argued that outright condemnation of pharmaceuticals per se is most often not a useful political or theoretical strategy. Instead, we suggested that

> Medications must be analysed ... in their specificity, and any connections with other health issues or generalisations about the action of medicine must be built *outwards* from each specific case – carefully and with close attention to difference. (Fraser, valentine and Roberts 2009: 127–8)

In tune with the work of many patient organisations, we advised that social scientists should engage in 'thoughtful unpacking rather than (or at least prior to) condemnation or hopeful approval' of particular pharmaceuticals (2009: 128). The histories I have told above start to do this in the case of GnRH analogues, but how might we go further to unpack and understand their actions in children's bodies?

Here, I want to build on my earlier work on hormone replacement therapies and think about GnRH analogues as actors engaged in

[7] For analyses of contemporary health activism, see Dumit (2012); Rabeharisoa, Moreira and Akrich (2014).

activities with bodies understood as situated, complex and lived (that is, as embodied subjectivities). I am inspired by Elizabeth Wilson's recent work on the use of SSRIs (selective serotonin reuptake inhibitors – a common form of anti-depressant medications) in children. As part of a wider project on depression, Wilson makes an argument that contrasts sharply with highly critical accounts of the prescription of SSRIs to children coming from authors such as Healy (2004), Tinimi (2002) and Moncrieff (2008). Their arguments, Wilson argues, are politically aligned with earlier anti-psychiatry accounts which focused on the physical and mental harms produced by psychiatric interventions, including drugs (Wilson 2011: 278). Figuring children as innocent and non-worldly and as consequently vulnerable to damage through medication, these accounts, Wilson argues, affirm a mind/body distinction that has been thoroughly critiqued within feminist and poststructuralist theory. They are also, in her view, too quick to dismiss the importance of biological processes in depression. Turning to authors from psychological and psychoanalytic traditions who 'are not primarily focused on biological explanations and ... not wedded to the disease model of depression' (most notably British psychoanalyst Peter Fonagy), however, Wilson finds that even these discussions figure children as innocent and non-worldly. However admirable, she suggests, Fonagy's attempts to rethink childhood depression ultimately 'lean on and silently promote' models of subjectivity and mental health that disarticulate mind from body through reducing mind to brain, thus rendering the rest of the body redundant (Wilson 2011: 278).

In contrast to both approaches, Wilson aims to develop a feminist account that troubles traditional mind/body and cause/effect distinctions (Wilson 2004: 278). Borrowing key terms from Karen Barad's (2007) theorising of materiality and causality, she conceptualises depressions as entanglements of moods and pharmaceuticals, describing the actions of SSRIs as intra-actions. Arguing against accounts that focus solely on anti-depressants' actions in the brain in which non-depressive ideation is figured as a neurological outcome of taking medication, Wilson emphasises the involvement of the whole body in consuming pills and articulating or 'calling forth' mental health:

> [A]n SSRI is not a pill that dissolves once it arrives in the stomach; rather it comes to be a psychopharmaceutical (it solidifies as a psychological agent) only through its dispersal by the gut and liver and circulatory system and

synapse. This pill – not melting but materializing – calls forth ideation not from one site (synapse) but from the body as a whole. (Wilson 2011: 286)

This argument disrupts mainstream biomedical and scientific ideas about what constitutes a body: pills, in this model, come into being, or materialise, with/through a 'system of mind-body-world intra-action' (2011: 289). Depressions (or depressive ideations), then, are not effects of isolated parts of the body or particular bodily systems nor are they effects of 'interactions' between such systems and their environments: instead they are 'phenomena that neuro-serotonergic-ideational intra-actions may become' (2011: 290).

Barad's conceptual distinction between intra-action and inter-action is key here. As introduced in Chapter 2, Barad's argument refigures practices as agentic and productive of worlds. Unlike inter-actions that presuppose at least two already existing factors, intra-actions constitute entities in real time. Wilson quotes Barad to this effect:

> Bodies do not simply take their places in the world. They are not situated in, or located in, particular environments. Rather 'environments' and 'bodies' are intra-actively co-constituted. Bodies ('human', 'environmental', or otherwise) are integral 'parts' of, or dynamic reconfigurations of, what is. (Barad, in Wilson 2011: 290)

This orientation allows Wilson to make an important claim about the 'causes' of depression, avoiding the dualistic 'mind or body' ('biological or social') causal arguments that she argues plague other accounts. In contrast to mainstream models that attempt to separate and calculate their actions, 'Genes and environments are demarcated as agents together, out of the same intra-active fabric. Genes and environment are siblings of coeval origin, not strangers who occasionally meet at scenes of pathology' (Wilson 2011: 291). This argument aligns closely with Chapter 5's discussions of the folded causes of early onset puberty, in which I suggested that genes, overweight, exposure to environmental toxins and adverse childhood experience might be theorised as folds rather than origins.

For Wilson, figuring pills, depressions and bodies in Baradian mode means understanding the 'geography of the mind ... as a diverse, interconnected system (a mutuality of moods-objects-neurotransmitters-hormones-cognitions-affects-attachments-tears-glands-images-words-gut)' (2011: 280). As such diverse interconnected systems, children cannot reasonably be figured as innocent cyphers of social or biological forces. 'Developing mind-bodies', she writes, 'are systems of intense reciprocity and agency; these mind-bodies are juvenile but they are no less accomplished and no less worldly than the mind-bodies of adults' (2011: 293). Arguments against medicating children with SSRIs, then, should not be based on claims about children's innocence. Nor, I would add, should arguments *for* particular medications (GnRH analogues in this case) be made on the grounds that children's bodies are relatively simple or not-yet-social entities. The appeal to innocence figured in the photographs of beautiful children on AbbVie's website should not be replicated in medical or policy discussions about whether or not to use GnRH analogues in early maturing children.

Via Barad, Wilson provides a language for talking about the intra-actions of bodies and medications that emphasises the worldliness of children and assumes that biological bodies cannot be extricated from subjectivities, feelings or environments. The SSRI mind-body-world systems she describes focus on experience and embodiment. Influenced by the STS and sociological literatures cited earlier, however, I take a somewhat wider view, including pharmaceutical company websites, medical publishing and doctors' prescribing behaviours in the 'mutualities' constituting children's health. Wilson highlights the importance of considering the material differences constituting such worldliness in any particular instance and resisting basing arguments either for or against medications on claims to children's physiological or psychological innocence.

I have argued in earlier chapters that public concerns about early onset puberty often articulate a discourse about innocence requiring protection and have aligned myself with critical feminist scholars protesting such figurations of girls within the 'sexualisation' debates. In thinking about medical treatments of early puberty similarly, I want to resist arguing to protect children's purity. Learning from the history of hormonal medications and endocrine disrupting chemicals, I feel it is important to explore the potential long-term *physiological* costs of hormonal medications taken at a young age. These seem to me both under-researched and potentially significant. Additionally, as outlined above, I want to highlight concerns about the *psychological* effects of becoming enrolled in medication networks: the pharmaceutical-consuming-child-system, to use Wilson's language, is substantially different from the unmedicated-child-system. But GnRH-analogue-consuming children are not all the same – no matter how uniformly middle class and beautiful they appear on AbbVie's Lupron website. In exploring discourses around one marginalised group of Lupron consumers in the following section, then, I want to open up these questions of difference.

Trans children and GnRH analogues

In July 2007, the SF Weekly published an article entitled 'Girl/Boy Interrupted' (see Figure 7). Illustrated by a curious photograph of a blonde-haired, blue-eyed white child dressed half in jeans and half in a

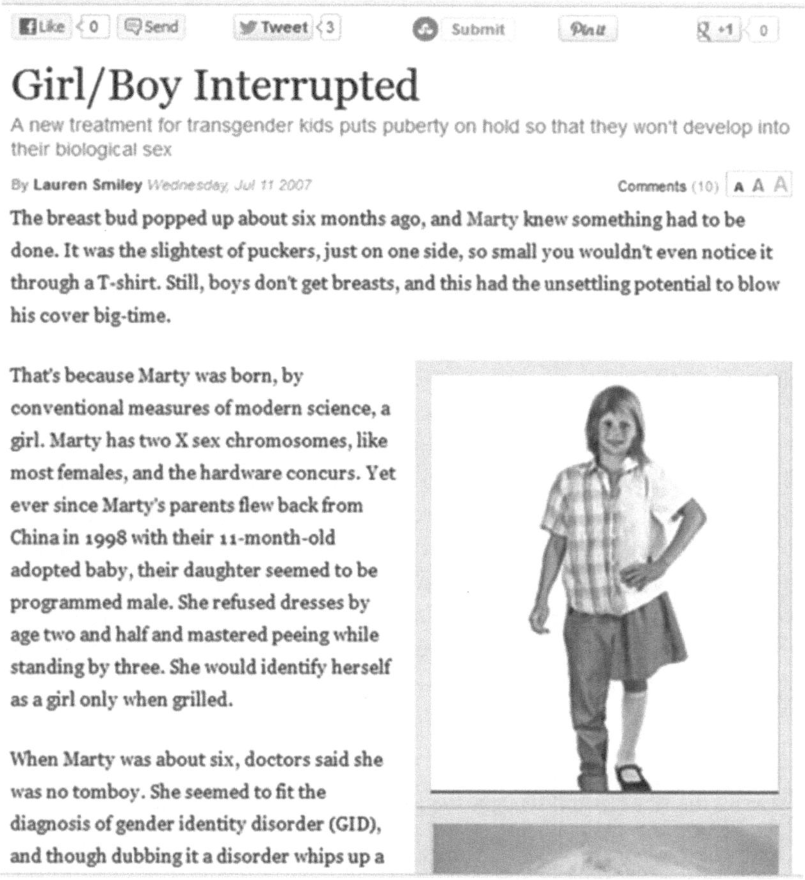

Like 0 Send Tweet 3 Submit Pin it +1 0

Girl/Boy Interrupted

A new treatment for transgender kids puts puberty on hold so that they won't develop into their biological sex

By **Lauren Smiley** *Wednesday, Jul 11 2007* Comments (10) A A A

The breast bud popped up about six months ago, and Marty knew something had to be done. It was the slightest of puckers, just on one side, so small you wouldn't even notice it through a T-shirt. Still, boys don't get breasts, and this had the unsettling potential to blow his cover big-time.

That's because Marty was born, by conventional measures of modern science, a girl. Marty has two X sex chromosomes, like most females, and the hardware concurs. Yet ever since Marty's parents flew back from China in 1998 with their 11-month-old adopted baby, their daughter seemed to be programmed male. She refused dresses by age two and half and mastered peeing while standing by three. She would identify herself as a girl only when grilled.

When Marty was about six, doctors said she was no tomboy. She seemed to fit the diagnosis of gender identity disorder (GID), and though dubbing it a disorder whips up a

Figure 7 Screenshot of SF Weekly, July 2007.

dress, the text highlights the difficulties experienced in puberty by children who identify as trans. In confusing contrast to the image, the opening lines introduce Marty, a child adopted from China as a baby girl. Diagnosed at six with 'Gender Identity Disorder' (GID), Marty has lived as a boy since toddlerhood.[8] The article begins:

> The breast bud popped up about six months ago, and *Marty knew something had to be done.* It was the slightest of puckers, just on one side, so small you wouldn't even notice it through a T-shirt. Still, boys don't get breasts, and this had the unsettling potential to blow his cover big-time. (Smiley 2007, emphasis added)

Unlike many internationally adopted girls, Marty's entry into puberty comes at a 'normal' age (9 years) but is figured here as a disaster. Describing his successful passing as male at school and elsewhere, Smiley writes:

> But the days when the only outward markers of gender lie in haircuts, clothes, and personality only last so long. Deep inside Marty's brain, a time bomb known as the hypothalamus waited to stage a hormone-armed mutiny. Breasts would sprout. Hips would widen. The uterus would shed blood on a monthly basis. Marty didn't want any of it. (Smiley 2007)

For children who identify as trans (many of whom are formally diagnosed with Gender Identity Disorder, now Gender Dysphoria), pubertal processes begin to emphasise a rupture between their self-identity and their bodily forms and processes. The claim that 'Marty knew something had to be done' frames a burgeoning response to this dilemma: rather than a trauma to be endured (see for example, Grossman and D'augeli 2008), pubertal transition into the 'wrong sex' is steadily becoming something to be avoided through GnRH analogue medication. This treatment has only very recently become accessible in some countries. First made available in the Netherlands, it has since become an option in many countries including the United States, Belgium, New Zealand, Sweden and Norway (Roen 2011: 61; Kreukels and Cohen-Kettenis 2011). In 2011, the only specialist UK clinic

[8] The diagnosis of Gender Identity Disorder (GID) was based on the American Psychiatric Association's *Diagnostic and Statistical Manual of Mental Disorders (DSM IV)*. This manual was revised in May 2013 and GID replaced by 'gender dysphoria', a potentially less stigmatising term. DSMV also removed this category from the group of sexual disorders. In this book I use the term 'trans' in an attempt to sidestep these medical classifications.

for trans-identified young people based at the Tavistock and Portman NHS Trust in London was granted approval by the National Research Ethics Service to prescribe hormone blockers to patients aged 12 and over. Children like Marty, as Smiley's article goes on to describe, can use such medication to 'interrupt' hormonal processes and delay puberty. Rather than materialising 'normal' development in the pathologically early developer, for these young people GnRH analogues prevent unwanted biological changes so that they can grow up (that is, become old enough to engage with medical transitioning practices) without gaining physical characteristics that are difficult to change.

The *San Francisco Weekly* article is highly positive about GnRH analogue treatments, framing them as a life-saving option that supports more 'successful' (that is, hidden) transition at a later stage:

> 'If you have someone who's 6–3, with broad shoulders like a football player and a deep voice, there's no amount of surgery or hormones in the world that's going to allow that person to pass and be safe,' says Nick Gorton, a doctor who treats transgender patients at Lyon-Martin Women's Health Services in San Francisco. 'If you treat them [young] then maybe at 25 they won't get raped, beaten, and killed.' (Smiley 2007).

Naming Lupron as 'the preferred drug for the controversial process' and quoting TAP's "Pause the child within" slogan, Smiley (2007) adds: 'It's potent, yet reversible, and incredibly expensive, and for transgender kids backed by increasingly supportive parents, it's ushering in a new era.' Although briefly citing fierce opponents like controversial Catholic psychiatrist Paul McHugh[9] – 'He calls the Lupron treatment "a modern form of child abuse"' – Smiley (2007) argues that the off-label use of Lupron to treat trans children is 'catching on' amongst American doctors. Returning to Marty's story, at the end of the article she describes taking Lupron both as a parental decision to 'leave the road open' and as a resistance to biology, ensuring that Marty's body does not act against his wishes:

> So they [Marty's parents] will ensure Marty's body doesn't do any deciding for him, leaving the road open with Lupron until Marty can better navigate to points female, trans-male, or somewhere in between. It's a decision, essentially, not to decide. But of course that's still a decision.

[9] McHugh famously argued in 1977 that sex reassignment surgery was also abusive and closed down the Johns Hopkins Gender Identity clinic in 1979.

So the Lupron has been ordered, and the family is waiting for the loaded syringe to arrive in the mail. Once it does, they'll climb into the car and drive to Children's Hospital Oakland, where Marty will steel himself and take the first shot. (Smiley 2007)

Engaging in off-label use of Lupron, children like Marty are not found on AbbVie's website.[10] A quick internet search for information on GnRH analogues in young trans people, however, leads directly to video blogs (vlogs) produced by teenagers about their own treatment. Ethical concerns prevent me from naming these vlogs here but several notable cases on YouTube painstakingly document years of treatment with puberty blockers and transitioning hormones, with young trans authors recording their experiences of treatment and their own bodily response. Watching these video blogs brings the politics of GnRH analogues to the fore: vloggers talk about family rejection and struggle with parents, complain about the high costs of medication and engage in sharp debate with each other about access to different kinds of medication (see also Raun 2012).[11]

In North America, as described by Dumit (2012), access to drugs is a fiercely contested business. Regulation is relatively weak (compared with the UK) and access to black market medications quite open. In this context, medical groups – notably the World Professional Association for Trans Health (WPATH) – have produced guidelines about the use of GnRH analogues, hoping to maximise safety. For young people undergoing gender transition, the WPATH outlines three categories of physical interventions: (1) fully reversible interventions (hormone blockers to delay the physical changes of puberty), (2) partially reversible (hormones used to masculinise or feminise the body) and (3) irreversible changes (i.e. surgeries). The WPATH recommends moving slowly and sequentially through the stages to give the adolescent and family members time to adapt:

A staged process is recommended to keep options open through the first two stages. Moving from one state to another should not occur until there has

[10] Off-label use of pharmaceuticals – taking them for indications, age groups, dosages or delivery methods other than those for which they were approved – is a widespread, legal and integral part of US biomedicine (see Dumit 2012). It is also legal in the United Kingdom.

[11] Debate about the use of vlogs as research materials is somewhat fraught. For a vlog about the use of trans vlogs in research and an interesting string of comments, see www.youtube.com/watch?v=pMOidZb2dpo.

been adequate time for adolescents and their parents to assimilate fully the effects of earlier interventions. (World Professional Association for Trans Health 2012: 19)

An earlier version of these guidelines, published in 2001, suggested that treatments to delay physical pubertal changes be initiated only after an adolescent reaches Tanner stage 2 of pubertal development, giving the young person an opportunity to 'experience puberty in his/her biologic sex' (World Professional Association for Trans Health 2001: 10). In the 2012 revisions, it was noted that 'some children may arrive at this stage at very young ages (e.g. 9 years of age) and that existing studies of these treatments have only included children of 12 and older (World Professional Association for Trans Health 2012: 18). Treatments to delay puberty are variously described in these guidelines as allowing a young person to pass as a member of their desired sex, as providing more time to explore gender identity and nonconformity, and as preventing the growth of sexual characteristics that may be difficult or impossible to alter in later transitioning. Masculinising or feminising hormones can be prescribed after age 16, and so, unlike puberty blockers, do not require parental agreement. Due to the permanent nature of the interventions, the guidelines suggest that young people should have reached the age of legal majority before undertaking surgery (World Professional Association for Trans Health 2012: 21). Similar guidelines were published in 1998 by the Royal College of Psychiatrists in Britain (di Ceghe, Sturge and Sutton 1988).

In 2005, the British Society for Paediatric Endocrinology and Diabetes (BSPED) also published guidelines for medical treatment of trans young people but these advised, in contrast, that puberty blockers should not be offered until Tanner stage 4 or 5 was reached, that is until pubertal development completed. These guidelines were criticised by the Gender Identity Research and Education Society, a British charity for trans people and their supporters, who argued that there was not sufficient evidence to justify this different approach which would, in their view, cause substantial suffering to some young people (www.gires.org.uk/treatment-BSPED.php). Having earlier removed these guidelines from their website, in 2009 the BSPED published a 'Position Statement' on the use of GnRH analogues in trans young people; revising this statement in November 2012 (www.bsped.org.uk/clinical/clinical_position.html). This very brief statement states that cases should be assessed on an individual basis and that treatment decisions should be made by a specialist multidisciplinary treatment team. Although vague, this statement seems to indicate a change of position towards a potentially more positive approach to providing puberty blocking drugs to younger people. The American Endocrine Society's (2009) draft guidelines, written by US and Dutch clinicians, go further, recommending that adolescents who meet clinical criteria 'undergo treatment to suppress pubertal development' (Hembree *et al.* 2009: 90). Although at time of writing these remained draft guidelines only, they do, as Roen argues, demonstrate 'that this practice is moving from being an isolated practice of a few clinicians sympathetic to the concerns of transsexual people to a practice that is publicly recommended and officially endorsed' (2011: 58). Roen (2011: 58) thus names contemporary times 'an era of puberty suppression' for trans young people. Although recognising the importance of these medications to some young people, Roen worries about the politics of this shift. In contrast to Smiley's (2007) claim that Lupron will allow Marty to 'better navigate to points female, trans-male, or somewhere in between', Roen (2011) argues that the prescription of these drugs confirms a medical model of gender variance in which 'health' is defined as belonging clearly to one sex and aligned with heterosexuality.

In academic literatures, young trans people's desire for puberty blockers is most often voiced by clinicians rather than by the young people themselves. In a response to Roen's partially critical piece, for example, leading Dutch clinician Peggy T. Cohen-Kettenis describes the young people she offers puberty blockers to as being 'unable to live with their gender issues without any medical intervention' (Cohen-Kettenis 2011: 260). The publicly accessible online video blogs provide more direct accounts. Here, young trans people detail their pursuit and use of GnRH analogues (specifically Lupron), speaking directly to camera and/or filming their own clinical encounters to provide rich documentation of their hopes and experiences around puberty blocking practices. In one prolific example, a 15-year-old woman speaks with great passion about Lupron, detailing its effects on every part of her body and mood in a long series of videos. Although terrified of the 3-monthly injections – in her first video it takes 20 minutes for her to allow the very patient care provider to inject her buttock – her general orientation towards Lupron is intensely positive. This blogger criticises those taking black market medications (hormones) during transition. Such criticism leads to counter blogs, which rail against the presumption of privilege underpinning the claim that people 'should' take puberty blockers and then hormones: as noted earlier, each injection of Lupron costs about US$1,800 or US$8,000 per year. Here, the class-based politics of drug availability is articulated and the difference between the North American experience and the UK or European one becomes clear (in the UK, for example, GnRH analogue treatment is available at no cost to some patients). The role of supportive families is also highlighted. Unlike Marty, some vloggers do not have parents who will order drugs through the post and then 'climb into the car to drive to ... hospital.'

Online testimonies, and those of clinicians like Cohen-Kettenis, figure puberty blocking medications as psychologically as well as materially life-saving. Building on historical accounts of trans people's struggles to access highly desired pharmaceutical and surgical interventions, these accounts represent GnRH analogues as the first step in the well-choreographed sequence (if often emotionally, financially and physically challenging) constituting contemporary trans lives in the medicalised North. The more critical approaches to pharmaceuticalisation found in other health fields are largely missing here, although Roen is a key exception.

The vlog testimonies clarify the significance of attending to difference when evaluating pharmaceuticals and their effects on bodies. Children's bodies, as Wilson argues, are worldly. They are articulated with race/ethnicity, class, location, age, , sexuality, sex/gender and dis/ability. Attending to trans accounts, I do not feel able to straightforwardly reject GnRH analogues and the work they do in children's bodies, despite serious worries about the potential physical harms that might occur and wider concerns, following Roen, about how a shift to a 'puberty blocking era' might, for both trans and cis young people, reinforce heteronormative articulations of health and ill health (see also Hird 2003).

Evaluating medications, exploring pharmaceuticalisation

> [M]any empirical studies of technoscience have disabled the notion that the word 'technical' designates a clean and orderly practical or epistemological space. Nothing so productive could be so simple. (Haraway 1997: 68)

Science studies' disabling of technical discourses, practices and spaces is one of the key contributions of the field as a whole. In relation to pharmaceuticals, science studies methods articulate medications as dense material-semiotic knots: actors that carry meanings *and* actively bring about physical changes in bodies and environments. Making a mess (Law 2004) of the 'clean and orderly ... space' of medications figured in the AbbVie website as I have done here, importantly, is not to question that GnRH analogues do hold off puberty – it seems that agreement on this is strong – but to open up critical reflection on what they produce in their productiveness.

Evaluating GnRH analogues in this broader sense means asking questions about the 'complex system' constituting early sexual development and understanding developing bodies as bio-psycho-social – or as Wilson, following Barad, would call intra-active – phenomena. How, to put it as simply as possible, do puberty blockers and children's sexed bodies intra-act to produce specific medicated-child-systems? As I have argued, these systems materialise articulations of sex/gender, age, parent–child relations and healthy, embodied subjectivities. The children taking puberty blockers are, to use Wilson's word, worldly in multiple ways.

Learning from Dumit, Healy and others, I have additionally suggested that such evaluation also requires paying sustained attention to the role of pharmaceutical companies in establishing and sustaining relations with clinicians, parents and patients through direct-to-consumer advertising, medical publishing and sponsorship of patient organisations in simultaneously enacting early onset puberty as a condition requiring treatment and producing treatments and treatment discourses. In the puberty field, pharmaceutical companies constitute, articulate and trade in crisis; meaning both 'the problem' and the demand for intervention as solutions. Such trade is arguably part of a wider processes of pharmaceuticalisation. Whilst resisting this crisis talk may not always neatly align with refusing GnRH analogues, the role of pharmaceutical companies in articulating early onset puberty cannot be ignored.

Exploring GnRH analogues, then, I find myself somewhat caught between a critical, sociological approach and what might be called a 'new materialist' attempt to consider the possibilities that pharmaceuticals might open up. This dilemma stems in part from the materials I have discussed here, which show that although the articulation of puberty as a potential site for medical intervention can provide immense relief to some trans children, such articulations may also have significant negative effects on cis girls' sense of their bodies and themselves. My response to this ethical, political and theoretical dilemma is, as I argued in Chapter 2, to refuse to align myself with either side of this debate; indeed to query the figuration of these positions as oppositions. Like Robyn Wiegman (2014), I am worried about contemporary demands to avoid critical or 'paranoid' readings in favour of positive or affectionate ones. For me, these kinds of approaches interpenetrate; they are not absolute positions but possible orientations to take up at different times and places (see also Lewis 2014). Focusing on the multiple bodies articulated with and through GnRH analogues allows me to keep moving and to explore a range of responses that might help find 'interpretations that can sustain us' (Wiegman 2014: 19).

Although cis girls going through early puberty and young trans people constitute quite different kinds of mind-body-worlds, their relation to GnRH analogues raises some shared questions: what is a livable pubescent life? How do norms of sex/gender, sexuality and age restrict young people's development and happiness? What are the costs and benefits of accessing medical treatments to address these restrictions? What are the politics of the pharmaceuticalisation of sexual development? Debating these questions, in my view, must involve detailed engagement with medical and pharmaceutical discourses around GnRH analogues and their intra-actions with developing bodies.

The epigraph to this chapter suggests that using GnRH analogues to treat early sexual development 'says [to young girls that] "Something is wrong with your body"' (Greenspan, in Weil 2012). Building on my earlier work on sex hormones (Roberts 2007), I would suggest that it is not just that prescribing GnRH analogues 'sends this message' in a psycho-social sense, but that the hormonal medication literally messages an articulation of 'normal girl'. As my colleagues working on the 'sexualisation' debates and on teenage motherhood have made abundantly clear, analysing and intervening in such articulations is core business for contemporary feminisms. It is these analyses and interventions that clear a space to tell new stories about sexual development, sex/gender and sexuality.

Conclusion
Folding puberty differently: changing findings, feelings and figurations

Dutch photographer Rineke Dijkstra's photographic series *Beach Portraits* (taken primarily between 1992 and 1996) comprises images of individual, pairs or groups of young people posing in swimming outfits on beaches in the United States, Poland, England, the Ukraine, Gabon and Croatia.[1] Subjects are photographed full length on a small stretch of sand or pebbles, the water line horizon at thigh or waist height, the sky a wider band of grey or blue. The subjects' gaze is directly to the camera and the camera angle low, enabling a 'monumental, confrontational' format (Visser, in Dijkstra 2004: 8). Dijskra's images depict puberty as a time of awkwardness, when nothing seems to fit: clothes are not right, limbs are too long and skinny, skin is sore, swimming costumes are baggy. Standing calmly if sometimes quite tentatively in front of flat seas, the young people seem resigned to waiting for something better – for the sun to come out, to finish this posing, or to grow a different body.

In his introductory essay to a book of Dijkstra's photographs, Hripsime Visser quotes the Freudian analogy that adolescents are like crabs waiting to grow their shells. Crabs at this developmental stage hide under rocks until the new shell has hardened,

> because if it is wounded in this defenceless stage it will bear the scars for life. The comparison with the way in which Rineke Dijkstra – who herself grew up in a neighbourhood by the sea – has hauled her 'shell-less' adolescents from their hiding places in order to display them in their vulnerable nakedness is seductive. The presence of the sea in these early images is, in this respect, of course remarkable. (Visser, in Dijkstra 1999: 9)

Although the crab analogy is compelling, Visser's use of 'hauled' seems unnecessarily negative. Whilst I agree that the photographs articulate

[1] Unfortunately, I was not granted permission to reproduce any of these images here. A Google Image search on 'Dijkstra Beach' is the fastest way to view them.

vulnerability, I find them more compassionate. For me, Dijkstra figures a patience and resignation in young people that is compelling and admirable; the young people wear their vulnerability with grace and strength.

I have attempted in this book to replicate this compassionate orientation. In my analysis of Tanner's historic study of pubertal timing and child growth in Chapter 3, for example, I explored what it might have meant – and may yet mean – for the children and young people (now adults) to participate in the study and to have their naked images circulating so widely across the internet. Learning from young trans people's accounts of using puberty blockers in Chapter 7 I suggested that simple condemnation of such medications would be ill advised. In Chapters 5 and 6's discussions of the causes and effects of early sexual development, similarly, I have questioned accounts that articulate young people's sexuality as inherently problematic, something to be controlled and contained. My aim in querying crisis narratives of early onset puberty has been to open up what it might mean to enter puberty, to make space for broader articulations of physical and sexual development.

Importantly for this kind of thinking about difference, Dijkstra's photographs also tell complex stories about 'race'/ethnicity, gender and class during puberty and adolescence. Although the beaches and environments are virtually identical, embodied and sartorial differences between the subjects speak of vastly different socio-material worlds: some of Dijkstra's subjects wear fashionable bikinis; others are in their underwear or clothing as if they do not own, or at least could not on that day access, swimming attire. Some pose in fashion magazine mode, others stand limply or at least less self-consciously. Whilst the young people remain nameless – the image titles present only place names, countries and dates – the embodied differences constituting their experiences of growing up are palpable.

In another series of images made between 1994 and 2003, Dijkstra records the adolescence of a particular child named Almerisa, a Bosnian refugee. Initially photographed in 1994 at about 6 years old, Almerisa poses for a portrait again in 1996, 1998, 2000, 2002 and 2003. In each subsequent photograph, she sits alone on a chair in a relatively blank interior space – only floor coverings, curtains and wallpapers give us any visual clues as to where she is now. The first image is taken in an 'Asylum seekers' centre, Leiden'. Almerisa sits on an institutional red plastic chair, her feet dangling above a rather scruffy floor covering. She is dressed in a formal tartan outfit with patent leather party shoes, socks and tights. The second image is set in a domestic setting in 'Wormer, The Netherlands'. Dressed in a flowery yellow summer dress, Almerisa seems to be at home – there is a glimpse of a Persian carpet along the edge of the image and patterned wallpaper on the wall behind her. Her feet, in another pair of black patent leather shoes, are still dangling, although she has grown a lot. By the third image, taken at around 9 or 10, she is still in Wormer but sitting on a different chair. Dressed in a black lacey top and black jeans, her hair in pigtails, she is without shoes. Her toes, in red patterned socks, have reached the ground. We see more of a Persian rug – half of her chair sits on it – and leaves from a pot plant emerge from the left-hand frame. Two years later, in 'Leidschendam, The Netherlands', Almerisa slouches in her seat. She is wearing a blue long-sleeved top and white jeans and socks and her legs have grown, and she is firmly planted in place. The carpet is shag pile and there is a picture of a fashion model pinned to the wall as decoration. In this and the final two images, both set in Leidschendam, Almerisa has become a teenager; she looks much more boldly at the camera. In 2002 and 2003 we are in the presence of a young adult who has physically and sartorially transitioned. As Visser writes, 'We are clearly dealing here with "rites of passage", to adulthood ... These are moments when a person enters into a new, different community, but before all else, into a new emotional phase: [in the Almerisa series] that of ... an erotic being' (Visser, in Dijkstra 2004: 14).

As in the *Beach Portraits*, Dijkstra uses a slightly low camera angle with the subject looking directly at the camera. In each image, Almerisa's expression is calm – she does not smile – but over time her gaze becomes more confident: in the 2002 image there is a faint half smile. In the 2002 picture, for the first time, Almerisa is sitting in front of a window, which although covered by a long lace curtain, lets in a square of sunlight. In 2003, the entire background is a curtained window. These last images convey a sense of possibility, an escape from the confinement of the earlier images in which Almerisa was enclosed by walls. As a series, then, these images depict puberty and adolescence as a time of ultimately hopeful change and growth.

For me, these images articulate the bio-psycho-social nature of pubertal development in a positive way. Almerisa's becoming teenage is inextricably both physical and cultural: psychological changes are hinted by her facial expression and gaze, whilst her changing body and clothes articulate the bio-social. Importantly, her direct gaze implicates both the photographer and the viewer, reminding us that sexual development is something that is observed and regulated as well as lived by young people. Dijkstra's somewhat clinical gaze – heightened by the starkness of the bare rooms and the unsmiling expressions and repetitive poses – is clearly an interested one. Like her nineteenth-century anthropometric predecessors, like Tanner and Whitehouse and contemporary scientists engaged in laboratory work, like policymakers engaged in policy writing and, indeed, like social scientists articulating an argument, Dijkstra is part of the apparatus enacting her subject-object: her self-portrait in a wet swimming costume (1991) – echoed in the beach series – heightens this sense of inclusion.

Through her art practice, Dijkstra stages an encounter with puberty that is complex, rich and provocative. Situating Dijkstra's work in a genealogy of photographic portraiture, Urs Stahel writes:

> All this means that we, the viewers, must gain an insight into the visual world of Rineke Dijsktra; that, used as we are to the extremes of our frequently insipid, colourless and stressful everyday world and the shrill, brash, colourful media world, we must once again learn to look at calm, apparently simple pictures that are nevertheless endowed with a high level of presence, to be aware of tiny yet highly meaningful changes, and to recognise and absorb a reduced and conspicuously subtle and at the same time rich colourfulness. (Stahel, in Dijkstra 1999: 149–50)

It is this invitation to 'look again' and to become 'aware of tiny yet highly meaningful changes' constituting sexual development that resonates with my project here. In theorising bodies as bio-psycho-social, I want to advocate the significance of paying attention to the details of findings, feelings and figurations. My ethnographic approach to the Literature chimes with this orientation: in reading about early puberty and retelling the stories I have read, I have tried to convey a sense of the rich, dense networks in which scientific and other stories are made and flow. Like feelings and figurations, findings do not come from thin air: they are made in relational, situated practice.

Interpreting findings; developing alternative figurations

Throughout this book I have theorised sexual development as a process of folding. In some critical accounts, unfolding is seen as a negative biologistic notion that sexual maturity simply flows from a set of genetic instructions. For me, in contrast, folding describes a more complex set of intra-actions in which a particular set of arrangements comes into being or congeals over time. Building on Deleuze's and Haraway's concepts of folding and infolding, I have emphasised the indeterminate and relational qualities of the material-semiotic, human–non-human relations at stake in the making of bodies.

The preceding chapters have discussed a range of intra-active forces involved in pubertal development: hormones, genes, early childhood experiences, social and cultural forces including language and patterns of discrimination and poverty, medical, scientific and cultural practices, including photographing, measuring, observing, injecting, dressing and eating. As Anne Fausto-Sterling (2005) argues in the case of bone accumulation in childhood, genes, hormones and social and cultural experiences (in her case, exposure to sunlight and cigarette smoke, activity levels, diet, gendered forms of childhood play) are all involved in the making of bodies. As discussed in Chapter 5, she theorises bodies as emergent. Borrowing Barad's term, I have articulated the interplay of forces in sexual development as intra-actions that disrupt or 'message across' (Roberts 2007) social/biological or nature/nurture divisions. Blending feminist notions of embodiment with science studies accounts of relational ontologies, I have argued that puberty is always bio-psycho-social.

Contemporary biomedical accounts of 'normal' sexual development describe genes as stimulating hormonal cascades and causing physiological change. As I noted in Chapter 5, this leads scientists to search for the specific genes that constitute what Palmert and Boepple (2001), for example, describe as a form of 'genetic control' underlying environmental and metabolic factors influencing the timing of puberty: such factors, they suggest are 'critical regulators' of the timing of puberty 'but their influence is superimposed on significant genetic control' (2001: 2366). Importantly, however, puberty is also widely viewed as riddled with complexities, mostly centring on the relations between individual biological factors (genes and hormonal systems) and 'other' or 'environmental' factors. Unlike scientific descriptions of other physiological changes (bone growth for example) that figure bodies as enclosed, homeostatic biological systems, then, contemporary biomedical texts describe the causes of puberty in ways that disrupt distinctions between the biological and the social. Ebling (2005: 683), for example, writes that 'the neurotransmitter and neuromodulatory systems that impact upon the GnRH secretory network convey information about metabolic fuels, energy stores and somatic development and, for many species, information about season and social environment'. Such disruptions, as discussed in Chapter 5, indicate spaces for developing more open and exploratory understandings of embodiment.

Unfortunately these spaces are often closed down through models that produce hierarchies of effects in which biological factors such as genes and hormones take priority over messy, less measurable social forces. Figure 8, taken from a paper by Parent *et al.* introduced in Chapter 4, provides a typical example. Whilst acknowledging a wide range of possible contributors to the timing of puberty, including genes, inter-uterine conditions, insulin sensitivity, diet, exposure to sunlight, environmental toxins and emotional and physical stress, the diagram figures a conventional ontology in which a 'cascade of genes' remains the most important determinant of pubertal timing (Parent *et al.*, 2003: 680). Observations and findings from twin studies, Parent *et al.* (2003: 679) write, 'indicate that 70–80% of the variance in pubertal timing can be explained by heritable factors'. At the centre of the concentric circles then, the genetic core affects the other 'factors' in an outward-pointing fashion. Encircling this 'genetic predisposition' are other individual biological factors (post-natal growth, weight, insulin sensitivity, possible malignancies), whilst 'environmental hits' (stress, endocrine disrupting chemicals and nutrition) are figured as inward-pointing arrows at the circle's boundary.

Somewhat surprisingly given her theoretical orientation, Fausto-Sterling (2008: 677) uses a set of embedded boxes to articulate the 'embedded systems' of bone development. Here, the 'individual system' lies at the centre and 'short- and long-term history' at the edge. Expanding the individual system box in a second set of boxes, Fausto-Sterling places 'genes' at the centre, 'organs' in the middle and 'routine activities' at the outer edge. Like Parent *et al.*'s diagram, this nested depiction repeats conventional narratives of surface and depth and inside/outside relations.

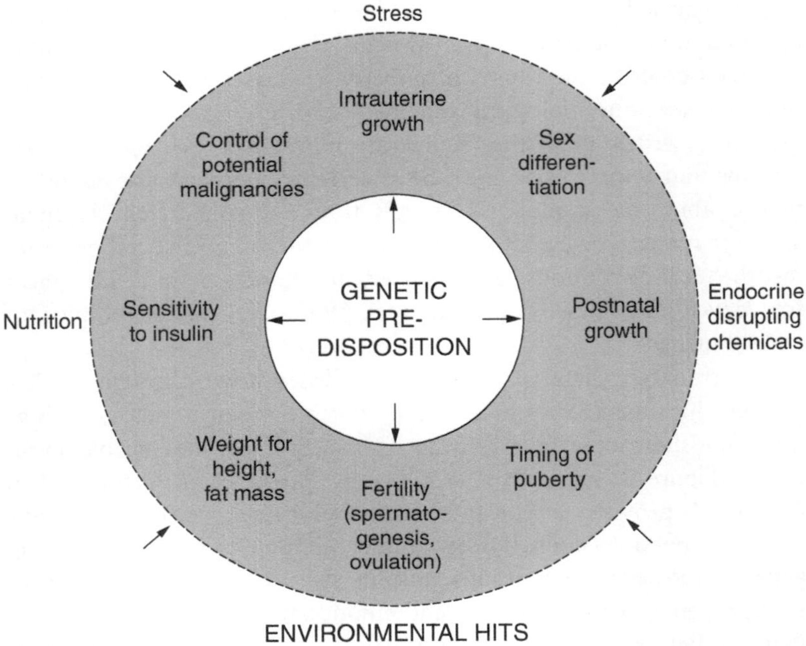

Figure 8 The concentric circles of sexual development. Integration of timing of puberty within a spectrum of processes that are influenced by both genetic and environmental factors.

Diagrams like Parent *et al.*'s, as feminist theorist Jackie Stacey (2000: 128–32) has argued in her analysis of alternative health discourses on cancer, position the individual and his or her susceptibilities within an environmental context of risk (in this case 'hits') that are more or less avoidable. They thus produce a set of responsibilities: the individual body is positioned as potentially pure, something that is overwhelmed or attacked by 'unnatural' forces that could and should be avoided. Although Fausto-Sterling is certainly not suggesting that individuals be held responsible for their own 'short- and long-term history', her modelling of internal and external factors as nested boxes also runs the risk of positing a version of health that involves defending a biological core against the dangers of social life.

This model of health is articulated in the distinction Parent *et al.* draw between timely and early onset puberty. In their model, timely puberty is *not* notably influenced by external factors; in the 'normal' case, these remain merely 'permissive' (Parent *et al.* 2003: 686). Early onset puberty, in contrast, is problematic because it is too open to these factors. In my view, such figurations fail to come to terms with the ways in which puberty disrupts distinctions between the biological, the psychological and the social. Resisting complexity (or trying to manage it), diagrams that use concentric circles or nested boxes maintain a genetically programmed, biological norm and figure 'other' (environmental or social) factors as abnormal, something 'outside' that should be prevented, resisted or treated. (The psychological is most often absent.)

In contrast, I have argued throughout this book that both timely and early onset puberty are bio-psycho-social. Understanding puberty as folding would, in both cases, disrupt the hierarchical nature of the circles or boxes, allowing for a more dynamic, intra-active flow between 'external' and 'internal' forces.

As Dijkstra's photographs so beautifully convey, puberty involves change over time. But time does not simply unfold sequentially within bodies: bio-psycho-social flows are multi- not uni-directional. This more complex sense of change over time is captured in Figure 9, a diagram depicting the life course of a tuberculosis patient, produced by Bowker and Star (1999: 191) to represent what they call 'the topology-typology twist' of a person's trajectory through an enduring illness. Building on the earlier work of Julia Corbin and Anselm Strauss (1988; 1991) and Stephan Timmermans (1996), this diagram successfully articulates the 'tensions among bodies, biographies and classifications' that I call the bio-psycho-social. Although moving forward in time, the 'body trajectory' is wiggly and intersected at various intervals by the lines of biography: careers, plans, work and relationships which may or may not continue during illness. In the case of a child progressing through puberty, this would include relationships with family and friends, schooling and other activities, as well as nutrition, experiences of racism, poverty, wealth, etc. Underlying these two personal trajectories, Bowker and Star introduce the discontinuous, sometimes overlapping lines of formal classification; that which forms scientific knowledge and practice. These lines impact on the individual's trajectory in moments of diagnosis, treatment and monitoring but do not correlate neatly with their lived experience. In the field of early puberty, and many others, one might wish to add another set of lines

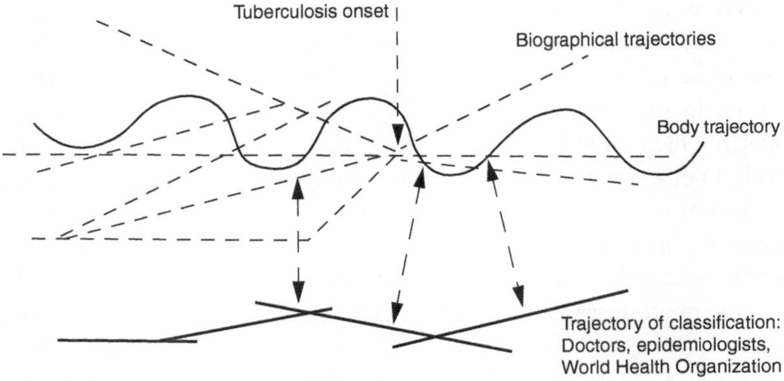

Figure 9 Bowker and Star's (1999) topology-typology twist.
Tensions among bodies, biographies and classification – the twisted landscape of multiple classifications. The topology created by the body-biography trajectory is pulled against the idealised, standardised typology of the global classification of tuberculosis, itself a broken and moving target. When standard classifications are added to the scheme, patients try to fit their experiences along both body and biographical trajectories to a standard picture of metric. Changing definitions, local arrangements and complex relations of all three trajectories contribute to torquing the typology/topography via the dotted lines, which represent negotiations.

depicting less formal but nonetheless shared knowledges, such as those produced by patient organisations or found in news media articles or vlogs.

Akin to Deleuze's notion of the fold, the twisting topology depicted here introduces a complex temporal texture: the diagram helps us to conceptualise 'the relationships between representations, work, body, and biography' that constitute an individual's life (Bowker and Star 1999: 192). My theorisation of sexual development as folding similarly articulates the temporal and relational entanglements of 'insides' and 'outsides'.

But even as folding, early onset puberty is sometimes a problem in a child's life. So what might be done to help? In Chapter 7 I discussed the use of GnRH analogues to delay puberty. This medication creates physiological changes and for some children (notably those who identify as trans) seems to be life-enhancing. Although altering hormonal messaging in the body, however, these drugs do not address other forces involved in sexual development. These need to be addressed in other ways: through activism, education, physical activities, forms of care.

In an article on racism and hypertension, Fausto-Sterling (2004) makes a similar point about blood pressure medications. Altering the diameter of blood vessels, these do nothing to change the higher brain regulation that sets the blood pressure 'thermostat'. This thermostat, she argues, is set in part by an individual's experience of racism and structural inequality and the biological stress caused by consequent hypervigilance. A more effective approach to treating hypertension, then, would focus on 'higher level interventions, adjusting entire systems of physiology and attending to the emotions and unmet needs that produce the negative physiological results of hypervigiliance' (Fausto-Sterling 2004: 29). This could include paying attention to diet and exercise but also directly addressing racism and inequality. Redirecting rage and psychological pain into political action, improving social connectedness and working towards necessary social change-would, Fausto-Sterling suggests, reduce hypertension.

In the case of early onset puberty I suggest that we need to consider childhood experience, environmental toxins and cultural figurations of sexuality and sex/gender. Toxins biologically accumulate alongside the physiological echoes of racism, poverty and sexism, potentially exacerbating their impacts on a child's development. As discussed in Chapter 6, internationally adopted or neglected or abused children may learn to function as if in danger, reacting to everyday social situations in ways usually reserved for more life-threatening events. The physiological patterns involved in such learning – higher levels of circulating cortisol for example – may intra-act with other hormonal messaging circuits, altering the timing of sexual development. As in the hypertension case, changing social patterns and figurations – through political action, vlogging, public debate – should have powerful effects here.

Worryingly, as we have seen throughout this book, a range of powerful forces act in a different direction, articulating sexual development in more limiting ways. Drug companies prioritise marketable pharmaceutical 'solutions'; social policy documents depict changes to childhood as 'crisis'; environmentalists describe early sexual development as a threat to our future. As crisis, early onset puberty becomes something to be diagnosed, worried about and treated pharmacologically. The main task of this book has been to challenge and problematise these articulations so that early sexual development can be thought of and treated differently.

The politics of technoscience and biomedicine

Technoscience and biomedicine are multiple phenomena: they comprise a wide set of practices that are not contained within laboratories, universities, pharmaceutical company offices or clinics. Policymakers, journalists, environmentalists, writers, teachers, children and their families all do the science of puberty and participate in the making of sexually developing bodies. Each of these groups is differently situated as actors in apparatuses. Their engagements with formal scientific knowledges – those made in laboratories for example – are also varied, but it is remarkable how widespread such engagement is. From teenage vloggers to journalists, from policymakers to parents, 'non-experts' like myself grapple with technical articulations of genes, hormones, statistics, organisms and environments in order to try to better understand and to intervene in bodily experiences.

Whilst not wanting to make a romantic claim about the democratising of science – untenable at a moment in which the British National Health Service is being steadily dismantled by a conservative government and the global pharmaceutical industry is making huge profits – I think it is important to note that this is a time in which biomedical and technoscientific findings, discourses and practices are open to public scrutiny and experimentation in a variety of new ways, including citizens' panels and focus groups, television documentaries and films, citizen science projects and public consultations (see papers in Haran and McNeil 2013). Such practices help a wide range of interested actors to articulate concerns and areas of interest and to speak across traditional divisions between 'experts' and 'non-experts'. Although subject to capture in the interests of governmental and corporate power, at their best these practices can open up a space for critical conversations about science, for thinking about the formulation of scientific questions, the directions of scientific research and the machinations of science policy and funding (see for example Kashefi and Mort 2004).

Discussing the science of human development, Evelyn Fox Keller calls for a recognition of a shared interest in 'maximisation ... of human potential', arguing that 'we' (for me, this would include social scientists, activists, citizens and young people) need to participate in the formulation of scientific questions:

> We may not share the interests of breeders in artificial selection, but as both scientists and citizens, we are surely committed to trying to maximize the development of human potential. And for this, we need a better understanding of what resources can contribute to such development, and of how they can best be deployed ... There is no shortage of scientific work that can productively inform us about the things we want to know, but we do need to pose our questions in ways that researchers can answer. (Keller 2010: 84)

In this call, Keller articulates a relationship in which science 'productively inform[s]' citizens about 'the things we want to know'.

In this book, I have repeatedly questioned the aims, logics and methods of current scientific work on sexual development, arguing that rather than telling us the things we want to know, this work helps to articulate pubertal bodies as problems and recent changes in pubertal timing as a crisis. In other places, I have suggested that scientific and biomedical discourses do help us to understand the complexities of sexually developing bodies and the risks that the contemporary circumstances of many children may pose. Locating myself within a lineage of feminist science studies that takes biological and biomedical research and findings seriously, I have navigated a path between paranoid criticism and reparative affirmation when engaging with all kinds of texts, including scientific and biomedical ones.

Although focusing on early sexual development, this book is also a contribution to feminist theories of the body more broadly. I hope it will encourage other feminists to keep exploring scientific and biomedical articulations of bodies and to continue thinking carefully about how these articulations challenge and develop our attempts to theorise bodily differences. Politically I consider it vital to open up these articulations to detailed engagement and debate within the social sciences and humanities, in various public spheres and in related professional fields, in medicine, paediatric endocrinology and gynaecology, public health, education and social work, to name a few key possibilities. Such interactions are rarely straightforward – they can sometimes be alienating and dispiriting – but they are worth pursuing in whatever way we can manage. I have been struck throughout my time working on this book by the intense interest that people from all walks of life have in early sexual development. Parents, teachers, scientists and social scientists have much to share in future conversations about the complexities of early onset puberty: I hope my mapping of the debates here will support these conversations.

Contemporary changes to pubertal timing do not constitute a crisis. We should, therefore, be wary of demands to act. But feminists interested in bodies, in childhood, in sex/gender and sexuality would do well to turn their attention to sexual development. Important changes are occurring, and we need to get involved in public and technical debates in this area. For feminist theorists, puberty also provides a rich and fascinating example of the complexities of embodiment, of sex/gender and of change over time. Ultimately, puberty is an unfolding of possibilities, a 'channelling into the future' as Pinto (2007: 536) put it. There is much to explore here, both to celebrate and to change.

References

Adams, V., Murphy, M. and Clarke, A.E. 2009. 'Anticipation: Technoscience, Life, Affect, Temporality', *Subjectivity* 28(1): 246–65.

Agaibi, C.E. and Wilson, J.P. 2005. 'Trauma, PTSD, and Resilience: A Review of the Literature', *Trauma, Violence, & Abuse* 6(3): 195–216.

Ahlgren, M., Melbye, M., Wohlfahrt, J. and Sørensen, T.I. 2004. 'Growth Patterns and the Risk of Breast Cancer in Women', *New England Journal of Medicine* 351(16): 1619–26.

Ahmed, S. 2008. 'Open Forum Imaginary Prohibitions: Some Preliminary Remarks on the Founding Gestures of the "New Materialism"', *European Journal of Women's Studies* 15(1): 23–39.

Ainsworth, M.D.S. 1978. 'The Bowlby-Ainsworth Attachment Theory', *Behavioural and Brain Sciences* 1: 436–8.

Aksglaede, L., Juul, A., Leffers, H., Skakkebaek, N.E. and Andersson, A.M. 2006. 'The Sensitivity of the Child to Sex Steroids: Possible Impact of Exogenous Estrogens', *Human Reproduction Update* 12(1): 341–9.

Aksglaede, L., Olsen, L.W., Sørensen, T.I.A. and Juul, A. 2008. 'Forty Years Trends in Timing of Pubertal Growth Spurt in 157,000 Danish School Children', *Public Library of Science One* 3(7): e2728.

Aksglaede, L., Sorensen, K., Petersen, J.H., Skakkebaek, N.E. and Juul, A. 2009. 'Recent Decline in Age at Breast Development: The Copenhagen Puberty Study', *Pediatrics* 123(5): e932–9.

Alaimo, S. 2010. *Bodily Natures: Science, Environment, and the Material Self*. Bloomington: Indiana University Press.

Albanese, A., Hall, C. and Stanhope, R. 1995. 'The Use of a Computerized Method of Bone Age Assessment in Clinical Practice', *Hormone Research* 44(3): 2–7.

Alcoff, L. 1988. 'Cultural Feminism versus Post-structuralism: The Identity Crisis in Feminist Theory', *Signs* 13: 405–36.

American Psychological Association (Task Force on the Sexualization of Girls). 2010. *Report of the APA Task Force on the Sexualization of Girls*. www.apa.org/pi/women/programs/girls/report-full.pdf.

Andrusiak, T. 2009. 'Finding the Courage to Get Real', in M.T. Reist (ed.), *Getting Real: Challenging the Sexualisation of Girls*, North Melbourne: Spinifex Press, pp. 171–8.

Anitai, S. 2007. 'Early Puberty Makes Girls Prone to Sex and Drugs. And to Relationships with Much Older Partners', http://news.softpedia.com/news/Early-Puberty-Makes-Girls-Prone-to-Sex-and-Drug-50131.shtml.

Ankarberg, C. and Norjavaara, E. 1999. 'Diurnal Rhythm of Testosterone Secretion before and throughout Puberty in Healthy Girls: Correlation with 17beta-estradiol and Dehydroepiandrosterone Sulfate', *Journal of Clinical Endocrinology and Metabolism* 84(3): 975–84.

Anon. 2005. 'So Much More to Know . . .', *Science* 309(5731): 78–102.

Aphramor, L. 2005. 'Is a Weight-centred Health Framework Salutogenic? Some Thoughts on Unhinging Certain Dietary Ideologies', *Social Theory & Health* 3(4): 315–40.

Apter, D. 1997. 'Development of the Hypothalamic-Pituitary-Ovarian Axis', *Annals of the New York Academy of Sciences* 816 (June 17): 9–21.

Arnett, J.J. 1999. 'Adolescent Storm and Stress, Reconsidered', *American Psychologist* 54(5): 317–26.

2006. 'G. Stanley Hall's *Adolescence*: Brilliance and Nonsense', *History of Psychology* 9(3): 186–97.

Attwood, F. 2011. 'Through the Looking Glass? Sexual Agency and Subjectification Online', in R. Gill and C. Scharff (eds.), *New Femininities: Postfeminism, Neoliberalism and Subjectivity*, Basingstoke: Palgrave Macmillan, pp. 203–14.

Bailey, R. 2011. *Letting Children Be Children: Report of an Independent Review of the Commercialisation and Sexualisation of Childhood*, vol. 8078. London: The Stationery Office.

Balkishori Team of VACHA Women's Resource Center with Jackie Kirk. 2009. 'Reclaiming Girlhood: Understanding the Lives of Balkishori in Mumbai', in C. Mitchell and J. Reid-Walsh (eds.), *Seven Going on Seventeen: Tween Studies in the Culture of Girlhood*, New York: Peter Lang, pp. 135–47.

Bar, A., Linder, E.H., Sobel, B. and Dimartinonardi, J. 1994. 'The Bayley-Pinneau (BP) Method for Height Prediction (HP) Is Accurate for Girls with Central Precocious Puberty (CPP)', *Pediatric Research* 35(4): A94–A94.

Barad, K.M. 2007. *Meeting the Universe Halfway: Quantum Physics and the Entanglement of Matter and Meaning*. Durham, NC: Duke University Press.

2010. 'Quantum Entanglements and Hauntological Relations of Inheritance: Dis/continuities, Spacetime Enfoldings, and Justice-to-Come', *Derrida Today* 3(2): 240–68.

2011. 'Erasers and Erasures: Pinch's Unfortunate "Uncertainty Principle"', *Social Studies of Science* 41(3): 443–54.

Bateman, A.J. 1948. 'Intra-sexual Selection in Drosophila', *Heredity* 2(3): 349–68.

Batsleer, J. 2008. *Informal Learning in Youth Work*, Los Angeles and London: Sage.

BBC News Health. 2010. 'Genes Give Clue to Early Puberty.' www.bbc.co.uk/news/health-11795645.

Belkin, L. 2000. 'The Making of an 8-Year-Old Woman.' www.nytimes.com/2000/12/24/magazine/the-making-of-an-8-year-old-woman.html?pagewanted=all&src=pm.

2012. 'How Parenting Is Like Groundhog Day And Mad Libs', *Huffington Post.* www.huffingtonpost.com/lisa-belkin/parenting-trends_b_1401513.html.

Bell, S.E. 2009. *DES Daughters, Embodied Knowledge, and the Transformation of Women's Health Politics in the Late Twentieth Century*, Philadelphia, PA: Temple University Press.

Belluck, P. 2012. 'Puberty Starting Earlier in Boys, New Study Suggests.' www.nytimes.com/2012/10/20/health/puberty-starting-earlier-in-boys-new-study-suggests.html.

Belsky, J. 1990. 'Parental and Nonparental Child Care and Children's Socio-emotional Development: A Decade in Review', *Journal of Marriage and the Family* 52(4): 885–903.

1997. 'Theory Testing, Effect-size Evaluation, and Differential Susceptibility to Rearing Influence: The Case of Mothering and Attachment', *Child Development* 68(4): 598–600.

2001. 'Emanuel Miller Lecture: Developmental Risks (Still) Associated with Early Child Care', *Journal of Child Psychology and Psychiatry* 42(7): 845–59.

2005. 'Differential Susceptibility to Rearing Influence', in B.J. Ellis and D.F. Bjorklund (eds.), *Origins of the Social Mind: Evolutionary Psychology and Child Development*, New York: Guilford Press, pp. 139–63.

2010. 'Childhood Experience and the Development of Reproductive Strategies', *Psicothema* 22(1): 28–34.

Belsky, J., Bakermans-Kranenburg, M.J. and Van Jzendoorn, M.H. 2007. 'For Better and for Worse: Differential Susceptibility to Environmental Influences', *Current Directions in Psychological Science* 16(6): 300–4.

Belsky, J. and Beaver, K.M. 2011. 'Cumulative-genetic Plasticity, Parenting and Adolescent Self-regulation', *Journal of Child Psychology and Psychiatry* 52(5): 619–26.

Belsky, J., Houts, R.M. and Pasco Fearon, R.M. 2010. 'Infant Attachment Security and the Timing of Puberty: Testing an Evolutionary Hypothesis', *Psychological Science* 21(9): 1195–1201.

Belsky, J. and Pluess, M. 2009. 'The Nature (and Nurture?) of Plasticity in Early Human Development', *Perspectives on Psychological Science* 4(4): 345–51.

Belsky, J., Steinberg, L. and Draper, P. 1991. 'Childhood Experience, Interpersonal Development, and Reproductive Strategy: An Evolutionary Theory of Socialization', *Child Development* 62(4): 647–70.

Belsky, J., Vandell, D.L., Burchinal, M., Clarke-Stewart, K.A., McCartney, K. and Owen, M.T. 2007. 'Are There Long-Term Effects of Early Child Care?', *Child Development* 78(2): 681–701.

Benatar, S.R., Gill, S. and Bakker, I. 2011. 'Global Health and the Global Economic Crisis', *American Journal of Public Health* 101(4): 646–53.

Berenbaum, S.A. and Beltz, A.M. 2011. 'Sexual Differentiation of Human Behavior: Effects of Prenatal and Pubertal Organizational Hormones', *Frontiers in Neuroendocrinology* 32(2): 183–200.

Berkson, L. 2000. *Hormonal Destiny: How Artificial Hormones from Everyday Products Are Sending Our Bodies the Wrong Messages – and How to Protect Yourself and Your Family*, Lincolnwood: Contemporary Books.

Biro, F.M., Galvez, M.P., Greenspan, L.C., Succop, P.A., Vangeepuram, N., Pinney, S.M., Teitelbaum, S., Windham, G.C., Kushi, L.H. and Wolff, M.S. 2010. 'Pubertal Assessment Method and Baseline Characteristics in a Mixed Longitudinal Study of Girls', *Pediatrics* 126(3): 583–90.

Biro, F.M., Khoury, P. and Morrison, J.A., 2006. 'Influence of Obesity on Timing of Puberty', *International Journal of Andrology* 29(1): 272–7.

Biro, F.M., McMahon, R.P., Striegel-Moore, R., Crawford, P.B., Obarzanek, E., Morrison, J.A., Barton, B.A. and Falkner, F. 2001. 'Impact of Timing of Pubertal Maturation on Growth in Black and White Female Adolescents: The National Heart, Lung, and Blood Institute Growth and Health Study', *Journal of Pediatrics* 138(5): 636–43.

Bland, L. 1995. *Banishing the Beast: English Feminism and Sexual Morality, 1885–1914*. London: Penguin.

Boepple, P.A. and Crowley, W.F. 1991. 'Gonadotropin-releasing-hormone Analogs as Therapeutic Probes in Human Growth and Development: Evidence from Children with Central Precocious Puberty', *Acta Paediatrica Scandinavica* 1(372): 33–8.

Boepple, P.A., Mansfield, M.J., Crawford, J.D., Crigler, J.F., Blizzard, R.M. and Crowley, W.F. 1991. 'Final Heights in Girls with Central Precocious Puberty (CPP) following GNRH Agonist (GnRHa)-induced Pituitary-gonadal Suppression', *Pediatric Research* 29(4): A74.

Borjesson, A.E., Lagerquist, M.K., Liu, C., Shao, R., Windahl, S.H., Karlsson, C., Sjogren, K., Moverare-Skrtic, S., Antal, M.C., Krust, A., Mohan, S., Chambon, P., Savendahl, L. and Ohlsson, C. 2010. 'The Role of Estrogen Receptor alpha in Growth Plate Cartilage for Longitudinal Bone Growth', *Journal of Bone and Mineral Research* 25(12): 2690–700.

Bourguignon, J-P., Gérard, A., Alvarez Gonzalez, M.L., Fawe, L. and Franchimont, P. 1992. 'Effects of Changes in Nutritional Conditions on Timing of Puberty: Clinical Evidence from Adopted Children and Experimental Studies in the Male Rat', *Hormone Research in Paediatrics* 38(Suppl. 1): 97–105.

Bowker, G.C. 2010. 'A Plea for Pleats' in C.P. Jensen and K. Rodje (eds.), *Deleuzian Intersections: Science, Technology, Anthropology*, New York and Oxford: Berghahn Books, pp. 123–38.

Bowker, G.C. and Star, L. 1999. *Sorting Things Out: Classification and its Consequences*, Cambridge, MA: MIT Press.

Bowlby, J. 1969. *Attachment and Loss*, New York: Basic Books.

Bradshaw, J. 2011. *The Well-being of Children in the UK*, Bristol: The Policy Press.

Bradshaw, J. and Richardson, D. 2009. 'An Index of Child Well-being in Europe', *Child Indicators Research* 2(3): 319–51.

Braidotti, R. 2013. *The Posthuman*, London: Polity.

Braithwaite, J. 1984. *Corporate Crime in the Pharmaceutical industry*, London: Routledge & Kegan Paul.

Braun, L. 2002. 'Race, Ethnicity, and Health: Can Genetics Explain Disparities?', *Perspectives in Biology and Medicine* 45(2): 159–74.

Braun, L., Fausto-Sterling, A., Fullwiley, D., Hammonds, E.M., Nelson, A., Quivers, W., Reverby, S.M. and Shields, A.E. 2007. 'Racial Categories in Medical Practice: How Useful Are They?', *PLoS Medicine* 4(9):1423–8.

Braun, L., Wolfgang, M. and Dickersin, K. 2013. 'Defining Race/Ethnicity and Explaining Difference in Research Studies on Lung Function', *European Respiratory Journal* 41(6): 1362–70.

Braun, M. 1994. *Picturing Time: The Work of Etienne-Jules Marey (1830–1904)*, University of Chicago Press.

1997. 'The Expanded Present: Photographing Movement', in A. Thomas (ed.), *Beauty of Another Order: Photography in Science*, New Haven and London: Yale University Press, pp. 150–85.

2010. *Eadweard Muybridge*, London: Reaktion Books.

2013. 'Muybridge, Authorship, Originality', *Early Popular Visual Culture* 11(1): 41–51.

Bray, A. 2008. 'The Question of Intolerance', *Australian Feminist Studies* 23(57): 323–41.

2009. 'Governing the Gaze', *Feminist Media Studies* 9(2): 173–91.

Brennan, T. 2004. *The Transmission of Affect*, Ithaca, NY: Cornell University Press.

Brierley, J. and Larcher, V. 2010. 'Lest We Forget ... Research Ethics in Children: Perhaps Onerous, yet Absolutely Necessary', *Archives of Disease in Childhood* 95(11): 863–6.

Briscoe, A.M. 1978. 'Hormones and Gender', in E. Tobach and B. Rosoff (eds.), *Genes and Gender 1*, New York: Gordon Press, pp. 31–50.

Brown, J., Cohen, P., Chen, H., Smailes, E. and Johnson, J.G. 2004. 'Sexual Trajectories of Abused and Neglected Youths', *Journal of Developmental & Behavioral Pediatrics* 25(2): 77–82.

Brown, J.D., Halpern, C.T. and L'Engle, K.L. 2005. 'Mass Media as a Sexual Super Peer for Early Maturing Girls', *Journal of Adolescent Health* 36(5): 420–7.

Brown, J.D., L'Engle, K.L., Pardun, C.J., Guo, G., Kenneavy, K. and Jackson, C. 2006. 'Sexy Media Matter: Exposure to Sexual Content in Music, Movies, Television, and Magazines Predicts Black and White Adolescents' Sexual Behavior', *Pediatrics* 117(4): 1018–27.

Bruinsma, F.J., Venn, A.J., Patton, G.C., Rayner, J.A., Pyett, P., Werther, G., Jones, P. and Lumley, J.M. 2006. 'Concern about Tall Stature during Adolescence and Depression in Later Life', *Journal of Affective Disorders* 91(2): 145–52.

Brulle, R. and Pellow, D.N. 2006. 'Environmental Justice: Human Health and Environmental Inequalities', *Annual Review of Public Health* 27: 103–24.

Brumberg, J. 1997. *The Body Project: An Intimate History of American Girls*, New York: Vintage Books.

Buckingham, D. 2000. *After the Death of Childhood: Growing Up in the Age of Electronic Media*, Cambridge: Polity Press.

2007. *The Impact of the Commercial World on Children's Wellbeing*, London: Department for Children, Schools and Families and the Department for Culture, Media and Sport.

2009. *The Impact of the Commercial World on Children's Wellbeing: Report of an Independent Assessment*. Available at http://publications.dcsf.gov.uk/default.aspx.

Buckingham, D., Willett, R., Bragg, S. and Russell, R. 2010. *Sexualised Goods Aimed at Children: A Report to the Scottish Parliament Equal Opportunities Committee*, Edinburgh: Scottish Parliament Equal Opportunities Committee.

Burman, E. 1994. Deconstructing Developmental Psychology, London: Routledge.

2008. Deconstructing Developmental Psychology, New York: Routledge.

Burman, E. and Stacey, J. 2010a. 'The Child and Childhood in Feminist Theory', *Feminist Theory* 11(3): 227–40.

(eds.) 2010b. *The Child and Childhood: A Special Issue of Feminist Theory* 11(3).

Bute, J.J. and Russell, L.D. 2012. 'Public Discourses about Teenage Pregnancy: Disruption, Restoration, and Ideology', *Health Communication* 27(7): 712–22.

Butland, B., Jebb, S., Kopelman, P., McPherson, K., Thomas, S., Mardell, J., Parry, V. *et al.* 2007. *Foresight. Tackling Obesities: Future Choices.* www.cabdirect.org/abstracts/20073277472.html.

Butler, J. 1990. *Gender Trouble and the Subversion of Identity*, London and New York: Routledge.

1993. *Bodies That Matter: On the Discursive Limits of Sex*, London and New York: Routledge.

Buyken, A.E., Karaolis-Danckert, N. and Remer, T. 2009. 'Association of Prepubertal Body Composition in Healthy Girls and Boys with the Timing of Early and Late Pubertal Markers', *American Journal of Clinical Nutrition* 89(1): 221–30.

Callon, M. and Rabeharisoa, V. 2008. 'The Growing Engagement of Emergent Concerned Groups in Political and Economic Life Lessons from the French Association of Neuromuscular Disease Patients', *Science, Technology & Human Values* 33(2): 230–61.

Cameron, N. 2002. *Human Growth and Development*, San Diego, CA: Academic Press.

Carel, J-C., Eugster, E.A., Rogol, A., Ghizzoni, L., Palmert, M.R., and on behalf of the members of the ESPE-LWPES GnRH Analogs Consensus Conference Group. 2009. 'Consensus Statement on the Use of Gonadotropin-Releasing Hormone Analogs in Children', *Pediatrics* 123(4): e752–62.

Carey, T. 2011. *Where Has My Little Girl Gone? How to Protect Your Daughter from Growing Up too Soon*, Oxford: Lion Books.

2012. 'The Little Girls Who Reach Puberty as Young as Six: Could Junk Food, Plastic Packaging and Computer Screens Be to Blame?' www.dailymail.co.uk/femail/article-2225986/The-little-girls-reach-puberty-young-Could-junk-food-plastic-packaging-screens-blame.html.

Cartwright, L. 1995. *Screening the Body: Tracing Medicine's Visual Culture*, University of Minnesota Press.

Caselli, D. 2010. 'Kindergarten Theory: Childhood, Affect, Critical Thought', *Feminist Theory* 11(3): 241–54.

Castañeda, C. 2002. *Figurations: Child, Bodies, Worlds*, Durham, NC: Duke University Press.

Castree, N. 2010. 'Crisis, Continuity and Change: Neoliberalism, the Left and the Future of Capitalism', *Antipode* 41: 185–213.

Cesario, S.K. and Hughes, L.A. 2007. 'Precocious Puberty: A Comprehensive Review of Literature', *Journal of Obstetric, Gynecologic, & Neonatal Nursing* 36(3): 263–74.

Chagin, A.S. and Sävendahl, L. 2007. 'Oestrogen Receptors and Linear Bone Growth', *Acta Paediatrica* 96(9): 1275–9.

Cheu, H.F. 2009. 'Imported Girl Fighters: Ripeness and Leakage', in C. Mitchell and J. Reid-Walsh (eds.), *Seven Going on Seventeen: Tween Studies in the Culture of Girlhood*, New York: Peter Lang, pp. 294–310.

Chisholm, J.S. 1996. 'The Evolutionary Ecology of Attachment Organization', *Human Nature* 7: 1–38.

1999. *Death, Hope and Sex: Steps to an Evolutionary Ecology of Mind and Morality*, Cambridge University Press.

Clarke, A.E., Mamo, L., Fishman, J.R. and Shim, J.K. 2003. 'Biomedicalization: Technoscientific Transformations of Health, Illness, and U.S. Biomedicine', *American Sociolological Review* 68(2): 161–94.

Clarke, A.E., Mamo, L., Fosket, J.R., Fishman, J.R. and Shim, J.K. (eds.) 2010. *Biomedicalization: Technoscience, Health, and Illness in the U.S.*, Durhman, NC: Duke University Press.

Clarke, A., Shim, J.K., Shostak, S. and Nelson, A. 2009. 'Biomedicalising Genetic Health, Diseases and Identities', in P. Atkinson and P. Glasner (eds.), *The Handbook of Genetics and Society*, London and New York: Routledge, pp. 21–40.

Coghlan, A. 2010. 'Early Puberty in Girls Doubles in a Decade', *New Scientist* 207(2773): 16.

Cohen, T. 2012. 'Stress of Family Breakdown and Rise of Obesity Levels Blamed as Girls' Puberty Age Falls to Ten', *Mail Online*. www.dailymail.co.uk/health/article-2159439/Stress-family-breakdown-rise-obesity-levels-blamed-girls-puberty-age-falls-ten.html.

Cohen-Kettenis, P.T. 2011. 'Response to the Discursive and Clinical Production of Trans Youth: Gender Variant Youth who Seek Puberty Suppression by Katrina Roen', *Psychology & Sexuality* 2(1): 58–68.

Colborn, T., Dumanoski, D. and Myers, J.P. 1996. *Our Stolen Future: Are We Threatening Our Fertility, Intelligence, and Survival? A Scientific Detective Story*, New York: Dutton.

Coleman, R. 2008. 'The Becoming of Bodies', *Feminist Media Studies* 8(2): 163–79.

Conrad, P. 2007. *The Medicalization of Society: On the Transformation of Human Conditions into Treatable Disorders*, 1st edition, Baltimore: Johns Hopkins University Press.

Coole, D. and Frost, S. (eds.) 2010. *New Materialisms: Ontology, Agency, and Politics*. Durham, NC: Duke University Press.

Cooper, E. 1995. *Fully Exposed: The Male Nude in Photography*, 2nd edn, London and New York: Routledge.

Corbin, J.M. and Strauss, A. 1988. *Unending Work and Care: Managing Chronic Illness at Home*. San Francisco: Jossey-Bass.

1991. 'Comeback: The Process of Overcoming Disability', in G. Albrecht and J. Levy (eds.), *Advances in Medical Sociology*, Greenwich, CT: JAI Press, pp. 137–58.

Creighton, S., Alderson, J., Brown, S. and Minto, C.L. 2002. 'Medical Photography: Ethics, Consent and the Intersex Patient', *BJU International* 89(1): 67–71.

Davis, K. 2007. *The Making of Our Bodies, Ourselves: How Feminism Travels across Borders*, Durham, NC: Duke University Press.

Davis, N. 2009. 'New Materialism and Feminism's Anti-biologism: A Response to Sara Ahmed', *European Journal of Women's Studies* 16(1): 67–80.

Davison, K.K., Birch, L.L. and Susman, E.J. 2003. 'Percent Body Fat at Age 5 Predicts Earlier Pubertal Development among Girls at Age 9', *Pediatrics* 111(4 Pt 1): 815–21.

Dawkins, R. 1976. *The Selfish Gene*, Oxford University Press.

De Semir, V., Ribas, C. and Reveulta, G. 1998. 'Press Releases of Science Journal Articles and Subsequent Newspaper Stories on the Same Topic', *Journal of the American Medical Association* 280(3): 294–5.

De Vries, A.L. and Cohen-Kettenis, P.T. 2012. 'Clinical Management of Gender Dysphoria in Children and Adolescents: The Dutch Approach', *Journal of Homosexuality* 59(3): 301–20.

Deardorff, J., Ekwaru, J.P., Kushi, L.H., Ellis, B.J., Greenspan, L.C., Mirabedi, A., Landaverde, E.G. and Hiatt, R.A. 2011. 'Father Absence, Body Mass Index, and Pubertal Timing in Girls: Differential Effects by Family Income and Ethnicity', *Journal of Adolescent Health* 48(5): 441–7.

Deleuze, G. 1988. *Spinoza: Practical Philosophy*, San Francisco: City Lights Books.

Deleuze, G. and Hand, S. 1988. *Foucault*, London: Athlone.

Demerath, E.W., Li, J., Sun, S.S., Chumlea, W.C., Remsberg, K.E., Czerwinski, S.A., Towne, B. and Siervogel, R.M. 2004a. 'Fifty-year Trends in Serial Body Mass Index during Adolescence in Girls: The Fels Longitudinal Study', *American Journal of Clinical Nutrition* 80(2): 441–6.

Demerath, E.W., Towne, B., Chumlea, W.C., Sun, S.S., Czerwinski, S.A., Remsberg, K.E. and Siervogel, R.M. 2004b. 'Recent Decline in Age at Menarche: The Fels Longitudinal Study', *American Journal of Human Biology* 16(4): 453–7.

Di Ceghe, D., Sturge, S. and Sutton, A. 1988. *Gender Identity Disorders in Children and Adolescents: Guidance for Management (Council Report No. CR63)*, London: Royal College of Psychiatrists.

Diamanti-Kandarakis, E. and Gore, A.C. (eds.) 2012. *Endocrine Disruptors and Puberty, Contemporary Endocrinology*, New York: Humana Press.

Diamanti-Kandarakis, E., Palioura, E. and Kandaraki, E.A. 2012. 'Developmental Exposure to Endocrine Disruptors and Ovarian Function', in E. Diamanti-Kandarakis and A.C. Gore (eds.), *Endocrine Disruptors and Puberty, Contemporary Endocrinology*, New York: Humana Press, pp. 177–99.

Dijkstra, R. 1999. *Portraits*, Mosel: Schirmer.

DiVall, S.A. and Radovick, S. 2009. 'Endocrinology of Female Puberty', *Current Opinion in Endocrinology, Diabetes and Obesity* 16(1): 1–4.

Dolphijn, R. and van der Tuin, I. 2012. *New Materialism: Interviews & Cartographies*, University of Michigan: Open Humanities Press.

Dorn, L.D. and Biro, F.M. 2011. 'Puberty and Its Measurement: A Decade in Review', *Journal of Research on Adolescence* 21(1):180–95.

Dorn, L.D. and Rotenstein, D. 2004. 'Early Puberty in Girls: The Case of Premature Adrenarche', *Women's Health Issues* 14(6): 177–83.

Downing, J. and Bellis, M.A. 2009. 'Early Pubertal Onset and its Relationship with Sexual Risk Taking, Substance Use and Anti-social Behaviour: A Preliminary Cross-sectional Study', *BMC Public Health* 9(1): 446–56.

Draper, P. and Harpending, H. 1982. 'Father Absence and Reproductive Strategy: An Evolutionary Perspective', *Journal of Anthropological Research* 38(3): 255–73.

1988. 'A Sociobiological Perspective on the Development of Human Reproductive Strategies', in K.B. Macdonald (ed.), *Sociobiological Perspectives on Human Development*, New York: Springer-Verlag, pp. 340–72.

Driscoll, C. 2002. *Girls: Feminine Adolescence in Popular Culture and Cultural Theory*, New York: Columbia University Press.

2009. 'Girl-Doll: Barbie as Puberty Manual', in C. Mitchell and J. Reid-Walsh (eds.), *Seven Going on Seventeen: Tween Studies in the Culture of Girlhood*, New York: Peter Lang, pp. 224–41.

Dumit, J. 2012. *Drugs for Life: How Pharmaceutical Companies Define our Health*, Durham, NC: Duke University Press.

Ebbeling, C.B., Pawlak, D.B. and Ludwig, D.S. 2002. 'Childhood Obesity: Public Health Crisis, Common Sense Cure', *The Lancet* 360(9331): 473–82.

Ebling, F.J. 2005. 'The Neuroendocrine Timing of Puberty', *Reproduction* 129(6): 675–83.

Ebony 2012. 'Relaxers Linked to Early Puberty: Long Term Affects Can also Cause Uterine Fibroids.' www.ebony.com/black-listed/wellness-empowerment/relaxers-linked-to-early-puberty.

Eckert, L. 2009. '"Diagnosticism": Three Cases of Medical Anthropological Research into Intersexuality', in M. Holmes (ed.), *Critical Intersex*, Farnham: Ashgate, pp. 41–71.

Edell, D., Brown, L.M. and Tolman, D. 2013. 'Embodying Sexualisation: When Theory Meets Practice in Intergenerational Feminist Activism', *Feminist Theory* 14(3): 275–84.

Edelman, L. 2004. *No Future: Queer Theory and the Death Drive*. Durham, NC: Duke University Press.

Egan, D. 2013. *Becoming Sexual*, London: Polity Press.

Egan, R.D. and Hawkes, G.L. 2008. 'Endangered Girls and Incendiary Objects: Unpacking the Discourse on Sexualization', *Sexuality & Culture* 12(4): 291–311.

Elders, M.J., Scott, C.R., Frindik, J.P. and Kemp, S.K. 1997. 'Clinical Workup for Precocious Puberty', *The Lancet* 350(9076): 457–8.

Elks, C.E., Perry, J.R.B., Sulem, P., Chasman, D.I., Franceschini, N., He, C. and Lunetta, K.L. *et al.* 2010. 'Thirty New Loci for Age at Menarche Identified by a Meta-analysis of Genome-wide Association Studies', *Nature Genetics* 42(12): 1077–85.

Ellis, B.J. 2004. 'Timing of Pubertal Maturation in Girls: An Integrated Life History Approach', *Psychological Bulletin* 130(6): 920–58.

Ellison, G.T.H., Smart, A., Tutton, R., Outram, S.M., Ashcroft, R. and Martin, P. 2007. 'Racial Categories in Medicine: A Failure of Evidence-based Practice?', *PLoS Medicine* 4(9): 1434–6.

Ellwood, D.T. and Jencks, C. 2004. 'The Uneven Spread of Single-Parent Families: What Do We Know? Where Do We Look for Answers?' in K.M. Neckerman (ed.), *Social Inequality*, New York: Russell Sage Foundation, pp. 3–78.

Endometriosis Research Center. 2003. *Use of GnRH Agonists Prior to an Endometriosis Diagnosis*. Delray, FL: Endometriosis Research Center.

Epstein, S. 1996. *Impure Science: AIDS, Activism, and the Politics of Knowledge*, Los Angeles: University of California Press.

2000. 'Democracy, Expertise, and AIDS Treatment Activism', in D.L. Kleinman (ed.), *Science, Technology and Democracy*, New York: SUNY Press, pp. 15–32.

2007. *Inclusion: The Politics of Difference in Medical Research*, University of Chicago Press.

2008. 'The Rise of Recruitmentology: Clinical Research, Racial Knowledge, and the Politics of Inclusion and Difference', *Social Studies of Science* 38(5): 801–32.

Euling, S.Y., Herman-Giddens, M.E., Lee, P.A., Selevan, S.G., Juul, A., Sorensen, T.I.A., Dunkel, L., Himes, J.H., Teilmann, G. and Swan, S.H. 2008. 'Examination of US Puberty-timing Data from 1940 to 1994 for Secular Trends: Panel Findings', *Pediatrics* 121(3): 172–91.

Evans, A. 2015. 'Age 10 the "New Norm" for Puberty in Girls Thanks to BPA', *Natural Society*. http://naturalsociety.com/age-10-the-new-norm-for-puberty-in-girls-thanks-to-bpa/.

Evans, C. 2012. 'New Study Links Relaxers to Fibroids', *BlackDoctor*. http://blackdoctor.org/2582/new-study-links-relaxers-to-fibroids-2/.

Eveleth, P.B. 1986. 'Timing of Menarche: Secular Trend and Population Differences', in J.B. Lancaster and B.A. Hamburg (eds.), *School-age Pregnancy and Parenthood: Biosocial Dimenisions*, New York: Aldine de Gruyter, pp. 39–52.

Fausto-Sterling, A. 1989. 'Life in the XY Corral', *Women's Studies International Forum* 12(3): 319–31.

1992. Myths of Gender: Biological Theories about Men and Women, New York: Basic Books.

1997. 'Feminism and Behavioral Evolution: A Taxonomy', in P. Gowaty (ed.), *Feminism and Evolutionary Biology: Boundaries, Intersections, and Frontiers*, New York: Springer, pp. 42–60.

2000. 'Beyond Difference: Feminism and Evolutionary Psychology', in H. Rose (ed.), *Alas Poor Darwin: Arguments against Evolutionary Psychology*, London: Vintage Press, pp. 174–89.

2004. 'Refashioning Race: DNA and the Politics of Health Care', *Differences: A Journal of Feminist Cultural Studies* 15(3): 1–37.

2005. 'The Bare Bones of Sex: Part 1—Sex and Gender', *Signs* 30(2): 1491–1527.

2008. 'The Bare Bones of Race', *Social Studies of Science* 38(5): 657–94.

2012a. 'Not Your Grandma's Genetics: Some Theoretical Notes', *Psychology of Women Quarterly* 36(4): 411–18.

2012b. *Sex/Gender: Biology in a Social World*. New York: Routledge.

Fausto-Sterling, A., Coll, C.G. and Lamarre, M. 2012a. 'Sexing the Baby: Part 1 – What Do We Really Know about Sex Differentiation in the First Three Years of Life?', *Social Science & Medicine* 74(11): 1684–92.

2012b 'Sexing the Baby: Part 2 Applying Dynamic Systems Theory to the Emergences of Sex-related Differences in Infants and Toddlers', *Social Science & Medicine* 74(11): 1693–1702.

Fausto-Sterling, A., Gowaty, P.A. and Zuk, M. 1997. 'Evolutionary Psychology and Darwinian Feminism (book review)', *Feminist Studies* 23(2): 403–17.

Felner, E.I. and White, P.C. 2000. 'Prepubertal Gynecomastia: Indirect Exposure to Estrogen Cream', *Pediatrics* 105: 55–7.

Feminist Webs. 2013. *The Exciting Life of Being a Woman: A Handbook for Women and Girls*. Manchester: Hammer/On Press.

Fernandez, M.F. and Olea, N. 2012. 'Developmental Exposure to Endocrine Disruptors and Male Urogenital Tract Malformations', in: E. Diamanti-Kandarakis and A.C. Gore (eds.), *Endocrine Disruptors and Puberty, Contemporary Endocrinology*, New York: Humana Press, pp. 225–39.

Fonagy, P. 2010. *Attachment Theory and Psychoanalysis*, New York: Other Press.

Foster, H., Hagan, J. and Brooks-Gunn, J. 2008. 'Growing Up Fast: Stress Exposure and Subjective "Weathering" in Emerging Adulthood', *Journal of Health and Social behavior* 49(2): 162–77.

Foucault, M. 1988. *The History of Sexuality: The Use of Pleasure*, trans. R. Hurley, New York: Vintage.

1990. *The History of Sexuality*, vol. I: *An Introduction*, trans. R. Hurley, New York: Vintage.

Franklin, S. 2007. *Dolly Mixtures: The Remaking of Genealogy*. Durham, NC: Duke University Press.

Franklin, S. and Lock, M.M. (eds.) 2003. *Remaking Life and Death: Toward an Anthropology of the Biosciences*, Santa Fe: School of American Research Press.

Franklin, S. and Roberts, C. 2006. *Born and Made: An Ethnography of Preimplantation Genetic Diagnosis*, Princeton University Press.

Franklin, S.L. and Geffner, M.E. 2003. 'Precocious Puberty Secondary to Topical Testosterone Exposure', *Journal of Pediatric Endocrinology & Metabolism* 16(1): 107–10.

Fraser, L. 2009. 'Psychotherapy in the World Professional Association for Transgender Health's Standards of Care: Background and Recommendations', *International Journal of Transgenderism* 11(2): 110–26.

Freedman, D.S., Kettel-Khan, L., Srinivasan, S.R. and Berenson, G.S. 2000. 'Black/White Differences in Relative Weight and Obesity among Girls: The Bogalusa Heart Study', *Preventive Medicine* 30(3): 234–43.

Freedman, D.S., Khan, L.K., Serdula, M.K., Dietz, W.H., Srinivasan, S.R. and Berenson, G.S. 2002. 'Relation of Age at Menarche to Race, Time Period, and Anthropometric Dimensions: The Bogalusa Heart Study', *Pediatrics* 110(4): e43.

Freyre, E.A., Llaza, G., Rebaza-Gonzalez, R. and Sami, S. 2002. 'Tanner's Pubic Hair Staging Is not Applicable to All Adolescents', *Journal of Adolescent Health* 30(3): 144–5.

Fry, V. and Stanhope, R. 2004. *Premature Sexual Maturation (Including Precocious Puberty), Series No. 4*, London: The Child Growth Foundation.

Furedi, F. 2008. *Paranoid Parenting: Why Ignoring the Experts May Be Best for your Child*, London: Continuum.

Gard, M. and Wright, J. 2005. *The Obesity Epidemic: Science, Morality and Ideology*, London: Routledge.

Garry, V.F. and Truran, P. 2012. 'Secular Trends in Pubertal Timing: A Role for Environmental Chemical Exposure?', in E. Diamanti-Kandarakis and A.C. Gore (eds.), *Endocrine Disruptors and Puberty, Contemporary Endocrinology*, New York: Humana Press, pp. 357–72.

Gerhardt, S. 2004. *Why Love Matters: How Affection Shapes a Baby's Brain*, Hove and New York: Brunner-Routledge.

Geronimus, A. 1994. 'The Weathering Hypothesis and the Health of African-American Women and Infants: Implications for Reproductive Strategies and Policy Analysis', in G. Sen and R.C. Snow (eds.), *Power and Decision: The Social Control of Reproduction*, Cambridge, MA: Harvard University, Center for Population, pp. 77–100.

Gill, R. and Scharff, C. (eds.) 2011. *New Femininities: Postfeminism, Neoliberalism and Subjectivity*, Houndmills: Palgrave Macmillan.

Giroux, H.A. 2012. *Disposable Youth, Racialized Memories, and the Culture of Cruelty*, New York: Routledge.

2013. *Youth in Revolt: Reclaiming a Democratic Future*, Boulder, CO: Paradigm.

Glantz, L.H. 1994. 'Conducting Research with Children: Legal and Ethical Issues', *Journal of the American Academy of Child & Adolescent Psychiatry* 35(10): 1283–91.

Goldstein, H. 1979. *The Design and Analysis of Longitudinal Studies: Their Role in the Measurement of Change*, London: Academic Press.

Goodman, J., McElligott, A. and Marks, L. (eds.) 2003. *Useful Bodies: Humans in the Service of Medical Science in the Twentieth Century*. Baltimore, MD: Johns Hopkins University Press.

Gowaty, P.A. 2003. 'Sexual Natures: How Feminism Changed Evolutionary Biology', *Signs* 28(3): 901–21.

Graber, J.A., Brooks-Gunn, J. and Warren, M.P. 1999. 'The Vulnerable Transition: Puberty and the Development of Eating Pathology and Negative Mood', *Women's Health Issues* 9(2): 107–14.

Graber, J.A., Lewinsohn, P.M., Seeley, J.R. and Brooks-Gunn J, 1997. 'Is Psychopathology Associated with the Timing of Pubertal Development?', *Journal of the American Academy of Child and Adolescent Psychiatry* 36(12): 1768–76.

Graber, J.A., Nichols, T.R. and Brooks-Gunn, J. 1995. 'The Antecedents of Menarcheal Age: Heredity, Family Environment, and Stressful Life Events', *Child Development* 66(2): 346–59.

2010. 'Putting Pubertal Timing in Developmental Context: Implications for Prevention', *Developmental Psychobiology* 52(3): 254–62.

Graber, J.A., Seeley, J.R., Brooks-Gunn, J. and Lewinsohn, P.M., 2004. 'Is Pubertal Timing Associated with Psychopathology in Young Adulthood?', *Journal of the American Academy of Child and Adolescent Psychiatry* 43(6): 718–26.

Graham, H. (ed.) 2009. *Understanding Health Inequalities*, 2nd edition, Maidenhead: Open University Press.

Gray, K. 2013. *Hormones in Food May Lead to Early Puberty*. Available at http://thegrio.com/2013/02/12/hormones-in-food-may-lead-to-early-puberty/.

Greulich, W.W. and Pyle, S.I. 1950. *Radiographic Atlas of Skeletal Development of the Hand and Wrist*. Stanford University Press.

Grinyer, A. 2007. 'The Ethics of Internet Usage in Health and Personal Narratives Research', *Social Research Update* 49: 1–4.

Grodin, M.A. and Glantz, L.H. 1994. *Children as Research Subjects: Science, Ethics, and Law*. Oxford University Press.

Grossman, A.H. and D'Augelli, A.R. 2006. 'Transgender Youth', *Journal of Homosexuality* 51(1): 111–28.

Grosz, E.A. 1994. *Volatile Bodies: Toward a Corporeal Feminism*, Indianapolis: Indiana University Press.

2005. *Time Travels: Feminism, Nature, Power*. Durham, NC: Duke University Press.

2010. 'The Untimeliness of Feminist Theory', *NORA – Nordic Journal of Feminist and Gender Research* 18(1): 48–51.

2012. 'The Nature of Sexual Difference: Irigaray and Darwin', *Angelaki* 17(2): 69–93.

Gupta, R., Patra, K., Dariya, V., Sankararaman, S., Reddy, S. and McVie, R. 2010. 'Spray It with Caution: Precocious Puberty from Maternal Transdermal Estradiol Spray', *Journal of Investigative Medicine* 58(2): 196

Hacking, I. 1990. *The Taming of Chance*. Cambridge University Press.

Hall, G.S. 1905. *Adolescence*, New York: Appleton.

Hall, Lesley A. 2000. *Sex, Gender and Social Change in Britain since 1880*, London: Macmillan.

Hall, S.S. 2005. *With His Bells and Curves, Human Growth Science Grew Up*. www.nytimes.com/2005/03/01/science/01tann.html.

2006. *Size Matters: How Height Affects the Health, Happiness, and Success of Boys – and the Men They Become*, Boston and New York: Houghton Mifflin Harcourt.

Halpern, C.T., Kaestle, C.E., Guo, G. and Hallfors, D.D. 2007. 'Gene-Environment Contributions to Young Adult Sexual Partnering', *Archives of Sexual Behavior* 36(4): 543–54.

Hamilton, A.S. and Mack, T.M. 2003. 'Puberty and Genetic Susceptibility to Breast Cancer in a Case-Control Study in Twins', *New England Journal of Medicine* 348(23): 2313–22.

Hamilton, M. 2009. 'The Seduction of Girls: The Human Cost', in M. Tankard Reist (ed.), *Getting Real: Challenging the Sexualisation of Girls*, Melbourne: Spinifex Press, pp. 55–66..

Hancock, A.-M. 2004. *The Politics of Disgust: The Public Identity of the Welfare Queen*, New York University Press.

Haran, J. and McNeil, M. (eds.) 2013. *Publics of Bioscience: Special Issue of Science as Culture* 224.

Haraway, D.J. 1988. 'Situated Knowledges: The Science Question in Feminism and the Privilege of Partial Perspective', *Feminist Studies* 14(3): 575–99.

1989. *Primate Visions: Gender, Race, and Nature in the World of Modern Science*, New York and London: Routledge.

1991. *Simians, Cyborgs and Women: The Reinvention of Nature.* London: Free Association Books.

1997. *Modest-Witness@Second-Millennium. FemaleMan-Meets-Onco-Mouse: Feminism and Technoscience.* New York and London: Routledge.

2003. *The Companion Species Manifesto: Dogs, People, and Significant Otherness*, Chicago: Prickly Paradigm Press.

2008. *When Species Meet*, Minneapolis: University of Minnesota Press.

Harding, S.G. 1993. *The 'Racial' Economy of Science: Toward a Democratic Future*, Bloomington: Indiana University Press.

Harris, A. 2004. *Future Girl: Young Women in the Twenty-first Century.* New York and London: Routledge.

2009. 'In a Girlie World: Tweenies in Australia', in C. Mitchell and J. Reid-Walsh (eds.), *Seven Going on Seventeen: Tween Studies in the Culture of Girlhood*, New York: Peter Lang, pp. 209–23.

Health and Social Care Information Centre. 2013. *Health Survey for England – 2012.* www.hscic.gov.uk/catalogue/PUB13218.

Healy, D. 2004. 'Shaping the Intimate: Influences on the Experience of Everyday Nerves', *Social Studies of Science* 34(2): 219–45.

Helmreich, S. 2008. 'Species of Biocapital', *Science as Culture* 17(4): 463–78.

Hembree, W.C., Cohen-Kettenis, P. Delemarre-van de Waal, H.A., Gooren, L.J., Meyer, W.J., Spack, N.P., Tangpricha, V. and Montori, V.M. 2009. 'Endocrine Treatment of Transsexual Persons: An Endocrine Society Clinical Practice Guideline', *Journal of Clinical Endocrinology & Metabolism* 94(9): 3132–54.

Hemmings, C. 2014. 'The Materials of Reparation', *Feminist Theory* 15(1): 27–30.

Herman-Giddens, M.E., Kaplowitz, P.B. and Wasserman, R. 2000. 'Current Age of Onset of Puberty – Reply', *Pediatrics 106: 622.*

2004. 'Navigating the Recent Articles on Girls' Puberty in Pediatrics: What Do We Know and Where Do We Go from Here?' *Pediatrics* 113(4): 911–17.

Herman-Giddens, M.E., Slora, E.J., Wasserman, R.C., Bourdony, C.J., Bhapkar, M.V., Koch, G.G. and Hasemeier, C.M. 1997. 'Secondary Sexual Characteristics and Menses in Young Girls Seen in Office Practice: A Study from the Pediatric Research in Office Settings Network', *Pediatrics* 99(4): 505–12.

Herman-Giddens, M.E., Steffes, J., Harris, D., Slora, E., Hussey, M., Dowshen, S.A., Wasserman, R., Serwint, J.R., Smitherman, L. and Reiter, E.O. 2012. 'Secondary Sexual Characteristics in Boys: Data from the Pediatric Research in Office Settings Network', *Pediatrics* 130(5): e1058–e1068.

Herndon, A.M. 2005. 'Collateral Damage from Friendly Fire? Race, Nation, Class and the "War Against Obesity"', *Social Semiotics* 15(2): 127–41.

Hiatt, R.A., Haslam, S.Z. and Osuch, J. 2009. 'The Breast Cancer and the Environment Research Centers: Transdisciplinary Research on the Role of the Environment in Breast Cancer Etiology', *Environmental Health Perspectives* 117(12): 1814–22.

Hird, M.J. 2003. 'A Typical Gender Identity Conference? Some Disturbing Reports from the Therapeutic Front Lines', *Feminism & Psychology* 13 (2): 181–99.

2009. *The Origins of Sociable Life: Evolution after Science Studies*, Basingstoke and New York: Palgrave Macmillan.

Hirsch, H., Gillis, D., Strich, D., Chertin, B., Farkas, A., Lindenberg, T., Gelber, H. and Spitz, I. 2005. 'The Histrelin Implant: A Novel Treatment for Central Precocious Puberty', *Pediatrics* 116(6): E798–E802.

Holland, J. and Thomson, R. 2010. 'Revisiting Youthful Sexuality: Continuities and Changes over Two Decades', *Sexual and Relationship Therapy* 25(3): 342–50.

Holmes, M. (ed.) 2009. *Critical Intersex*. Farnham: Ashgate

Hooper, J. 2004. *'Scientists Say Watching TV Hastens Puberty'*. www.theguardian.com/media/2004/jun/28/italy.broadcasting.

Hopkins P.E. and Hill, M. 2010. 'Contested Bodies of Asylum-seeking Children', in K. Horschelmannm and R. Colls (eds.), *Contested*

Bodies of Childhood and Youth, Basingstoke: Palgrave Macmillan, pp. 136–47.

Hughes, C. and Lury, C. 2013. 'Re-turning Feminist Methodologies: From a Social to an Ecological Epistemology', *Gender and Education* 25(6): 786–99.

Hughes, D.A. 2006. *Building the Bonds of Attachment: Awakening Love in Deeply Troubled Children*. New York: Jason Aronson.

2009. *Attachment-focused Parenting: Effective Strategies to Care for Children*, New York: W.W. Norton & Co.

Hughes, D.A. and Baylin, J.F. 2012. *Brain-based Parenting: The Neuroscience of Caregiving for Healthy Attachment*, New York: W.W. Norton & Co.

Hughes, I.A., Houk, C., Ahmed, S.F. and Lee, P.A. 2006. 'Consensus Statement on Management of Intersex Disorders', *Journal of Pediatric Urology* 2(3): 148–62.

Imperato-McGinley, J., Peterson, R.E., Gautier, T. and Sturla, E., 1979. 'Male Pseudohermaphroditism Secondary to 5α-reductase Deficiency: A Model for the Role of Androgens in both the Development of the Male Phenotype and the Evolution of a Male Gender Identity', *Journal of Steroid Biochemistry* 11(1): 637–45.

Inhelder, B. and Tanner, J.M. (eds.) 1960. *Discussions on Child Development: A Consideration of the Biological, Psychological, and Cultural Approaches to the Understanding of Human Development and Behaviour*, vol. IV: *The Proceedings of the Fourth Meeting of the World Health Organization Study Group on the Psychobiological Development of the Child*, London: Tavistock Publications.

Jackson, M. 1995. 'Images of Deviance: Visual Representations of Mental Defectives in Early-twentieth Century Medical Texts', *British Journal for the History of Science* 28(3): 319–37.

Jamieson, A. 2010. '*Food and Chemicals Could* Be *Linked to Early Puberty in Girls*'. Available at www.telegraph.co.uk/foodanddrink/foodanddrinknews/7561878/Food-can-chemicals-could-be-linked-to-early-puberty-in-girls.html.

Janson-Smith, D. 1980. 'What Is Socio-biology?', in L. Birke, W. Faulkner, S. Best, D. Janson-Smith and K. Overfield (eds.), *Alice Through the Microscope: The Power of Science over Women's Lives*, New York: Virago, pp. 62–88.

Jaruratanasirikul, S. and Thaiwong, M. 2011. 'Outcome of Gonadotropin-releasing Analog Treatment for Children with Central Precocious Puberty: 15-year Experience in Southern Thailand', *Journal of Pediatric Endocrinology & Metabolism* 24(7–8): 519–23.

Jaruratanasirikul, S., Thongkum, K., Krisaneepaiboon, S. and Sriplung, H. 2011. 'Girls with Early Puberty Attain a Near-final Height Similar to their Target Height', *Journal of Pediatric Endocrinology & Metabolism* 24(5–6): 339–45.

Jasik, C.B. and Lustig, R.H. 2008. 'Adolescent Obesity and Puberty: The "Perfect Storm"', *Annals of the New York Academy of Sciences* 1135 (1): 265–79.

Jenks, C. 2005. *Childhood*, London and New York: Routledge.

Jensen, T. 2010. 'Warmth and Wealth: Re-imagining Social Class in Taxonomies of Good Parenting', *Studies in the Maternal* 2(1): 1–13.

2012. 'Tough Love in Tough Times', *Studies in the Maternal* 4(2): 1–26.

Johansson, T. and Ritzén, E.M. 2005. 'Very Long-term Follow-up of Girls with Early and Late Menarche', *Endocrine Development* 8: 126–36.

Jordan-Young, R.M. 2012. 'Hormones, Context, and Brain Gender: A Review of Evidence from Congenital Adrenal Hyperplasia' *Social Science & Medicine* 74(11): 1738–44.

Jurewicz, J. and Hanke, W. 2011. 'Exposure to Phthalates: Reproductive Outcome and Children Health. A Review of Epidemiological Studies', *International Journal of Occupational Medicine and Environmental Health* 24(2): 115–41.

Juul, A., Magnusdottir, S., Scheike, T., Prytz, S. and Skakkebaek, N.E. 2007. 'Age at Voice Break in Danish Boys: Effects of Pre-pubertal Body Mass Index and Secular Trends', *International Journal of Andrology* 30(6): 537–42.

Kaltiala-Heino, R., Marttunen, M., Rantanen, P. and Rimpelä, M. 2003. 'Early Puberty Is Associated with Mental Health Problems in Middle Adolescence', *Social Science & Medicine* 57(6): 1055–64.

Kaltiala-Heino, R., Rimpelä, M., Rissanen, A. and Rantanen, P. 2001. 'Early Puberty and Early Sexual Activity Are Associated with Bulimic-type Eating Pathology in Middle Adolescence', *Journal of Adolescent Health* 28(4): 346–52.

Kaplowitz, P. 2004. *Early Puberty in Girls: The Essential Guide to Coping with this Common Problem*. New York: Ballantine Books.

2008. 'Link between Body Fat and the Timing of Puberty', *Pediatrics* 121 (3): 208–17.

2011. 'Update on Precocious Puberty: Girls Are Showing Signs of Puberty Earlier, but Most Do Not Require Treatment', *Advances in Pediatrics* 58(1): 243–58.

Kaplowitz, P.B., Oberfield, S.E. and The Drug Society, Therapeutics, and Executive Committees of the Lawson Wilkins Pediatric Endocrine Society. 1999. 'Reexamination of the Age Limit for Defining When Puberty

Is Precocious in Girls in the United States: Implications for Evaluation and Treatment', *Pediatrics* 104(4): 936–41.

Kaplowitz, P.B., Slora, E.J., Wasserman, R.C., Pedlow, S.E. and Herman-Giddens, M.E. 2001. 'Earlier Onset of Puberty in Girls: Relation to Increased Body Mass Index and Race', *Pediatrics* 108(2): 347–53.

Karkazis, K.A. 2008. *Fixing Sex: Intersex, Medical Authority, and Lived Experience*, Durham, NC: Duke University Press.

Karlberg, J. 2002. 'Secular Trends in Pubertal Development', *Hormone Research in Paediatrics* 5 (suppl. 2):19–30.

Kashefi, E. and Mort, M. 2004. 'Grounded Citizens' Juries: A Tool for Health Activism?', *Health Expectations* 7(4): 290–302.

Katsnelson, A. 2011. 'Life Sciences: Biomarkers on the Brain', *Nature* 479 (7371): 139–40.

Kay, L.E. 2000. *Who Wrote the Book of Life? A History of the Genetic Code*, Stanford University Press.

Keller, E.F. 1984. *A Feeling for the Organism: The Life and Work of Barbara McClintock. 10th Anniversary Edition*, New York: W.H. Freeman and Company.

2000. *The Century of the Gene*, Cambridge, MA: Harvard University Press.

2010. *The Mirage of a Space between Nature and Nurture*. Durham, NC: Duke University Press.

Kellett, M. 2011. *Children's Perspectives on Integrated Services: Every Child Matters in Policy and Practice*, London: Palgrave Macmillan.

Kelty, C. and Landecker, H. 2009. 'Ten Thousand Journal Articles Later: Ethnography of "The Literature" in Science', *Empiria: Revista de metodología de ciencias sociales* 18: 173–92.

Kemp, M. 1997. 'A Perfect and Faithful Record: Mind and Body in Medical Photography before 1900', in A. Thomas (ed.), *Beauty of Another Order: Photography in Science*, New Haven, London: Yale University Press, pp. 120–49.

Kempers, M.J.E. and Otten, B.J. 2002. 'Idiopathic Precocious Puberty versus Puberty in Adopted Children: Auxological Response to Gonadotrophin-releasing Hormone Agonist Treatment and Final Height', *European Journal of Endocrinology* 147(5): 609–16.

Kim, H.K., Kee, S.J., Seo, J.Y., Yang, E.M., Chae, H.J. and Kim, C.J. 2011. 'Gonadotropin-releasing Hormone Stimulation Test for Precocious Puberty', *Korean Journal of Laboratory Medicine* 31(4): 244–9.

Kim, J., Kim, S., Huh, K., Kim, Y., Joung, H. and Park, M. 2011. 'High Serum Isoflavone Concentrations Are Associated with the Risk of Precocious Puberty in Korean Girls', *Clinical Endocrinology* 75(6): 831–5.

Kim, S.H. and Park, M.J. 2012. 'Effects of Phytoestrogen on Sexual Development', *Korean Journal of Pediatrics* 55(8): 265–71.

King, S. 2006. *Pink Ribbons, Inc: Breast Cancer and the Politics of Philanthropy*, Minneapolis: University of Minnesota Press.

Kirby, V. 2011. *Quantum Anthropologies: Life at Large*, Durham, NC: Duke University Press.

Kirby, V. and Wilson, E.A. 2011. 'Feminist Conversations with Vicki Kirby and Elizabeth A. Wilson', *Feminist Theory* 12(2): 227–34.

Kirk, J. and the British Society for Pediatric Endocrinology and Pediatrics. 2004. *Shared Care Protocol for the Use of GnRH Agonists in Central Precocious Puberty (CPP)*. London: The British Society for Pediatric Endocrinology and Pediatrics.

Klawiter, M. 2008. *The Biopolitics of Breast Cancer: Changing Cultures of Disease and Activism*. Minneapolis: University of Minnesota Press.

Kolata, G. 2001a. 'Doubters Fault Theory Finding Earlier Puberty'. www.nytimes.com/2001/02/20/us/doubters-fault-theory-finding-earlier-puberty.html?pagewanted=all&src=pm.

2001b. '2 Endocrinology Groups Raise Doubt on Earlier Onset of Girls' Puberty'. www.nytimes.com/2001/03/03/us/2-endocrinology-groups-raise-doubt-on-earlier-onset-of-girls-puberty.html.

Koselleck, R. 2006. 'Crisis', trans. M. W. Richter, *Journal of the History of Ideas* 67(2): 617–50.

Kreukels, B.P. and Cohen-Kettenis, P.T. 2011. '*Puberty Suppression in Gender Identity Disorder: The Amsterdam Experience*', Nature Reviews Endocrinology 7(8): 466–72.

Krieger, N. and Fee, E. 1994a. 'Social Class: The Missing Link in US Health Data', *International Journal of Health Services* 24(1): 25–44.

1994b. 'Man-made Medicine and Women's Health: The Biopolitics of Sex/Gender and Race/Ethnicity', *International Journal of Health Services* 24(2): 265–83.

Krimsky, S. 2000. *Hormonal Chaos: The Scientific and Social Origins of the Environmental Endocrine Hypothesis*, Baltimore: Johns Hopkins University Press.

Krstevska-Konstantinova, M., Charlier, C., Craen, M., Du Caju, M., Heinrichs, C., De Beaufort, C., Plomteux, G. and Bourguignon, J.-P. 2001. 'Sexual Precocity after Immigration from Developing Countries to Belgium: Evidence of Previous Exposure to Organochlorine Pesticides', *Human Reproduction* 16(5): 1020–6.

Kunz, G., Klein, K., Clemons, R., Gottschalk, M. and Jones, K. 2004. 'Virilization of Young Children after Topical Androgen Use by Their Parents', *Pediatrics* 114(1): 282–4.

Landecker, H. 2007. *Culturing Life: How Cells Became Technologies*, Cambridge, MA: Harvard University Press.

Langston, N. 2010. *Toxic Bodies: Hormone Disruptors and the Legacy of DES*, New Haven: Yale University Press.

Laqueur, T.W. 1990. *Making Sex: Body and Gender from the Greeks to Freud*, Cambridge, MA: Harvard University Press.

Larcher, V. 2009. 'The Development and Function of Clinical Ethics Committees (CECs) in the United Kingdom', *Diametros* 22: 47–63.

Latour, B. 1988. *The Pasteurization of France*, trans. A. Sheridan and J. Law, Cambridge, MA: Harvard University Press.

Law, J. 2004. *After Method: Mess in Social Science Research*. London: Routledge.

Lederer, S.E. 1992a. 'Orphans as Guinea Pigs: American Children and Medical Experimenters', in R. Cooper (ed.), *In the Name of the Child: Health and Welfare, 1880–1940*, pp. 96–123. London: Routledge.

1992b. 'Political Animals: The Shaping of Biomedical Research Literature in Twentieth-century America', *Isis* 83(1): 61–79.

1995. *Subjected to Science: Human Experimentation in America before the Second World War*, Baltimore, MD: Johns Hopkins University Press.

2003. 'Children as Guinea Pigs: Historical Perspectives', *Accountability in Research: Policies and Quality Assurance* 10(1):1–16.

Lederer, S.E. and Davis, A.B. 1995. 'Subjected to Science: Human Experimentation in America before the Second World War', *History: Reviews of New Books* 24(1): 1–13.

Lederer, S.E. and Grodin, M.A. 1994. 'Historical Overview: Pediatric Research', in M.A. Grodin and L.H. Glantz (eds.), *Children as Research Subjects: Science, Ethics and Law*, Oxford University Press, pp. 3–28.

Lederer, S.E. and More, E. 1996. 'Subjected to Science: Human Experimentation in America before the Second World War', *Journal of the History of Medicine and Allied Sciences* 51(1): 104–5.

Lee, J.M., Appugliese, D., Kaciroti, N., Corwyn, R.F., Bradley, R.H. and Lumeng, J.C. 2007. 'Weight Status in Young Girls and the Onset of Puberty', *Pediatrics* 119(3): 624–30.

Lemonick, M.D., Cray, D., Fowler, D, Grace, J., Jones, A. and Thompson, D. 2000. 'Teens before their Time'. *Available at* http://content.time.com/time/magazine/article/0,9171,58388,00.html.

Lesko, N. 2012. *Act Your Age: A Cultural Construction of Adolescence*, 2nd edn, New York and London: Routledge.

Lesnik-Oberstein, K. 2010. 'Childhood, Queer Theory, and Feminism', *Feminist Theory* 11(3): 309–21.

Levin, D.E. and Kilbourne, J. 2008. *So Sexy So Soon: The New Sexualized Childhood and What Parents Can Do to Protect their Kids*, New York: Ballantine.

Levin, D. and Linn, S. 2003. 'The Commercialization of Childhood: Understanding the Problem and Finding Solutions', in T. Kasser and A. Kanner (eds.), *Psychology and Consumer Culture: The Struggle for a Good Life in a Materialistic World*, Washington, DC: American Psychological Association, pp. 213–32.

Lewis, G. 2014. 'Not by Criticality Alone', *Feminist Theory* 15(1): 31–8.

Lien, L., Dalgard, F., Heyerdahl, S., Thoresen, M. and Bjertness, E. 2006. 'The Relationship between Age of Menarche and Mental Distress in Norwegian Adolescent Girls and Girls from Different Immigrant Groups in Norway: Results from an Urban City Cross-sectional Survey', *Social Science & Medicine* 63(2): 285–95.

Lien, L., Haavet, O.R. and Dalgard, F. 2010. 'Do Mental Health and Behavioural Problems of Early Menarche Persist into Late Adolescence? A Three Year Follow-up Study among Adolescent Girls in Oslo, Norway', *Social Science & Medicine* 71(3): 529–33.

Linn, S. 2005. *Consuming Kids: Protecting our Children from the Onslaught of Marketing and Advertising*, New York: Anchor Books (Random House).

Loder, R.T., Estle, D.T., Morrison, K., Eggleston, D., Fish, D.N., Greefield, M.L. and Kuire, K.E. 1993. 'Applicability of the Greulich and Pyle Skeletal Age Standards to Black and White Children of Today', *American Journal of Disorders of Childhood* 147(12): 1329–33.

Louis, G.M.B., Gray, L.E., Marcus, M., Ojeda, S.R., Pescovitz, O.H., Witchel, S.F., Sippell, W., Abbott, D.H., Soto, A., Tyl, R.W., Bourguignon, J.-P., Skakkebaek, N.E., Swan, S.H., Golub, M.S., Wabitsch, M., Toppari, J. and Euling, S.Y. 2008. 'Environmental Factors and Puberty Timing: Expert Panel Research Needs', *Pediatrics* 121 (suppl. 3): S192–S207.

Ma, H.M., Du, M.-L., Luo, X.-P., Chen, S.-K., Liu, L., Chen, R.-M., Zhu, C., Xiong, F., Tang, L., Wang, W. and Liu, G.-L. 2009. 'Onset of Breast and Pubic Hair Development and Menses in Urban Chinese Girls', *Pediatrics* 124(2): 269–77.

Maehle, A.-H. 1993. 'The Search for Objective Communication: Medical Photography in the Nineteenth Century', in R. Mazzolini (ed.), *Non-verbal Communication in Science Prior to 1900*, Florence: Leo S. Olschki, pp. 563–86.

2009. *Doctors, Honour, and the Law: Medical Ethics in Imperial Germany*, Basingstoke and New York: Palgrave Macmillan.

Mamo, L., Nelson, A. and Clark, A. 2010. 'Producing and Protecting Risky Girlhoods', in A.E. Clarke, L. Mamo, J.R. Fosket, J.R. Fishman and J.K. Shim (eds.), *Biomedicalization: Technoscience, Health and Illness in the US*, Durham, NC: Duke University Press, pp. 121–45.

Mansfield, M.J., Beardsworth, D.E., Loughlin, J.S., Crawford, J.D., Bode, H.H., Rivier, J., Vale, W., Kushner, D.C., Crigler, J.F., Jr and Crowley, W.F., Jr, 1983. 'Long-term Treatment of Central Precocious Puberty with a Long-acting Analogue of Luteinizing Hormone-releasing Hormone. Effects on Somatic Growth and Skeletal Maturation', *New England Journal of Medicine* 309(21): 1286–90.

Mantovani, A. 2012. 'Endocrine Disruptors and Puberty Disorders from Mice to Men (and Women)', in E. Diamanti-Kandarakis and A.C. Gore (eds.), *Endocrine Disruptors and Puberty*, New York: Humana Press, pp. 119–37.

Marcus, G.E. 1995. 'Ethnography in/of the World System: The Emergence of Multi-sited Ethnography', *Annual Review of Anthropology* 24: 95–117.

Marshall, B.L. 2009. 'Sexual Medicine, Sexual Bodies and the "Pharmaceutical Imagination"', *Science as Culture* 18(2): 133–49.

Marshall, W.A. and Tanner, J.M. 1969. 'Variations in the Pattern of Pubertal Changes in Girls', *Archives of Disease in Childhood* 44(235): 291–303.

1970. 'Variations in the Pattern of Pubertal Changes in Boys', *Archives of Disease in Childhood* 45(239): 13–23.

Massart, F., Federico, G., Harrell, J.C. and Saggese, G. 2009. 'Growth Outcome during GnRH Agonist Treatments for Slowly Progressive Central Precocious Puberty', *Neuroendocrinology* 90(3): 307–14.

Maudsley, H. 1874. *Sex in Mind and in Education*. London: J. Miller.

Mayall, B. (ed.) 1995. *Children's Childhoods: Observed and Experienced*, London and Bristol, PA: The Falmer Press.

McGarth, R. 2002. *Seeing her Sex: Medical Archives and the Female Body*, University of Manchester Press.

M'charek, A. 2005. *The Human Genome Diversity Project: An Ethnography of Scientific Practice,* Cambridge University Press.

2010. 'Fragile Differences, Relational Effects: Stories about the Materiality of Race and Sex', *European Journal of Women's Studies* 17(4): 307–22.

McNeil, M. 2010. 'Post-Millennial Feminist Theory: Encounters with Humanism, Materialism, Critique, Nature, Biology and Darwin', *Journal for Cultural Research* 14(4): 427–37.

McNeil, M. and Roberts, C. 2011. 'Feminist Science and Technology Studies', in R. Buikema, G. Griffin and N. Lykke (eds.), *Theories and Methodologies in Postgraduate Feminist Research: Researching Differently*, London and New York: Routledge.

McRobbie, A. 1991. *Feminism and Youth Culture: From 'Jackie' to 'Just Seventeen'*, London: Macmillan.

2009. *The Aftermath of Feminism: Gender, Culture and Social Change*. London: Sage.

Midyett, L.K., Moore, W.V. and Jacobson, J.D. 2003. 'Are Pubertal Changes in Girls before Age 8 Benign?' *Pediatrics* 111(1): 47–51

Mintzes, B. 2002. 'For and Against: Direct to Consumer Advertising Is Medicalising Normal Human Experience', *British Medical Journal* 324(7342): 908–11.

Mintzes, B., Barer, M.L., Kravitz, R.L., Kazanjian, A., Bassett, K., Lexchin, J., Evans, R.G., Pan, R. and Marion, S.A. 2002. 'Influence of Direct to Consumer Pharmaceutical Advertising and Patients' Requests on Prescribing Decisions: Two Site Cross Sectional Survey', *British Medical Journal* 324: 278–9.

Mitchell, C. and Reid-Walsh, J. (eds.) 2009. *Seven Going on Seventeen: Tween Studies in the Culture of Girlhood*, New York and London: Peter Lang.

Moffitt, T.E. and Belsky, J. 1992. 'Childhood Experience and the Onset of Menarche: A Test of a Sociobiological Model', *Child Development* 63(1): 47–58.

Mol, A. 2002. *The Body Multiple: Ontology in Medical Practice*, Durham, NC: Duke University Press.

2008. *The Logic of Care: Health and the Problem of Patient Choice*, London and New York: Routledge.

2012. 'Mind Your Plate! The Ontonorms of Dutch Dieting', *Social Studies of Science* 43(3): 379–96.

Moletsane, R. 2009. '"I Do Know Who I Am"': Writing, Consciousness, and Reflection', in C. Mitchell and J. Reid-Walsh (eds.), *Seven Going on Seventeen: Tween Studies in the Culture of Girlhood*, New York: Peter Lang, pp. 148–62.

Moncrieff, J. 2008. 'The Creation of the Concept of an Antidepressant: An Historical Analysis', *Social Science and Medicine* 66(11): 2346–55.

Monk, D. 2001. 'New Guidance/Old Problems: Recent Developments in Sex Education', *Journal of Social Welfare and Family Law* 23(3): 271–91.

Montgomery, K.C. 2009. *Generation Digital: Politics, Commerce, and Childhood in the Age of the Internet*. Cambridge, MA: MIT Press

Montoya, M.J. 2007. 'Bioethnic Conscription: Genes, Race, and Mexicana/o Ethnicity in Diabetes Research' *Cultural Anthropology* 22: 94–128.

Moorhead, J. 2010. 'Should We Be Worried about Early Puberty?' www.guardian.co.uk/lifeandstyle/2010/oct/19/worried-about-early-puberty.

Mora, S., Boechat, M.I., Pietka, E., Huang, H.K. and Gilsanz, V. 2001. 'Skeletal Age Determinations in Children of European and African

Descent: Applicability of the Greulich and Pyle Standards', *Pediatric Research* 50(5): 624–8.

Moran, J. 2000. *Teaching Sex: The Shaping of Adolescence in the 20th Century*, Cambridge, MA: Harvard University Press.

Morris, D.H., Jones, M.E., Schoemaker, M.J., Ashworth, A. and Swerdlow, A.J. 2010. 'Determinants of Age at Menarche in the UK: Analyses from the Breakthrough Generations Study', *British Journal of Cancer* 103 (11): 1760–4.

2011a. 'Secular Trends in Age at Menarche in Women in the UK Born 1908–93: Results from the Breakthrough Generations Study', *Paediatric and Perinatal Epidemiology* 25(4): 394–400.

2011b. 'Familial Concordance for Age at Menarche: Analyses from the Breakthrough Generations Study', *Paediatric and Perinatal Epidemiology* 25(3): 306–11.

Morrison, M. 2008. '*Beyond Therapy? Investigating Biomedical Enhancement in the Case of Human Growth Hormone*', unpublished PhD thesis, University of Nottingham.

Mort, F. 1987. *Dangerous Sexualities: Medico-Moral Politics in England since 1830*, London: Routledge & Kegan Paul.

Mort, M., Roberts, C., Pols, J., Domenech, M. and Moser, I. 2013. 'Ethical Implications of Home Telecare for Older People: A Framework Derived from a Multisited Participative Study', *Health Expectations*. http://onlinelibrary.wiley.com/doi/10.1111/hex.12109/full.

Mouritsen, A., Aksglaede, L., Sorensen, K., Mogensen, S. S., Leffers, H., Main, K.M., Frederiksen, H., Andersson, A.-M., Skakkebaek, N. E., and Juul, A. 2010. 'Hypothesis: Exposure to Endocrine-disrupting Chemicals May Interfere with Timing of Puberty', *International Journal of Andrology* 33(2): 346–59.

Mul, D., Bertelloni, S., Carel, J.C., Saggese, G., Chaussain, J.L. and Oostdijk, W. 2002. 'Effect of Gonadotropin-releasing Hormone Agonist Treatment in Boys with Central Precocious Puberty: Final Height Results', *Hormone Research* 58(1): 1–7.

Mul, D. and Hughes, I.A. 2008. 'The Use of GnRH Agonists in Precocious Puberty', *European Journal of Endocrinology* 159(suppl. 1): 3–9.

Mul, D., Oostdijk, W. and Drop, S.L.S. 2002. 'Early Puberty in Girls', *Best Practice & Research Clinical Endocrinology & Metabolism* 16(1): 153–63.

Mul, D., Oostdijk, W., Otten, B.J., Rouwe, C., Jansen, M., Delemarre-van de Waal, H.A., Waelkens, J.J.J. and Drop, S.L.S. 2000. 'Final Height after Gonadotrophin Releasing Hormone Agonist Treatment for Central Precocious Puberty: The Dutch Experience', *Journal of Pediatric Endocrinology & Metabolism* 13(1): 765–72.

Murphy, M. 2012. *Seizing the Means of Reproduction: Entanglements of Feminism, Health, and Technoscience*, Durham, NC: Duke University Press.

Murray, S. 2008. 'Pathologizing Fatness: Medical Authority and Popular Culture', *Sociology of Sport Journal* 25(1): 7–21.

Nadeem, E. and Graham, S. 2005. 'Early Puberty, Peer Victimization, and Internalizing Symptoms in Ethnic Minority Adolescents', *Journal of Early Adolescence* 25(2): 197–222.

Negriff, S., Dorn, L.D. and Huang, B. 2010. 'Pubertal Timing and Smoking Initiation in Adolescent Females: Differences by Race', *Nicotine and Tobacco Research* 12(7): 748–55.

Newbold, R.R. 2004. 'Lessons Learned from Perinatal Exposure to Diethylstilbestrol', *Toxicology and Applied Pharmacology* 199(2):142–50.

Newbold, R.R., Hanson, R.B., Jefferson, W.N., Bullock, B.C., Haseman, J. and McLachlan, J.A. 1998. 'Increased Tumors but Uncompromised Fertility in the Female Descendants of Mice Exposed Developmentally to Diethylstilbestrol', *Carcinogenesis* 19(9): 1655–63.

News Services, the University of North Caroline at Chapel Hill. 2007. 'Girls with Early Puberty, Older Boyfriends at Greater Risk for Drugs, Sex, Alcohol (News Release)', Minneapolis: University of North Carolina at Chapel Hill.

Novas, C. and Rose, N. 2000. 'Genetic Risk and the Birth of the Somatic Individual', *Economy and Society* 29(4): 485–513.

O'Connor, E. 1995. 'Medical Photography and the Emergence of Anorexia Nervosa', *Journal of the History of Sexuality* 5(4): 535–72.

Odone, C. 2002. 'Sexy Kids', *New Statesman*, 5 July: 18.

Ong, K.K., Ahmed, M.L. and Dunger, D.B. 2006. 'Lessons from Large Population Studies on Timing and Tempo of Puberty (Secular Trends and Relation to Body Size): The European Trend', *Molecular and Cellular Endocrinology* 254: 8–12.

Ofsted 2013. *Not Good Enough Yet: Personal, Social, Health and Economic Education in Schools. Personal, Social and Health Education in English Schools in 2012*, Manchester: Office for Standards in Education.

Opelka, M. 2011. 'Why Are British Women Taking Chicken Fattening Pills?' www.theblaze.com/stories/2011/02/15/why-are-british-women-taking-chicken-fattening-pills/.

O'Sullivan, E. and O'Sullivan, M. 2002. 'Precocious Puberty: A Parent's Perspective', *Archives of Disorders of Childhood* 86: 320–1.

Oudshoorn, N. 1994. *Beyond the Natural Body: An Archaeology of Sex Hormones*, London: Routledge.

Palmert, M.R. and Boepple, P.A. 2001. 'Variation in the Timing of Puberty: Clinical Spectrum and Genetic Investigation', *Journal of Clinical Endocrinology & Metabolism* 86(6): 2364–8.

Palmert, M.R., Hayden, D.L., Mansfield, M.J., Crigler, J.F., Crowley, W.F., Chandler, D.W. and Boepple, P.A. 2001. 'The Longitudinal Study of Adrenal Maturation during Gonadal Suppression: Evidence that Adrenarche Is a Gradual Process', *Journal of Clinical Endocrinology & Metabolism* 86(9): 4536–42.

Papadopoulos, L. 2010. *Sexualisation of Young People*, London: The Home Office.

Parent, A., Teilmann, G., Juul, A., Skakkebaek, N., Toppari, J. and Bourguignon, J. 2003. 'The Timing of Normal Puberty and the Age Limits of Sexual Precocity: Variations around the World, Secular Trends, and Changes after Migration', *Endocrine Reviews* 24(5): 668–93.

Pathomvanich, A. and Merke, D.P. 2000. 'Early Puberty: A Cautionary Tale', *Pediatrics* 105(1): 115.

Patton, C. 1995. 'Between Innocence and Safety: Epidemiologic and Popular Constructions of Young People's Need for Safe Sex', in J. Terry and J. Urla (eds.), *Deviant Bodies: Critical Perspectives on Difference in Science and Popular Culture*, Indianapolis: Indiana University Press, pp. 338–57.

Pearson, C. 2012. 'Boys Entering Puberty Up To 2 Years Earlier, Study Says'. www.huffingtonpost.com/2012/10/20/boys-puberty_n_1987979.html.

Pedwell, C. and Whitehead, A. (eds.) 2012. *Affecting Feminism: Questions of Feeling in Feminist Theory: A Special Issue. Feminist Theory* 13(2).

Penny, L. 2011. *Meat Market: Female Flesh under Capitalism.* Winchester and Washington, DC: Zero Books.

Phoenix, A. 2011. *Review of Recent Literature for the Bailey Review of Commercialisation and Sexualisation of Childhood*, Loughborough: Childhood Wellbeing Research Centre.

Pilcher, J. 2005. 'School Sex Education: Policy and Practice in England 1870 to 2000', *Sex Education* 5(2): 153–70.

Pinto, K. 2007. 'Growing Up Young', *Journal of Early Adolescence* 27(4): 509–44.

Pollock, L.A. 1983. *Forgotten Children: Parent–Child Relations from 1500 to 1900.* Cambridge University Press.

Pols, J. 2012. *Care at a Distance: On the Closeness of Technology*, Amsterdam University Press.

Posner, R.B. 2006. 'Early Menarche: A Review of Research on Trends in Timing, Racial Differences, Etiology and Psychosocial Consequences', *Sex Roles* 54(5): 315–22.

Postman, N. 1994. *The Disappearance of Childhood*, New York: Vintage.

Pringle, R. 2004. 'Adoption in Britain: Reflexive Modernity?', *Australian Feminist Studies* 19(44): 225–40.

Proos, L.A., Lonnerholm, T., Jonsson, B. and Tuvemo, T. 2006. 'Can Bone Age Determination Provide Criteria for Growth Hormone Treatment in Adopted Girls with Early Puberty? A Comparison of the Greulich-Pyle and the Tanner-Whitehouse 2 Methods', *Upsala Journal of Medical Sciences* 111(1): 117–29.

2010. 'Can the TW3 Bone Age Determination Method Provide Additional Criteria for Growth Hormone Treatment in Adopted Girls with Early Puberty? A Comparison of the Tanner-Whitehouse 3 Method with the Greulich-Pyle and the Tanner-Whitehouse 2 Methods', *Hormone Research in Paediatrics* 73(1): 35–40.

Pyett, P., Rayner, J., Venn, A., Bruinsma, F., Werther, G. and Lumley, J. 2005. 'Using Hormone Treatment to Reduce the Adult Height of Tall Girls: Are Women Satisfied with the Decision in Later Years?', *Social Science and Medicine* 61(8): 1629–39.

Rabeharisoa, V., Moreira, T. and Akrich, M. 2014. 'Evidence-based Activism: Patients', Users' and Activists' Groups in Knowledge Society', *BioSocieties* 9(2): 111–28.

Rabinow, P. and Rose, N. 2006. 'Biopower Today', *BioSocieties* 1: 195–217.

Race, K. 2009. *Pleasure Consuming Medicine: The Queer Politics of Drugs.* Durham, NC: Duke University Press.

Rajan, K.S. 2006. *Biocapital: The Constitution of Postgenomic Life.* Durham, NC: Duke University Press.

Raman, S. and Tutton, R. 2010. 'Life, Science, and Biopower', *Science, Technology & Human Values* 35(5): 711–34.

Rapp, R. 2000. *Testing Women, Testing the Fetus: The Social Impact of Amniocentesis in America*, New York and London: Routledge.

Raun, T. 2012. 'DIY Therapy: Exploring Affective Aspects of Trans Video Blogs on YouTube', in A. Kuntsman and A. Karatzogianni (eds), *Digital Cultures and the Politics of Emotion: Feelings, Affect and Technological Change*, London: Palgrave Macmillan, pp. 165–80.

Rayner, J. 2008. 'Cosmetic Endocrinology: (Re)constructing Femininity in "Tall" Girls', unpublished PhD manuscript, LaTrobe University.

Rayner, J.-A., Pyett, P. and Astbury, J. 2010. 'The Medicalisation of "Tall" Girls: A Discourse Analysis of Medical Literature on the Use of Synthetic Oestrogen to Reduce Female Height', *Social Science and Medicine* 71(6): 1076–83.

Reardon, J. 2004. 'Decoding Race and Human Difference in a Genomic Age', *Differences: A Journal of Feminist Cultural Studies* 15(3): 38–65.

2005. *Race to the Finish: Identity and Governance in an Age of Genomics*, Princeton University Press.

Reist, M.T. (ed.) 2009. *Getting Real: Challenging the Sexualisation of Girls*, North Melbourne: Spinifex Press.

Renold, E. and Ringrose, J. 2011. 'Schizoid Subjectivities? Re-theorizing Teen Girls' Sexual Cultures in an Era of "Sexualization"', *Journal of Sociology* 47(4): 389–409.

2013. 'Feminisms Re-figuring "Sexualisation," Sexuality and "the Girl"', *Feminist Theory* 14(3): 247–54.

Rich, E., Monaghan, L. and Aphramor, L. 2010. *Debating Obesity: Critical Perspectives*, London: Palgrave Macmillan.

Roberts, C. 2003. 'Drowning in a Sea of Estrogens: Sex Hormones, Sexual Reproduction and Sex', *Sexualities* 6(2): 195–213.

2006. 'What Can I Do to Help Myself? Somatic Individuality and Contemporary Hormonal Bodies', *Science Studies* 19(2): 54–76.

2007. *Messengers of Sex: Hormones, Biomedicine, and Feminism*, Cambridge University Press.

2013. 'Evolutionary Psychology, Feminism and Early Sexual Development', *Feminist Theory* 14(3): 295–304.

Roberts, C. and Hird, M. (eds.) 2011. 'Nonhuman Feminisms', a Special Issue of *Feminist Theory* 12(2).

Roberts, C., Kippax, S., Waldby, C. and Crawford, J. 1995. 'Faking It: The Story of 'Ohh!'', *Women's Studies International Forum*, 18(5/6): 523–32.

Roberts, C. and Mackenzie, A. 2006. 'Science', *Theory, Culture and Society* 23(2–3): 157–63.

Roberts, C., valentine, k. and Fraser, S. 2009. 'Rationalities and Nonrationalities in Clinical Encounters', *Science as Culture* 18(2): 165–81.

Roen, K. 2009. 'Clinical Intervention and Embodied Subjectivity: Atypically Sexed Children and their Parents', in M. Holmes (ed.) *Critical Intersex*, Farnham and Burlington, VT: Ashgate, pp. 15–40.

Roen, K. 2011. 'Reply to Peggy Cohen-Kettenis', *Psychology and Sexuality* 2(3): 261–2.

Rogers, I.S., Northstone, K., Dunger, D.B., Cooper, A.R., Ness, A.R. and Emmett, P.M. 2010. 'Diet throughout Childhood and Age at Menarche in a Contemporary Cohort of British Girls', *Public Health Nutrition* 13(12): 2052–63.

Rogers, L. 2007. 'The Girls Who Started Going through Puberty at THREE', *Mail Online*. www.dailymail.co.uk/femail/article-508020/The-girls-started-going-puberty-THREE.html.

Rose, N. 2007a. 'Molecular Biopolitics, Somatic Ethics and the Spirit of Biocapital', *Social Theory & Health* 5(1): 3–29.

2007b. *The Politics of Life Itself: Biomedicine, Power, and Subjectivity in the Twenty-first Century*, Princeton University Press.

2013. 'The Human Sciences in a Biological Age', *Theory, Culture & Society* 30(1): 3–34.

Rosenfield, R.L., Bachrach, L.K., Chernausek, S.D., Gertner, J.M., Gottschalk, M., Hardin, D.S., Pescovitz, O.H. and Saenger, P. 2000. 'Current Age of Onset of Puberty', *Pediatrics* 106(3): 622–3.

Rosengarten, M. 2010. *HIV Interventions: Biomedicine and the Traffic between Information and Flesh*, University of Washington Press.

Rosengarten, M. and Michael, M. 2009. 'Rethinking the Bioethical Enactment of Medically Drugged Bodies: Paradoxes of Using Anti-HIV Drug Therapy as a Technology for Prevention, *Science as Culture* 18(2): 183–99.

Rossouw, J.E., Anderson, G.L., Prentice, R.L., LaCroix, A.Z., Kooperberg, C., Stefanick, M.L., Jackson, R.D., Beresford, S.A., Howard, B.V. and Johnson, K.C. (Writing Group for the Women's Health Initiative Investigators). 2002. 'Risks and Benefits of Estrogen plus Progestin in Healthy Postmenopausal Women: Principal Results from the Women's Health Initiative Randomized Controlled Trial', *Journal of the American Medical Association* 288(3): 321–33.

Rubin, C., Maisonet, M., Kieszak, S., Monteilh, C., Holmes, A., Flanders, D., Heron, J., Golding, J., McGeehin, M. and Marcus, M. 2009. 'Timing of Maturation and Predictors of Menarche in Girls Enrolled in a Contemporary British Cohort', *Paediatric and Perinatal Epidemiology* 23(5): 492–504.

Rush, E. and La Nauze, A. 2006a. *Corporate Paedophilia: Sexualisation of Children in Australia*, Canberra: The Australia Institute.

2006b. *Letting Children Be Children: Stopping the Sexualisation of Children in Australia*, Canberra: The Australia Institute.

2006b. *Letting Children Be Children*, Canberra: The Australia Institute.

Rutter, M. 2006. 'Implications of Resilience Concepts for Scientific Understanding', *Annals of the New York Academy of Sciences* 1094(1): 1–12.

Sanghavi, D.M. 2006. 'Preschool Puberty, and a Search for the Causes'. www.nytimes.com/2006/10/17/science/17puberty.html.

Sauerteig, L. 2012. 'Puberty and the Making of Gender: Explaining Changes in Body and Mind', paper presented at European Social Science History Conference, Glasgow, April.

Savage, J. 2008. *Teenage: The Creation of Youth Culture, 1875–1945*, London: Pimlico.

Schiebinger, L. 1991. *The Mind Has No Sex? Women in the Origins of Modern Science*, Cambridge, MA: Harvard University Press.

Schofield, G. and Beek, M. 2006. *Attachment Handbook for Foster Care and Adoption*, London: British Association for Adoption & Fostering.

Schreck, C.J., Burek, M.W., Stewart, E.A. and Miller, J.M. 2007. 'Distress and Violent Victimization among Young Adolescents: Early Puberty and the Social Interactionist Explanation', *Journal of Research in Crime and Delinquency* 44(4): 381–405.

Seaman, B. 2003. *The Greatest Experiment Ever Performed on Women: Exploding the Estrogen Myth*, New York: Hyperion.

Seaton, E. 2005. 'Tween Social and Biological Reproduction: Early Puberty in Girls', in C. Mitchell and J. Reid-Walsh (eds.), *Seven Going on Seventeen: Tween Studies in the Culture of Girlhood*, New York: Peter Lang, pp. 25–45.

2009. ''Tween Social and Biological Reproduction: Early Puberty in Girls', in C. Mitchell and J. Reid-Walsh (eds.), *Seven Going on Seventeen: Tween Studies in the Culture of Girlhood*, New York: Peter Lang, pp. 25–41.

Sengoopta, C. 2006. *The Most Secret Quintessence of Life: Glands, Sex, and Bodies, 1850–1950*, University of Chicago Press.

Sharpe, S. 1984. *Double Identity: The Lives of Working Mothers*, London: Penguin.

Sherwood, L. 2013. *Human Physiology: From Cells to Systems*, Belmont, CA: Brooks/Cole, Cengage Learning.

Shim, J.K. 2000. 'Bio-power and Racial, Class, and Gender Formation in Biomedical Knowledge Production', *Research in the Sociology of Health Care* 17: 173–95.

Shostak, Sara. 2010. 'Marking Populations and Persons at Risk', in Adele E. Clarke, Laura Mamo, Jennifer Ruth Fosket, Jennifer R. Fishman and Janet K. Shim (eds.), *Biomedicalization: Technoscience, Health and Illness in the U.S.*, Durham, NC: Duke University Press, pp. 242–62.

Shuttleworth, F.K. 1938. 'The Adolescent Period: A Graphic and Pictorial Atlas', *Monographs of the Society for Research in Child Development* 3 (3): 233–46.

Sieben, A. 2011. 'Heteronormative Pheromones? A Feminist Approach to Human Chemical Communication', *Feminist Theory* 12(3): 263–80.

Sloboda, D.M., Hickey, M. and Hart, R. 2011. 'Reproduction in Females: The Role of the Early Life Environment', *Human Reproduction Update* 17(2): 210–27.

Smiley, L. 2007. 'Girl/Boy Interrupted. www.sfweekly.com/2007-07-11/news/girl-boy-interrupted/.

Smith, R. 2010. 'Early Puberty and Obesity Are Linked in Young Girls, Genetic Research Finds.' www.telegraph.co.uk/health/healthnews/8149785/Early-puberty-and-obesity-are-linked-in-young-girls-genetic-research-finds.html.

Sontag, L.M. and Graber, J.A. 2010. 'Coping with Perceived Peer Stress: Gender-specific and Common Pathways to Symptoms of Psychopathology', *Developmental Psychology* 46(6): 1605.

Soriano-Guillen, L. and Argente, J. 2011. 'Central Precocious Puberty: Epidemiology, Etiology, Diagnosis and Treatment', *Anales de Pediatria* 74(5): 336.

Soriano-Guillén, L., Corripio, R., Labarta, J.I., Cañete, R., Castro-Feijóo, L., Espino, R. and Argente, J. 2010. 'Central Precocious Puberty in Children Living in Spain: Incidence, Prevalence, and Influence of Adoption and Immigration', *Journal of Clinical Endocrinology and Metabolism* 95(9): 4305–13.

Spongberg, M. 2008. 'The Child', *Australian Feminist Studies* 23(57): 287.

Spurgas, A.K. 2009. '(Un)Queering Identity: The Biosocial Production of Intersex/DSD', in M. Holmes (ed.), *Critical Intersex*, Farnham and Burlington: Ashgate, pp. 97–122.

Spurgeon, D. 1999. 'Doctors Feel Pressurised by Direct to Consumer Advertising', *British Medical Journal* 319(7221): 1321.

Stacey, J. 2000. 'The Global Within: Consuming Nature, Embodying Health', in J. Stacey, S. Franklin and C. Lury (eds.), *Global Nature, Global Culture*, London: Sage, pp. 97–145.

2014. 'Wishing Away Ambivalence', *Feminist Theory* 15(1): 39–49.

Star, S.L. 1990. 'Power, Technology and the Phenomenology of Conventions: On Being Allergic to Onions', *Sociological Review* 38(S1): 26–56.

Steingraber, S. 2007. *The Falling Age of Puberty in US girls: What We Know, What We Need to Know*. San Francisco: The Breast Cancer Fund

2011. *Raising Elijah: Protecting Our Children in an Age of Environmental Crisis*, New York: Da Capo Press.

Stengers, I. 2000. 'God's Heart and the Stuff of Life', *Pli* 9: 86–118.

2010. *Cosmopolitics 1*. Minneapolis: University of Minnesota Press.

Strange, J. 2001. 'The Assault on Ignorance: Teaching Menstrual Etiquette in England, c. 1920s to 1960s', *Social History of Medicine* 14(2): 247–65.

Styne, D.M. 2004. 'Puberty, Obesity and Ethnicity', *Trends in Endocrinology and Metabolism* 15(10): 472–8

Tagg, J. 1988. *The Burden of Representation: Essays on Photographies and Histories*, Minneapolis: University of Minnesota Press.

Tanner, J.M. 1962. *Growth at Adolescence*, 2nd edn, Springfield, MA: Thomas.

1981a. 'Catch-up Growth in Man', *British Medical Bulletin* 37(3): 233–8.

1981b. *A History of the Study of Human Growth*, Cambridge University Press.

1986. 'Use and Abuse of Growth Standards', *Human Growth* 3: 95–109.

1998. 'A Brief History of the Study of Human Growth', in S.J. Ulijaszek, F.E. Johnston and M.A. Preece (eds.), *The Cambridge Encyclopedia of Human Growth and Development*, Cambridge University Press, pp. 2–13.

Tanner, J.M. and Inhelder, B. (eds.) 1956. *Discussions on Child Development: A Consideration of the Biological, Psychological, and Cultural Approaches to the Understanding of Human Development and Behaviour*, vol. I: *The Proceedings of the First Meeting of the World Health Organization Study Group on the Psychobiological Development of the Child Geneva, 1953–1956*, London: Tavistock.

(eds.) 1957. *Discussions on Child Development: A Consideration of the Biological, Psychological, and Cultural Approaches to the Understanding of Human Development and Behaviour*, vol. II: *The Proceedings of the Second Meeting of the World Health Organization Study Group on the Psychobiological Development of the Child, London, 1954*, New York: International Universities Press.

(eds.) 1958. *Discussions on Child Development: A Consideration of the Biological, Psychological, and Cultural Approaches to the Understanding of Human Development and Behaviour*, vol. III: *The Proceedings of the Third Meeting of the World Health Organization Study Group on the Psychobiological Development of the Child, Geneva, 1955*, London: Tavistock.

Tanner, J.M. and Whitehouse, R.H. 1982. *Atlas of Children's Growth: Normal Variation and Growth Disorders*, London: Academic Press.

Tanner, J.M., Whitehouse, R.H. and Takaishi, M. 1966. 'Standards from Birth to Maturity for Height, Weight, Height Velocity, and Weight Velocity: British Children, 1965. II', *Archives of Disease in Childhood* 41(220): 613–35.

Teilmann, G., Pedersen, C.B., Skakkebaek, N.E. and Jensen, T.K. 2006. 'Increased Risk of Precocious Puberty in Internationally Adopted Children in Denmark', *Pediatrics* 118(2): 391–9.

Teilmann, G., Petersen, J.H., Gormsen, M., Damgaard, K., Skakkebaek, N.E and Jensen, T.K. 2009. 'Early Puberty in Internationally Adopted Girls: Hormonal and Clinical Markers of Puberty in 276 Girls Examined Biannually over Two Years', *Hormone Research* 72(4): 236–46.

Terry, J. 1997. *An American Obsession: Science, Medicine, and Homosexuality in Modern Society*, University of Chicago Press.

The Kitchen Sisters. 2010. 'Chicken Pills on All Things Considered', www.kitchensisters.org/girlstories/hidden-world-of-girls-launches-monday-march-22/.

Thomas, A. 1997. *Beauty of Another Order: Photography in Science*, New Haven and London: Yale University Press.

Throsby, K. 2007. 'How Could You Let Yourself Get Like That? Stories of the Origins of Obesity in Accounts of Weight Loss Surgery' *Social Science and Medicine* 65(8): 1561–71.

2008. 'Happy Re-birthday: Weight Loss Surgery and the New Me', *Body and Society* 14(1): 117–33.

Throsby, K. and Roberts, C. 2010. 'Getting Bigger: Children's Bodies, Genes and Environments', *Sociological Review* 58(1): 73–92.

Timimi, S. 2002 *Pathological Child Psychiatry and the Medicalization of Childhood*, New York: Brunner-Routledge.

Timmermans, S. 1996. 'Saving Lives or Saving Multiple Identities? The Double Dynamic of Resuscitation Scripts', *Social Studies of Science* 26(4): 767–97.

Tiwary, C.M. 1998. 'Premature Sexual Development in Children Following the Use of Estrogen- or Placenta-containing Hair Products', *Clinical Pediatrics* 37(12):733–9.

Tolman, D. 2002. *Dilemmas of Desire: Teenage Girls Talk about Sexuality*, Cambridge, MA: Harvard University Press.

Toulalan, S. (ed.) 2007. *Imagining Sex: Pornography and Bodies in Seventeenth-Century England*, Oxford University Press.

2011. '"Unripe" Bodies: Children and Sex in Early Modern England', in K. Fisher and S. Toulalan (eds.), *Bodies, Sex and Desire from the Renaissance to the Present*, Basingstoke: Palgrave.

Tremblay, L. and Frigon, J.-Y. 2005. 'Precocious Puberty in Adolescent Girls: A Biomarker of Later Psychosocial Adjustment Problems', *Child Psychiatry and Human Development* 36(1): 73–94.

Triandafyllidou, A., Wodak, R. and Krzyzanowski, M. (eds.) 2009. *The European Public Sphere and the Media: Europe in Crisis*. London: Palgrave.

Trivers, R.L. 1972. 'Parental Investment and Sexual Selection', in B. Campbell (ed.), *Sexual Selection and the Descent of Man, 1871–1971*, London: Aldine Selection, pp. 136–79.

Tyler, I. 2008. '"Chav Mum, Chav Scum": Class Disgust in Contemporary Britain', *Feminist Media Studies* 8(1): 17–34.

2013. *Revolting Subjects: Social Abjection and Resistance in Neoliberal Britain*, London: Zed Books.

Ulijaszek, S.J., Johnston, F.E. and Preece, M.A. (eds.) 1998. *The Cambridge Encyclopedia of Human Growth and Development*, Cambridge University Press.

van der Tuin, I. 2008. 'Deflationary Logic: Response to Sara Ahmed's "Imaginary Prohibitions: Some Preliminary Remarks on the Founding Gestures of the 'New Materialism'"', *European Journal of Women's Studies* 15(4): 411–16.

Vanderschueren, D. and Bouillon, R. 1995. 'Androgens and Bone', *Calcified Tissue International* 56(5): 341–6.

Virdis, R., Street, M.E, Zampolli, M., Radetti, G., Pezzini B., Benelli, M., Ghizzoni, L. and Volta, C. 1998. 'Precocious Puberty in Girls Adopted from Developing Countries', *Archives of Disease in Childhood* 78(2): 152–4.

Wacharasindhu, S., Srivuthana, S., Aroonparkmongkol, S., Supornsilchai, V., Hiranrat, P. and Yodvisitsak, V. 2003. 'Final Adult Height in "Early Normal Pubertal Girls" Treated with Gonadotropin Releasing Hormone Agonists', *Journal of the Medical Association of Thailand* 86 (Suppl. 2): 170–3.

Wacharasindhu, S., Srivuthana, S., Aroonparkmongkol, S. and Trinavarat, P. 2001. Does GnRH analog Improve the Final Height in Thai Girls with Idiopathic Central Precocious Puberty?, *Journal of the Medical Association of Thailand* 84(Suppl. 1):S51–S56.

Walkerdine, V. 1998. *Daddy's Girl: Young Girls and Popular Culture*, Cambridge, MA: Harvard University Press.

Walkerdine, V., Lucey, H. and Melody, J. 2001. *Growing Up Girl: Psychosocial Explorations of Gender and Class*, London: Palgrave.

Walvoord, E.C. 2010. 'The Timing of Puberty: Is It Changing? Does It Matter?', *Journal of Adolescent Health* 47(5): 433–9.

Wang, C. 2009. *Alert to Parents: Real Dangers of Early Puberty*. www.action3news.com/Global/story.asp?S=11534030.

Watson-Verran, H. and Turnbull, D. 1995. 'Knowledge Systems as Assemblages of Local Knowledge', in S. Jasanoff (ed.), *Handbook of Science and Technology Studies*, London: Sage, pp. 115–39.

Way, N. and Stauber, H. 1996. 'Are Absent Fathers Really Absent? Urban Adolescent Girls Speak out about their Fathers', in N.J.R. Leadbeater and N. Way (eds.), *Urban Girls: Resisting Stereotypes, Creating Identities*, New York University Press, pp. 132–48.

Wehkalampi, K., Päkkilä, K., Laine, T. and Dunkel, L. 2011. 'Adult Height in Girls with Delayed Pubertal Growth', *Hormone Research in Paediatrics* 76(2):130–5.

Wehkalampi, K., Silventoinen, K., Kaprio, J., Dick, D.M., Rose, R.J., Pulkkinen, L. and Dunkel, L. 2008. 'Genetic and Environmental Influences on Pubertal Timing Assessed by Height Growth', *American Journal of Human Biology: The Official Journal of the Human Biology Council* 20(4): 417–23.

Weil, E. 2012. 'Puberty before Age 10: A New "Normal"?'. www.nytimes.com/2012/04/01/magazine/puberty-before-age-10-a-new-normal.html.

Westphal, S.P. 2002. 'Early Puberty Linked to Shampoos', www.newscientist.com/article/dn2119-early-puberty-linked-to-shampoos.html#.UqTvuOKgZZJ.

Whincup, P.H., Gilg, J.A., Odoki, K., Taylor, S.J.C. and Cook, D.G. 2001. 'Age of Menarche in Contemporary British Teenagers: Survey of Girls born between 1982 and 1986', *British Medical Journal* 322(7294): 1095–6.

Wiegman, R. 2014. 'The Times We're In: Queer Feminist Criticism and the Reparative "Turn"', *Feminist Theory* 15(1): 4–25.

Willems, D. and Pols, J. 2010. 'Goodness! The Empirical Turn in Health Care Ethics', *Medische Antropologie* 22(1): 161–70.

Williams, G.C. 1966. *Adaptation and Natural Selection*, Princeton University Press.

Williams, S.J., Gabe, J. and Davis, P. 2008. 'The Sociology of Pharmaceuticals: Progress and Prospects', *Sociology of Health and Illness* 30(6): 813–24.

Wilson, E.A. 1998. Neural Geographies: Feminism and the Microstructure of Cognition, New York: Routledge

2004. Psychosomatic: Feminism and the Neurological Body, Durham, NC: Duke University Press.

2010. *Affect and Artificial Intelligence*, University of Washington Press.

2011. 'Neurological Entanglements: The Case of Paediatric Depressions, SSRIs and Suicidal Ideation', *Subjectivity* 4(3): 277–7.

Wilson, E.E., Word, R.A., Byrd, W. and Carr, B.R. 1991. 'Effect of Superovulation with Human Menopausal Gonadatropins on Growth-hormone Levels in Women', *Journal of Clinical Endocrinology & Metabolism* 73(3): 511–15.

Wilson, J.D., Foster, D.W., Kronenberg, H.M. and Larsen, P.R. 1998. *Williams Textbook of Endocrinology*, 9th edition, Philadelphia: Saunders.

Wilson, M.E., Chikazawa, K., Fisher, J., Mook, D. and Gould, K.G. 2004. 'Reduced Growth Hormone Secretion Prolongs Puberty but Does Not Delay the Developmental Increase in Luteinizing Hormone in the Absence of Gonadal Negative Feedback', *Biology of Reproduction* 71 (2): 588–97.

Woloshin, S. and Schwartz, L.M. 2002. 'Press Releases', *JAMA: The Journal of the American Medical Association* 287(21): 2856–8.

World Professional Association for Trans Health. 2001. *Standards of Care for the Health of Transsexual, Transgender, and Gender-Nonconforming People*, Minneapolis: World Professional Association for Trans Health. www.wpath.org/uploaded_files/140/files/Standards%20of%20Care,%20V7%20Full%20Book.pdf.

2012. *Standards of Care for the Health of Transsexual, Transgender, and Gender-nonconforming People*, 7th version, Minneapolis: World Professional Association for Trans Health.

Wright, C.M., Booth, I.W., Buckler, J.M.H., Cameron, N., Cole, T.J., Healy, M.J.R., Hulse, J.A., Preece, M.A., Reilly, J.J. and Williams, A.F. 2002. 'Growth Reference Charts for Use in the United Kingdom', *Archives of Disease in Childhood* 86(1): 11–14.

Wu, T., Mendola, P. and Buck, G.M. 2002. 'Ethnic Differences in the Presence of Secondary Sex Characteristics and Menarche among US Girls: The Third National Health and Nutrition Examination Survey, 1988–1994', *Pediatrics* 110(4): 752–7.

Wu, X., Zhang, N. and Lee, M.M. 2012. 'The Influence of Endocrine Disruptors on Male Pubertal Timing', in E. Diamanti-Kandarakis and A.C. Gore (eds.), *Endocrine Disruptors and Puberty*, New York: Humana Press, pp. 339–55.

Yu, Y.M., Punyasavatsu, N., Elder, D. and D'Ercole, A.J. 1999. 'Sexual Development in a Two-Year-old Boy Induced by Topical Exposure to Testosterone', *Pediatrics* 104(2): e23–e23.

Zachmann, M., Sobradillo, B., Frank, M., Frisch, H. and Prader, A. 1978. 'Bayley-Pinneau, Roche-Wainer-Thissen, and Tanner Height Predictions in Normal Children and in Patients with Various Pathologic Conditions', *Journal of Pediatrics* 93(5):749–55.

Zola, I.K. 1972. 'Medicine as an Institution of Social Control', *Sociological Review* 20: 487–504.

Index

NOTE: Page numbers in italic type refer to figures.

WHAT IS A MATHEMATICAL CONCEPT?

Responding to widespread interest within cultural studies and social inquiry, this book addresses the question of what a mathematical concept is by using a variety of vanguard theories in the humanities and post-humanities. Tapping into historical, philosophical, sociological and psychological perspectives, each chapter explores the question of how mathematics comes to matter. Of interest to scholars across the usual disciplinary divides, this book tracks mathematics as a cultural activity, drawing connections with empirical practice. Unlike other books in this area, it is highly interdisciplinary, devoted to exploring the ontology of mathematics as it plays out in different contexts. This book will appeal to scholars who are interested in particular mathematical habits – creative diagramming, structural mappings, material agency, interdisciplinary coverings – that shed light on both mathematics and other disciplines. Chapters are also relevant to social sciences and humanities scholars, as each one offers philosophical insight into mathematics and how we might live mathematically.

Elizabeth de Freitas is a professor in the Education and Social Research Institute at Manchester Metropolitan University. Her research focuses on philosophical investigations of mathematics, science and technology, and pursuing the implications and applications of this work within cultural studies. She is a co-author of the book *Mathematics and the Body: Material Entanglements in the Classroom*, associate editor of the journal *Educational Studies in Mathematics* and has written more than 50 chapters and articles on diverse topics.

Nathalie Sinclair is the Canada Research Chair in Tangible Mathematics Learning at Simon Fraser University. She is the author of several books, including co-author of *Mathematics and the Body: Material Entanglements in the Classroom* and co-editor of *Mathematics and the Aesthetic: New Approaches to an Ancient Affinity*, as well as more than 50 articles. She has also led the design of educational technologies, including the touchscreen app TouchCounts and dynamic geometry microworlds for young learners (www.sfu.ca/geometry4yl). She is the founding editor of the journal *Digital Experiences in Mathematics Education*.

Alf Coles' recently published *Engaging in School Mathematics: Symbols and Experiences* draws on more than 20 years of work as a teacher-researcher at both primary and secondary levels. He is on the executive committee of the British Society for Research into Learning Mathematics and is an active member of the Mathematics Education Special Interest Group of the British Educational Research Association. His current interests include drawing his work in mathematics education into closer dialogue with issues of sustainability.

What Is a Mathematical Concept?

Edited by

Elizabeth de Freitas
Manchester Metropolitan University

Nathalie Sinclair
Simon Fraser University

Alf Coles
University of Bristol

CAMBRIDGE
UNIVERSITY PRESS

CAMBRIDGE
UNIVERSITY PRESS

One Liberty Plaza, 20th Floor, New York, NY 10006, USA

Cambridge University Press is part of the University of Cambridge.

It furthers the University's mission by disseminating knowledge in the pursuit of education, learning, and research at the highest international levels of excellence.

www.cambridge.org
Information on this title: www.cambridge.org/9781107134638
DOI: 10.1017/9781316471128

First published 2017

A catalogue record for this publication is available from the British Library.

Library of Congress Cataloging-in-Publication Data
Names: De Freitas, Elizabeth. | Sinclair, Nathalie. | Coles, Alf.
Title: What is a mathematical concept? / [edited by] Elizabeth de Freitas, Manchester Metropolitan University, Nathalie Sinclair, Simon Fraser University, Alf Coles, University of Bristol.
Description: Cambridge: Cambridge University Press, 2017. | Includes bibliographical references and index.
Identifiers: LCCN 2016059487 | ISBN 9781107134638 (hard back)
Subjects: LCSH: Mathematics – Social aspects. | Mathematics – Philosophy.
Classification: LCC QA10.7.W43 2017 | DDC 510.1–dc23
LC record available at https://lccn.loc.gov/2016059487

ISBN 978-1-107-13463-8 Hardback

CONTENTS

IMAGES

NOTES ON CONTRIBUTORS

YASMINE ABTAHI is a part-time professor at the Faculty of Education, University of Ottawa and post-doctoral research fellow at the Université du Québec à Montréal. Her research includes work on mathematical tools and artefacts.

MICHAEL J. BARANY is a postdoctoral fellow in the Dartmouth College Society of Fellows. He recently completed his PhD in Princeton University's Program in History of Science with a dissertation on the globalization of mathematics as an elite scholarly discipline in the mid-twentieth century. His research on the relationship between abstract knowledge and the modern world has led to articles (all available at http://mbarany.com) on such topics as dots, numbers, rigour, blackboards, basalt, bureaucracy, communism and internationalism, from the sixteenth century to the present.

RICHARD BARWELL is Professor of Mathematics Education at the Faculty of Education, University of Ottawa. His research includes work on language, multilingualism and discourse analysis in mathematics education. He was educated in the United Kingdom before moving to Canada in 2006. Prior to his academic career, he taught mathematics in the United Kingdom and Pakistan.

TONY BROWN is Professor of Mathematics Education at Manchester Metropolitan University, where he also leads research in teacher education. Brown's work explores how contemporary theory provides new insights into educational contexts. He has written seven books including three volumes for Springer's prestigious Mathematics Education Library series. He convenes the Manchester-based conference on Mathematics Education and Contemporary Theory.

ALF COLES is Senior Lecturer in Education (Mathematics) at the University of Bristol. He gained a research council scholarship for his PhD study that was adapted as a book: *Being Alongside: For the Teaching and Learning of Mathematics* (2013). His research covers early number development, creativity in learning mathematics, working on video with teachers and links between mathematics education and sustainability education. His latest book, *Engaging in School Mathematics* was published by Routledge in 2015.

DAVID CORFIELD is Senior Lecturer in Philosophy at the University of Kent. He works in the philosophy of science and mathematics and is a co-director of the Centre for Reasoning at Kent. He is one of the three owners of the blog The n-category Café, where the implications for philosophy, mathematics and physics of the new language of higher-dimensional category theory are discussed. In 2007, Corfield published *Why Do People Get Ill?* (co-authored with Darian Leader), which aims to revive interest in the psychosomatic approach to medicine.

BRENT DAVIS is Professor and Distinguished Research Chair in Mathematics Education in the Faculty of Education at the University of Calgary. He is the author of two books on pedagogy and co-author of three books on learning, teaching and research. He has served as editor of *For the Learning of Mathematics* (2008–2010), co-editor of *JCT: Journal of Curriculum Theorizing* (1995–1999), and founding co-editor of *Complicity: An International Journal of Complexity and Education* (2004–2007).

SIMON B. DUFFY received a PhD in Philosophy from the University of Sydney in 2003 after a Diplôme d'Etudes Approfondies (MPhil equivalent) in Philosophy from the Université de Paris X-Nanterre (1999). He has taught at the University of Sydney, the University of New South Wales and the University of Queensland, where he was a postdoctoral fellow in Philosophy at the Centre for the History of European Discourses. Dr Duffy is the author of *Deleuze and the History of Mathematics: In Defense of the New* (2013) and *The Logic of Expression: Quality, Quantity and Intensity in Spinoza, Hegel and Deleuze* (2006). He is editor of *Virtual Mathematics: The Logic of Difference* (2006), and co-editor with Sean Bowden of *Badiou and Philosophy* (2012). He is also translator of Albert Lautman's *Mathematics, Ideas and the Physical Real* (2011).

ELIZABETH DE FREITAS is a professor at the Education and Social Research Institute at Manchester Metropolitan University. She is the co-author of *Mathematics and the Body: Material Entanglements in the Classroom* (Cambridge University Press, 2014) and *Alternative Theoretical Frameworks for Mathematics Education Research: Theory meets Data* (2016). Her work focuses on the philosophy and history of mathematics and its implications for theories of learning and pedagogy. She is an associate editor of the journal *Educational Studies in Mathematics*.

MICHAEL HARRIS is a professor of mathematics at the Université de Paris Diderot and Columbia University. He is the author or co-author of more than seventy mathematical books and articles and has received a number of prizes, including the Clay Research Award, which he shared in 2007 with Richard Taylor. His most recent book is *Mathematics without Apologies: Portrait of a Problematic Vocation* (2014).

JULIETTE KENNEDY is Professor of Mathematics at the University of Helsinki. Her research interests include set theory and set-theoretic model theory, foundations and philosophy of mathematics, history of logic and aesthetics and art history. She has published several books including, most recently, *Interpreting Gödel: Critical Essays* (2014). She also co-organised the Simplicity, Ideals of Practice in Mathematics and the Arts conference in New York.

HEATHER MENDICK is a sociologist and a former mathematics teacher who currently works as a freelance academic. She is the author of *Masculinities in Mathematics* (2006), the co-author of *Urban Youth and Schooling* (2010) and the co-editor of *Mathematical Relationships in Education* (2009) and *Debates in Mathematics Education* (2014). Her most recent research project focused on the role of celebrity in young people's classed and gendered aspirations and was funded by the Economic and Social Research Council (www.celebyouth.org). She tweets about work, politics, darts and pop culture @helensclegel.

RICARDO NEMIROVSKY is Professor at Manchester Metropolitan University and a faculty member of the Education and Social Research Institute. Dr. Nemirovsky's research focuses on informal STEM education, museum pedagogy and embodied cognition. He has acted as PI on a number of National Science Foundation grants, including projects focusing on art- science museum collaborations. He has designed numerous interactive tools and manipulatives for mathematics learning and is the author of many seminal articles pertaining to mathematics and cognition, such as the co-authored Mathematical Imagination and Embodied Cognition (2009).

REVIEL NETZ is the Patrick Suppes Professor of Greek Mathematics and Astronomy at the Department of Classics, Stanford University. He has written widely on Greek mathematics, and among his books are *The Shaping of Deduction in Greek Mathematics: A Study in Cognitive History* (Cambridge University Press, 1999) and *The Archimedes Palimpsest* (co-edited with W. Noel., 2011).

DAVID PIMM is Professor Emeritus at the University of Alberta. He is the author of *Speaking Mathematically* (1987) and *Symbols and Meanings in School Mathematics* (1995) and a co-author of *Developing Essential Understanding of Geometry* (2012). He is a former editor of the journal *For the Learning of Mathematics* (1997–2003) and has written extensively on mathematics and mathematics education, drawing on both the history and the philosophy of mathematics.

ARKADY PLOTNITSKY is Professor of English and Theory and Cultural Studies, director of the Theory and Cultural Studies Program and co-director of the Philosophy and Literature Program at Purdue University. He earned his PhD in comparative literature and literary theory from the University of Pennsylvania and his MSc in mathematics from the Leningrad (St. Petersburg) State University in Russia. He has published several books including *Niels Bohr and Complementarity: An Introduction* (2012), *Epistemology and Probability: Bohr, Heisenberg, Schrödinger, and the Nature of Quantum-Theoretical Thinking* (2009) and *Complementarity: Anti-Epistemology after Bohr and Derrida* (1994).

WOLFF-MICHAEL ROTH is Lansdowne Professor of Applied Cognitive Science at the University of Victoria. He conducts research on how people across their lifespan know and learn mathematics and science. He is a Fellow of the American Association for the Advancement of Science, the American Educational Research Association (AERA) and the British Society. He received a Significant Contribution award from AERA and an Honorary Doctorate from the University of Ioannina, Greece.

NATHALIE SINCLAIR is a professor in the Faculty of Education, an associate member in the Department of Mathematics and the Canada Research Chair in Tangible Mathematics Learning at Simon Fraser University. She is also the editor of *Digital Experiences in Mathematics Education*. She is the author of *Mathematics and Beauty: Aesthetic Approaches to Teaching Children* (2006), and co-author of *Mathematics and the Body: Material Entanglements in the Classroom* (Cambridge University Press, 2014) and *Developing Essential Understanding of Geometry* (2012), among other books.